Household Safety Sourcebook
Hypertension Sourcebook
Immune System Disorders Sou_
Infant & Toddler Health Sourcebook
Infectious Diseases Sourcebook
Injury & Trauma Sourcebook
Kidney & Urinary Tract Diseases &
  Disorders Sourcebook
Learning Disabilities Sourcebook,
  2nd Edition
Leukemia Sourcebook
Liver Disorders Sourcebook
Lung Disorders Sourcebook
Medical Tests Sourcebook, 2nd Edition
Men's Health Concerns Sourcebook,
  2nd Edition
Mental Health Disorders Sourcebook,
  3rd Edition
Mental Retardation Sourcebook
Movement Disorders Sourcebook
Muscular Dystrophy Sourcebook
Obesity Sourcebook
Osteoporosis Sourcebook
Pain Sourcebook, 2nd Edition
Pediatric Cancer Sourcebook
Physical & Mental Issues in Aging
  Sourcebook
Podiatry Sourcebook
Pregnancy & Birth Sourcebook,
  2nd Edition
Prostate Cancer
Public Health Sourcebook
Reconstructive & Cosmetic Surgery
  Sourcebook
Rehabilitation Sourcebook
Respiratory Diseases & Disorders
  Sourcebook
Sexually Transmitted Diseases
  Sourcebook, 2nd Edition
Skin Disorders Sourcebook
Sleep Disorders Sourcebook,
  2nd Edition

Stroke Sourcebook
Substance Abuse Sourcebook
Surgery Sourcebook
Thyroid Sourcebook
Transplantation Sourcebook
Traveler's Health Sourcebook
Vegetarian Sourcebook
Women's Health Concerns Sourcebook,
  2nd Edition
Workplace Health & Safety Sourcebook
Worldwide Health Sourcebook

Teen Health Series

Alcohol Information for Teens
Asthma Information for Teens
Cancer Information for Teens
Diet Information for Teens
Drug Information for Teens
Eating Disorders Information
  for Teens
Fitness Information for Teens
Mental Health Information
  for Teens
Sexual Health Information
  for Teens
Skin Health Information for
  Teens
Sports Injuries Information
  for Teens
Suicide Information for Teens

Asthma
SOURCEBOOK

Second Edition

KINGSVILLE PUBLIC LIBRARY
6006 Academy Street
Kingsville, OH 44048-0057

Health Reference Series

Second Edition

Asthma
SOURCEBOOK

Basic Consumer Health Information about the Causes, Symptoms, Diagnosis, and Treatment of Asthma in Infants, Children, Teenagers, and Adults, Including Facts about Different Types of Asthma, Common Co-Occurring Conditions, Asthma Management Plans, Triggers, Medications, and Medication Delivery Devices

Along with Asthma Statistics, Research Updates, a Glossary, a Directory of Asthma-Related Resources, and More

KINGSVILLE PUBLIC LIBRARY
6006 Academy Street
Kingsville, OH 44048-0057

Edited by
Karen Bellenir

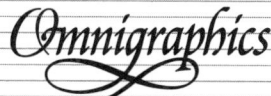

615 Griswold Street • Detroit, MI 48226

Bibliographic Note

Because this page cannot legibly accommodate all the copyright notices, the Bibliographic Note portion of the Preface constitutes an extension of the copyright notice.

Edited by Karen Bellenir

Health Reference Series

Karen Bellenir, *Managing Editor*
David A. Cooke, M.D., *Medical Consultant*
Elizabeth Barbour, *Research and Permissions Coordinator*
Cherry Stockdale, *Permissions Assistant*
Laura Pleva Nielsen, *Index Editor*
EdIndex, Services for Publishers, *Indexers*

* * *

Omnigraphics, Inc.

Matthew P. Barbour, *Senior Vice President*
Kay Gill, *Vice President—Directories*
Kevin Hayes, *Operations Manager*
Leif Gruenberg, *Development Manager*
David P. Bianco, *Marketing Director*

* * *

Peter E. Ruffner, *Publisher*
Frederick G. Ruffner, Jr., *Chairman*

Copyright © 2006 Omnigraphics, Inc.
ISBN 0-7808-0866-5

Library of Congress Cataloging-in-Publication Data

Asthma sourcebook : basic consumer health information about the causes, symptoms, diagnosis, and treatment of asthma in infants, children, teenagers, and adults, including facts about different types of asthma, common co-occurring conditions, asthma management plans, triggers, medications, and medication delivery devices; along with asthma statistics, research updates, a glossary, a directory of asthma-related resources, and more / edited by Karen Bellenir. -- 2nd ed.
   p. cm. -- (Health reference series)
  Summary: "Provides basic consumer health information about causes, triggers, treatment, and management of asthma. Includes index, glossary of related terms, and other resources"--Provided by publisher.
  Includes bibliographical references and index.
  ISBN 0-7808-0866-5 (hardcover : alk. paper)
  1. Asthma--Popular works.   I. Bellenir, Karen. II. Series: Health reference series (Unnumbered)
  RC591.A84 2006
  616.2'38--dc22

2006008844

Electronic or mechanical reproduction, including photography, recording, or any other information storage and retrieval system for the purpose of resale is strictly prohibited without permission in writing from the publisher.

The information in this publication was compiled from the sources cited and from other sources considered reliable. While every possible effort has been made to ensure reliability, the publisher will not assume liability for damages caused by inaccuracies in the data, and makes no warranty, express or implied, on the accuracy of the information contained herein.

This book is printed on acid-free paper meeting the ANSI Z39.48 Standard. The infinity symbol that appears above indicates that the paper in this book meets that standard.

Printed in the United States

Table of Contents

Visit www.healthreferenceseries.com to view *A Contents Guide to the Health Reference Series*, a listing of more than 12,000 topics and the volumes in which they are covered.

Preface xi

Part I: Asthma: An Introduction

Chapter 1—Basic Facts about Asthma 3
Chapter 2—Questions and Answers about Asthma 17
Chapter 3—Can You Prevent Asthma? 45
Chapter 4—What Happens during an Asthma Attack? 49
Chapter 5—How to Identify an Asthma Emergency 53
Chapter 6—Asthma in Infants 57
Chapter 7—Childhood Asthma 63
Chapter 8—Asthma and Teenagers 71
Chapter 9—Adult Onset Asthma 75
Chapter 10—Asthma and Older People 81
Chapter 11—Asthma and Pregnancy 89

Part II: Understanding Types of Asthma and Common Co-Occurring Conditions

Chapter 12—What Causes Asthma? 97
Chapter 13—Recognizing and Diagnosing Asthma 107
Chapter 14—Allergic Asthma 113

Chapter 15—Exercise-Induced Asthma 119
Chapter 16—Occupational Asthma 127
Chapter 17—Steroid-Resistant Asthma 131
Chapter 18—Status Asthmaticus 135
Chapter 19—Heart Disease and Asthma:
    A Complex Combination 141
Chapter 20—Asthma and Chronic Obstructive
    Pulmonary Disease (COPD) 147
Chapter 21—Rhinitis and Its Impact on Asthma 151
Chapter 22—Sinusitis and Asthma 163
Chapter 23—Food Allergies and Asthma 173
Chapter 24—Gastroesophageal Reflux Disease
    (GERD) and Asthma 179
Chapter 25—Influenza Information
    for People with Asthma 183
Chapter 26—Asthma and Bone Health 189

Part III: Asthma Management: Working with Your Doctor

Chapter 27—Finding a Doctor for Asthma Care 195
Chapter 28—You and Your Asthma Doctor:
    Roles, Rights, and Responsibilities 199
Chapter 29—Use of Asthma Diaries 203
Chapter 30—Developing an Asthma Action Plan 207
Chapter 31—Using a Peak Flow Meter
    to Monitor Asthma 211
Chapter 32—What Makes Asthma Worse? 217
Chapter 33—Exercise and Sports: Guidelines
    for People with Asthma 221
Chapter 34—Nutrition and Asthma 231
Chapter 35—The Weather and Asthma 237
Chapter 36—Asthma and Outdoor Air Pollution 243
Chapter 37—Indoor Environmental Asthma Triggers 247

Chapter 38—Air Filters: What People
   with Asthma Should Know 255
Chapter 39—How to Create a Dust-Free Bedroom 261
Chapter 40—Smoking and Asthma 265
Chapter 41—Traveling with Asthma... 269

Part IV: Treating Asthma: Medications and Delivery Devices

Chapter 42—How Is Asthma Treated? 275
Chapter 43—What Medications Are
   Used to Treat Asthma? 281
Chapter 44—Why People Don't Take
   Their Asthma Medication 295
Chapter 45—What's the Difference Between
   Rescue and Controller Medications? 299
Chapter 46—What You Should Know about
   Corticosteroids 303
Chapter 47—Asthma and Bronchodilators 309
Chapter 48—What You Should Know about
   Asthma Medication Delivery Devices 313
Chapter 49—Anti-IgE Therapy: A New Class
   of Asthma Medication 329
Chapter 50—Can Asthma Be Treated with Acupuncture? 331

Part V: Special Concerns about Asthma Management in Children

Chapter 51—The Art of Treating Childhood Asthma 339
Chapter 52—Your Child's Cough: Is It Asthma? 347
Chapter 53—Monitoring Your Child's Asthma 353
Chapter 54—Warning Signs that May Precede
   an Asthma Flare-Up 359
Chapter 55—Control Your Child's Asthma Triggers 361

Chapter 56—If Your Child Has Asthma,
　　　　　　Can You Keep Your Pet? 365

Chapter 57—When to Seek Emergency Care
　　　　　　for a Child with Asthma 369

Chapter 58—Emotional Problems in
　　　　　　Young People with Asthma 373

Chapter 59—Is Your Child-Care Setting or
　　　　　　School Asthma Friendly? 375

Chapter 60—Combatting Frequent School
　　　　　　Absenteeism in Children with Asthma 379

Chapter 61—Animals in School: A Concern
　　　　　　for Children with Asthma 387

Chapter 62—Chickenpox and Corticosteroids:
　　　　　　Is Your Child at Risk? 393

Part VI: Asthma Statistics and Research

Chapter 63—Asthma Prevalence, Health
　　　　　　Care Use, and Mortality 399

Chapter 64—Global Burden of Asthma 407

Chapter 65—Asthma: A Concern for
　　　　　　Minority Populations 413

Chapter 66—Asthma in Children Remains
　　　　　　Significantly Out of Control in the U.S. 419

Chapter 67—Studying Strategies to Improve Care
　　　　　　for Low-Income Children with Asthma 425

Chapter 68—Asthma Research Highlights from the
　　　　　　U.S. Environmental Protection Agency 435

Chapter 69—Asthma Research Updates from
　　　　　　the National Institutes of Health 457

Chapter 70—Researchers Find Obesity
　　　　　　Is Associated with Asthma 481

Chapter 71—Researchers Discover Gene
　　　　　　that Determines Asthma Susceptibility 487

Chapter 72—Discovery of Gene Clusters Could
             Lead to New Asthma Treatment
             Based on Genetic Profiles 489

Chapter 73—Do Hormonal Cycles Affect Asthma? 493

Chapter 74—Are All Aerosol Therapy Devices
             Equally Effective? 497

Chapter 75—Inhaled Steroids and the Risk of Glaucoma 501

Chapter 76—Studying Ways to Improve
             Asthma Treatment Outcomes 503

Chapter 77—Studying the Long-Term
             Effects of Asthma Therapy 515

Part VII: Additional Help and Information

Chapter 78—Asthma-Related Terms 525

Chapter 79—Directory of Asthma-Related Resources 537

Chapter 80—Health Insurance and
             Asthma-Related Services 547

Chapter 81—Asthma Prescription Medications:
             Assistance Programs and Online Purchasing 555

Index **561**

Preface

About This Book

In the United States, more than 30 million people have been diagnosed with asthma, including nearly nine million children. Worldwide, an estimated 300 million people suffer from asthma. The Global Initiative for Asthma predicts that by the year 2025, the number will increase to 400 million. Asthma symptoms, including shortness of breath, coughing, and wheezing, can vary from mild to life-threatening, and although medical researchers have identified some of the factors that can contribute to its development or trigger a worsening of symptoms, its ultimate cause remains a mystery. Asthma can often be controlled with medications and lifestyle modifications, but current medical science does not offer a cure.

Asthma Sourcebook, Second Edition provides updated information about asthma causes, triggers, and treatments. It explains the complex relationship between asthma and conditions that often occur with it, including allergies, rhinitis, sinusitis, and gastroesophageal reflux disease. A section on asthma management describes the steps that can be taken to reduce the number and severity of asthma flares, and a section on asthma treatment describes the different types of medications and delivery devices used to combat asthma. Special concerns about asthma management in children, including school-related issues, are described. Current research findings are discussed, and the book concludes with a glossary, directory of resources, and other information for people who need additional assistance.

How to Use This Book

This book is divided into parts and chapters. Parts focus on broad areas of interest. Chapters are devoted to single topics within a part.

Part I: Asthma: An Introduction begins with a general description of asthma and provides answers to commonly asked questions. It describes what is involved during an asthma flare and describes the signs that may indicate a health emergency. Facts about the different ways asthma affects people throughout the lifespan—from infants to senior citizens—are also included.

Part II: Understanding Types of Asthma and Common Co-Occurring Conditions discusses what is known about the things that may cause asthma and how the disorder is diagnosed. It provides information about the various types of asthma, including allergic asthma, exercise-induced asthma, and occupational asthma. It also describes disorders that commonly occur with asthma or complicate asthma treatment. For example, a chapter on heart disease explains the differences between bronchial asthma (the type of asthma people mean when they simply say "asthma") and cardiac asthma (a disorder with similar symptoms caused by heart disease) and the challenges of treating asthma in heart patients. Other chapters address concerns such as chronic obstructive pulmonary disease, rhinitis, sinusitis, food allergies, and gastroesophageal reflux disease.

Part III: Asthma Management: Working with Your Doctor describes the ways a doctor and patient can work together to keep asthma under control. It includes facts about developing an asthma action plan, using a peak flow meter, and identifying things that can exacerbate asthma. It offers facts about common asthma triggers—such as exercise, weather changes, and air quality—and provides tips about reducing asthma flares that result from being exposed to them.

Part IV: Treating Asthma: Medications and Delivery Devices explains bronchodilators, corticosteroids, and other commonly used medications and therapies for asthma treatment. It discusses the differences between the types of medications used for long-term asthma control and those used to provide immediate relief when asthma symptoms worsen. The various types of devices used with inhaled medications is also explained.

Part V: Special Concerns about Asthma Management in Children talks to parents and guardians about helping control asthma symptoms in children. It discusses ways to recognize that a child's asthma may be worsening, steps that can be taken to help a child avoid his or her asthma triggers, issues that impact whether or not the family of a child with asthma can keep a pet, and school-related concerns, such as absenteeism and animals in the classroom.

Part VI: Asthma Statistics and Research provides facts and figures about the occurrence of asthma in the United States and around the world. It also summarizes recent research initiatives, describes new discoveries about genetic factors involved in asthma, and explains studies that are helping improve the delivery of asthma care.

Part VII: Additional Help and Information includes a glossary of asthma-related terms, a directory of asthma resources, facts about health insurance for asthma-related services, and tips about obtaining prescription medications.

Bibliographic Note

This volume contains documents and excerpts from publications issued by the following U.S. government agencies: Agency for Healthcare Quality and Research; Centers for Disease Control and Prevention; National Asthma Education and Prevention Program; National Center for Environmental Health; National Center for Health Statistics; National Guideline Clearinghouse; National Heart, Lung, and Blood Institute; National Institute of Allergy and Infectious Diseases; National Institute of Environmental Health Sciences; National Institutes of Health; Osteoporosis and Related Bone Diseases National Resource Center; U.S. Environmental Protection Agency; and the U.S. Food and Drug Administration.

In addition, this volume contains copyrighted documents from the following organizations and individuals: A.D.A.M. Inc.; Alberta Medical Association; Allergy and Asthma Network Mothers of Asthmatics; American College of Allergy, Asthma, and Immunology; American College of Chest Physicians; American Lung Association; American Physiological Society; Asthma and Allergy Foundation of America; Asthma and Schools; Asthma Partners; Asthma Society of Canada; Better Health Channel (Victoria, Australia); Children's Asthma Respiratory and Exercise Specialists; Children's Hospital of Eastern Ontario; Cincinnati Children's Hospital Medical Center; Cleveland Clinic; Ellie Goldberg, M.Ed.; Elsevier, Inc.; eMedicine.com, Inc.; Global Initiative for Asthma (GINA); Healthology, Inc.; International Food

Information Council Foundation; Johns Hopkins Bloomberg School of Public Health; Miles Weinberger, M.D.; National Jewish Medical and Research Center; National Lung Health Education Program; Nemours Foundation; and the University of Iowa's Virtual Hospital.

Full citation information is provided on the first page of each chapter. Every effort has been made to secure all necessary rights to reprint the copyrighted material. If any omissions have been made, please contact Omnigraphics to make corrections for future editions.

Acknowledgements

In addition to the organizations, agencies, and individuals who have contributed to this *Sourcebook*, special thanks go to editorial assistant Elizabeth Bellenir, research and permissions coordinator Liz Barbour, and permissions assistant Cherry Stockdale.

About the Health Reference Series

The *Health Reference Series* is designed to provide basic medical information for patients, families, caregivers, and the general public. Each volume takes a particular topic and provides comprehensive coverage. This is especially important for people who may be dealing with a newly diagnosed disease or a chronic disorder in themselves or in a family member. People looking for preventive guidance, information about disease warning signs, medical statistics, and risk factors for health problems will also find answers to their questions in the *Health Reference Series*. The *Series*, however, is not intended to serve as a tool for diagnosing illness, in prescribing treatments, or as a substitute for the physician/patient relationship. All people concerned about medical symptoms or the possibility of disease are encouraged to seek professional care from an appropriate health care provider.

Locating Information within the Health Reference Series

The *Health Reference Series* contains a wealth of information about a wide variety of medical topics. Ensuring easy access to all the fact sheets, research reports, in-depth discussions, and other material contained within the individual books of the *Series* remains one of our highest priorities. As the *Series* continues to grow in size and scope, however, locating the precise information needed by a reader may become more challenging.

A Contents Guide to the Health Reference Series was developed to direct readers to the specific volumes that address their concerns. It presents an extensive list of diseases, treatments, and other topics of general interest compiled from the Tables of Contents and major index headings. To access *A Contents Guide to the Health Reference Series*, visit www.healthreferenceseries.com.

Medical Consultant

Medical consultation services are provided to the *Health Reference Series* editors by David A. Cooke, M.D. Dr. Cooke is a graduate of Brandeis University, and he received his M.D. degree from the University of Michigan. He completed residency training at the University of Wisconsin Hospital and Clinics. He is board-certified in Internal Medicine. Dr. Cooke currently works as part of the University of Michigan Health System and practices in Brighton, MI. In his free time, he enjoys writing, science fiction, and spending time with his family.

Our Advisory Board

We would like to thank the following board members for providing guidance to the development of this *Series*:

- Dr. Lynda Baker,
  Associate Professor of Library and Information Science,
  Wayne State University, Detroit, MI
- Nancy Bulgarelli,
  William Beaumont Hospital Library, Royal Oak, MI
- Karen Imarisio,
  Bloomfield Township Public Library, Bloomfield Township, MI
- Karen Morgan, Mardigian Library,
  University of Michigan-Dearborn, Dearborn, MI
- Rosemary Orlando,
  St. Clair Shores Public Library, St. Clair Shores, MI

Health Reference Series *Update Policy*

The inaugural book in the *Health Reference Series* was the first edition of *Cancer Sourcebook* published in 1989. Since then, the *Series* has been enthusiastically received by librarians and in the medical community. In order to maintain the standard of providing high-quality health information for the layperson the editorial staff at Omnigraphics felt it was necessary to implement a policy of updating volumes when warranted.

Medical researchers have been making tremendous strides, and it is the purpose of the *Health Reference Series* to stay current with the most recent advances. Each decision to update a volume is made on an individual basis. Some of the considerations include how much new information is available and the feedback we receive from people who use the books. If there is a topic you would like to see added to the update list, or an area of medical concern you feel has not been adequately addressed, please write to:

Editor
Health Reference Series
Omnigraphics, Inc.
615 Griswold Street
Detroit, MI 48226
E-mail: editorial@omnigraphics.com

Part One

Asthma:
An Introduction

Chapter 1

Basic Facts about Asthma

What is asthma?

Asthma occurs because the airways in the lungs overreact to various stimuli, resulting in narrowing with obstruction to air flow. This recurrently results in one or more of the following symptoms:

- Tightness in the chest
- Labored breathing
- Coughing
- Noises in the chest heard particularly during a prolonged forced expiration (wheezing)

As a result of these symptoms, asthmatics may not tolerate exertion. They may be awakened frequently at night. More severe symptoms may result in requirements for urgent medical care and hospitalization. For a very few with particularly severe asthma, there is a risk of fatality.

Asthma affects the airways, which begin just below the throat as a single tube called the trachea. The trachea is situated immediately in front of the esophagus, the passageway that connects the throat with the stomach. The trachea divides into two slightly narrower tubes

---

From "Managing Asthma for Patients and Families," by Miles Weinberger, MD, September 2004. Copyright protected material used with permission of the author and the University of Iowa's Virtual Hospital, www.vh.org.

called the main bronchi (each one is called a bronchus). Each main bronchus then divides into progressively smaller tubes—the smallest are called bronchioles—to carry air to and from microscopic air spaces called alveoli. It is in the alveoli that the important work of the lung occurs, exchanging oxygen in the air for carbon dioxide in the blood. The airways (trachea, bronchi, bronchioles) are surrounded by a type of involuntary muscle known as smooth muscle. The airways are lined with a mucus membrane that secretes a fine layer of mucus and fluid. This mucus washes the airways to remove any bacteria, dirt,

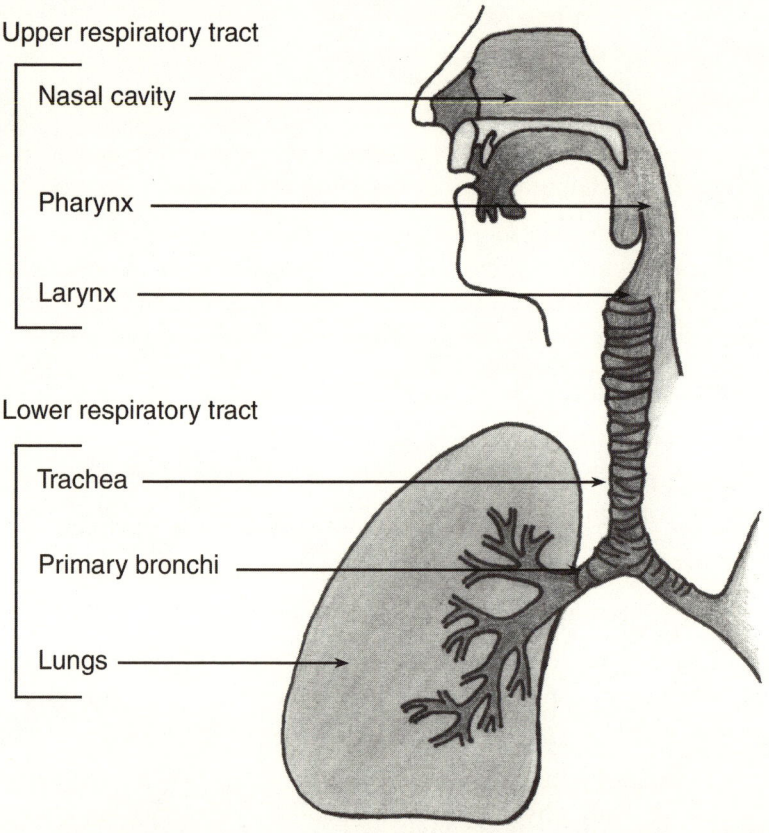

Figure 1.1. Conducting Passages (Source: From "Introduction to the Respiratory Sytem," an on-line training module produced by Surveillance, Epidemiology, and End Results (SEER), a program of the National Cancer Institute, 2000. Image re-drawn for Omnigraphics by Alison DeKleine).

Basic Facts about Asthma

or other foreign material that might get into our lungs. The overreaction or hyper-responsiveness of the airways results in bronchospasm, which is excessive contraction or spasm of the bronchial smooth muscle. The airways also become inflamed with swelling of the bronchial mucous membrane (mucosa) and secretion of excessive thick mucus that is difficult to expel. It is part of the evaluation process to identify the role of each of these physiologic components in asthma. This is important because bronchospasm (constriction of the muscle surrounding the airways) and inflammation respond to different medications.

The airway hyper-responsiveness leading to obstruction of the airways occurs from one or more of various stimuli that vary with the individual patient. These include the following:

- viral (but not bacterial) respiratory infections (common colds)
- inhaled irritants (cigarette smoke, wood burning stoves and fireplaces, strong odors, and chemical fumes)
- inhaled allergens (pollens, dusts, molds, and animal dander)
- cold air
- exercise
- occasional ingested substances (aspirin, sulfite preservatives, and specific foods)

Sometimes these exposures just act as triggers of brief symptoms with rapid relief once exposure ends. Sensitivity of the airway may be increased, however, following even brief exposure to one of these. This causes a longer period of asthmatic symptoms.

The obstruction of the airways decreases the rate at which air can flow. This is felt as tightness in the chest and labored breathing (dyspnea). The obstruction and inflammation causes coughing. Obstruction to air flow can be measured with pulmonary function tests, which can detect even degrees of airway obstruction not yet causing symptoms. Pulmonary function measurements can be an extremely valuable tool for your physician to make decisions regarding treatment.

The increased mucus in the airways stimulates coughing as the body attempts to clear the airways. The unusually thick (viscous) mucus is difficult to expel, however, resulting in continued coughing that fails to adequately expel the mucus. General irritability of the airways also causes coughing. The coughing and mucus production may cause some physicians to diagnose bronchitis. However, the term

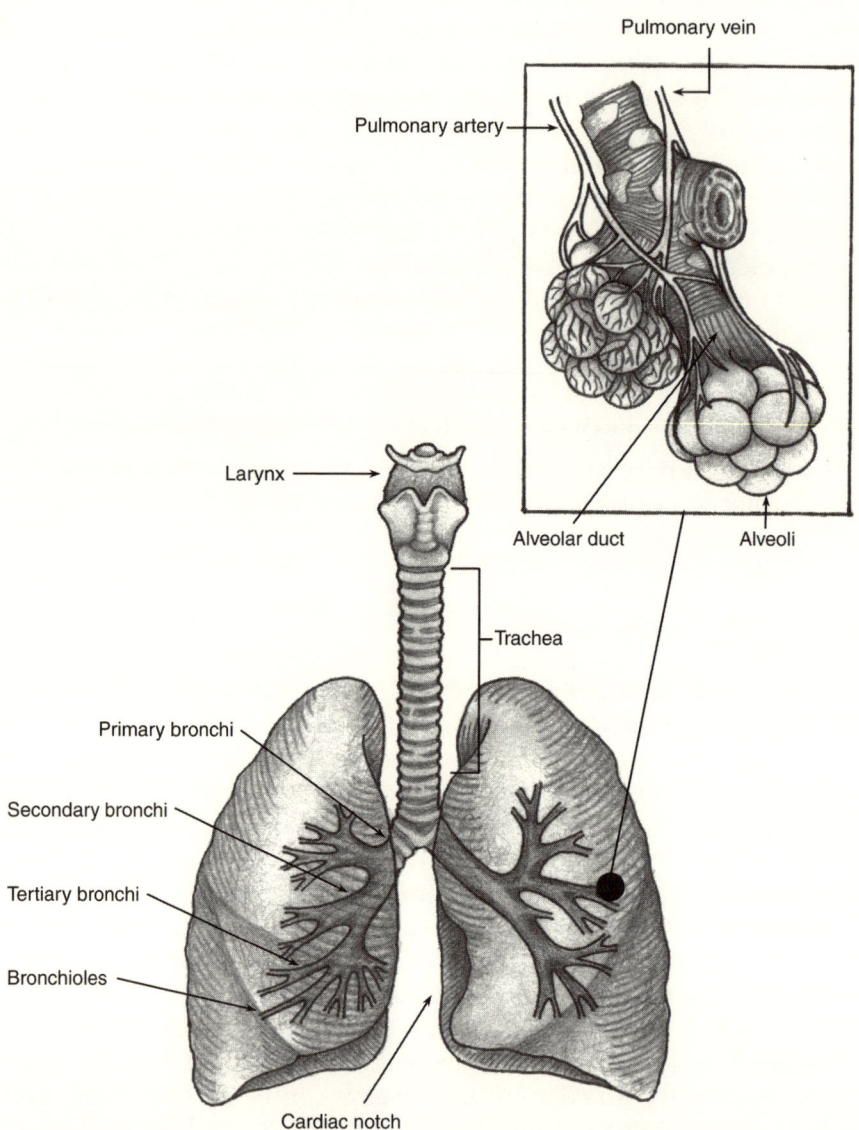

Figure 1.2. Bronchi, Bronchial Tree, and Lungs (Source: From "Introduction to the Respiratory Sytem," an on-line training module produced by Surveillance, Epidemiology, and End Results (SEER), a program of the National Cancer Institute, 2000. Image re-drawn for Omnigraphics by Alison DeKleine).

Basic Facts about Asthma

"bronchitis" simply means inflammation of the airways, and asthma causes airway inflammation. Consequently, anti-asthmatic medication, and not antibiotics, are the appropriate treatment. (Of course an asthmatic can, on occasion, have an infectious bronchitis that does not respond to anti-asthmatic medication, but this is usually viral and usual antibiotics are still not generally of any value—although there are exceptions to this generality).

Narrowing of the airway causes noises when air passes through them with sufficient speed. This typical high-pitched noise is called wheezing. Mucus in the airway causes a rattling sound. Complete obstruction of some airways can cause absorption of air from the alveoli (air sacks at the end of the airways in the lungs). This causes portions of the lung to appear more dense and cast more of a shadow on a chest x-ray (this is called atelectasis). The rattling sounds or increased shadows on the x-ray are often misinterpreted as indicating pneumonia. The inappropriate diagnoses of bronchitis and pneumonia cause much unnecessary use of antibiotics, which are ineffective both for asthma in general and for most of the infections, such as the common cold viruses, that trigger asthma.

Is all asthma the same?

Asthma is quite variable. Symptoms can range from trivial and infrequent in some to severe, unrelenting, and dangerous in others. Even when severe, however, the airway obstruction is usually fully reversible, either spontaneously or as a result of treatment. This means that symptoms can be relieved, airway obstruction can be reversed, and pulmonary function can be made normal.

There are different patterns of asthma. Some people have only an intermittent pattern of disease. They have self-limited episodes of varying severity followed by extended symptom-free periods. The individual episodes are frequently triggered by viral respiratory infections (causes of the common cold). This is particularly common in young children in whom viral respiratory infections are frequent (as many as 8 to 12 per year during the toddler and preschool age group). Others have these intermittent symptomatic periods brought on by vigorous exertion, cold air, or specific environmental exposures. This pattern is intermittent asthma.

More prolonged periods of symptoms occur in people who have asthma from seasonal outdoor inhalant allergens. This may be from grass pollen on the west coast or mold spores from molds that grow on decaying vegetation in the midwest. Through a knowledge of the

Before an Asthma Episode

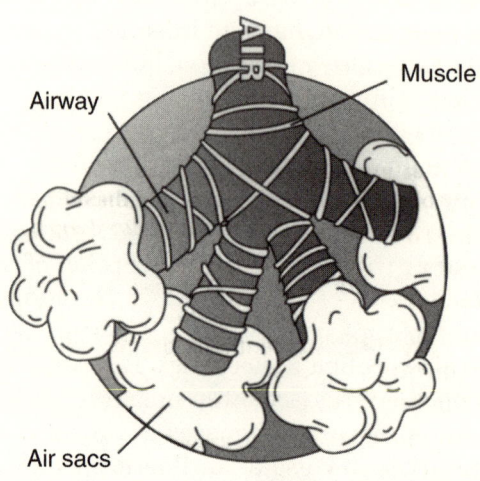

After an Asthma Episode

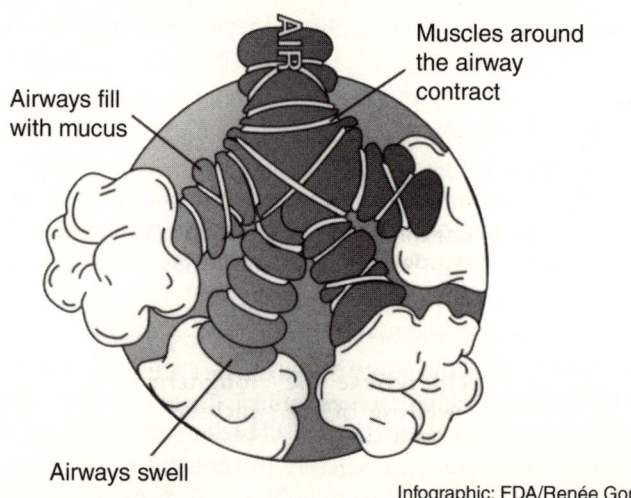

Figure 1.3. *In people with asthma, inflamed airways react to triggers such as smoke, dust, or pollen. The airways become narrow, making it difficult to breathe. (Source: Infographic by Renée Gordon,* FDA Consumer, *U.S. Food and Drug Administration, March–April 2003.)*

aerobiology in your area and allergy skin testing, your physician can attempt to identify whether the symptoms fit into this pattern of disease. This pattern is seasonal allergic asthma.

Some patients have daily or very frequently recurring symptoms. Although variable in severity, these patients do not have extended periods free of chest tightness, labored breathing, exertional intolerance, or cough. They may additionally have acute exacerbations triggered by the same factors that cause symptoms with an intermittent or seasonal allergic pattern of disease. Thus, viral respiratory infections (common colds) or specific environmental exposures may further increase the severity of symptoms in these patients. This pattern is chronic asthma (sometimes called persistent asthma).

All patterns of disease are associated with varying degrees of severity ranging from mild to severe. It is your doctor's job, with your help, to identify the pattern and severity of disease and provide effective intervention measures to rapidly relieve acute symptoms and determine appropriate maintenance measures for those with extended symptomatic periods.

Why does someone get it?

Over 10% of people have some history of asthma. It often runs in families. The heritable nature of asthma is not well understood, however, and geneticists cannot define the precise manner in which it is passed from parents to children. All we can say is that families with asthma are more likely to have children with asthma. Although there appears to be an inherited predisposition to develop asthma, severity varies considerably among asthmatics, even among members in the same family. If asthma is present in both parents, the likelihood of a child having asthma is even greater, but even then not all of the children will have asthma. Even among identical twins, both do not necessarily have asthma, although this is more likely than if they were just siblings or non-identical twins. This suggests that there is some additional factor that we do not yet fully understand, other than inheritance, that influences the development of asthma.

Asthma commonly begins early in childhood, even in infancy. But it can begin at any time, even among the elderly. In many cases, asthma runs in families; sometimes it does not. Sometimes it goes away with time; sometimes it does not. We do not know what causes asthma to start nor can we predict who will lose it with time. We do know that people with asthma can be provided with the means to control the disease and prevent symptoms that interfere with daily living. Rather than ask, "Why do I have asthma?" it is better to ask: "How can I control asthma so as to go about my usual activities without having interference from asthma?"

What can be done about it?

Asthma can be controlled. Moreover, it can be controlled by those who have asthma. The role of the physician is to provide the means for the patient to control asthma and to teach the patient to use provided measures (this is called physician-directed self-management).

Since asthma varies greatly in pattern of symptoms and severity, the treatment plan needs to be individualized. This should be done in a systematic manner. Goals of therapy must be realistically attainable and explicitly defined for you. The plan for attaining the treatment goals must be understood. Once the measures needed for control of asthma are identified, they can be placed in the hands of the patient with appropriate instructions for usage. Parental supervision is needed for young children, but progressive responsibility for self-management is given with advancing maturity.

Treatment may consist of medication, environmental changes, and life-style changes. The more the patient (or family for young children) understands the disease and its treatment, the better the outcome is likely to be. The patient (and family) should therefore be an active partner in making decisions about treatment. Be wary, however, of superstitions and misinformation regarding asthma. More than almost any other medical problem, asthma is associated with a wide diversity of medical and non-medical opinion. Both the physician and the patient therefore need to exercise judgment. Four common sense measures to remember include the following:

- ineffective measures should not be continued
- effective measures should be continued as long as they are needed unless risk exceeds benefit
- treatment should not be worse than the problem being treated
- treatment should be the simplest that is adequate

Remember that it is not sufficient just to do what is prescribed. You must also understand why measures are used so that you can be an active partner in learning what measures are required and when they should be applied. Learn the names of your medications (both the brand name and the generic name). Be critical in your observations.

Basic Facts about Asthma

Report observations and concerns regarding asthma to your physician. Ask questions. Answering your questions is part of the physician's job in providing you with the skills to manage your (or your child's) asthma. The final goal is for you, not the physician, to be treating the asthma. After all, you are there when it occurs. Your physician should try to determine the most appropriate therapeutic measures. However, these measures are not optimally effective until they are implemented by you.

Will it ever go away?

Asthma has a variable course. Many children with asthma see it improve or appear to go away as they get older. This can happen any time in childhood or adolescence. If asthma was only intermittent in nature and triggered by viral respiratory infections (a particularly common form of asthma in young children), there is an excellent likelihood that asthma will be much less of a problem as the child gets older. Sometimes the nature of the asthma changes with age. A young child may have asthma initially only from viral infections. As the child ages, asthma may occur less from viral infections (because older children get fewer viral respiratory infections than younger children), but inhalant allergy may become an important contributor to the asthma. If asthma persists into adult life, or returns later in adult life after a period of remission, persisting asthmatic symptoms may not be readily explainable by any environmental factors.

Approximately half of children with chronic asthma have little or no problem after adolescence. There appears to be no way to predict who will "outgrow" their asthma and who will not. This does not relate to severity, however. Very severe asthma often goes away, and mild asthma may persist. Even when asthmatic symptoms cease to be a problem for a awhile, this is not an assurance that asthma will not return later in life. We should therefore not talk about "growing out of asthma" in children but should instead refer to extended periods of remission when asthma becomes quiescent. Asthma that persists into adult life, returns in an adult, or begins later in life, is much less likely to go into remission, although some waxing and waning of severity may occur.

Whatever the course, however, asthma is virtually always controllable with acceptably safe measures. While ongoing medical evaluation of asthma should assess whether the disease is still active and continues to need treatment, it is not wise to withhold treatment in the hope that asthma will go away by itself. That may indeed occur, but it may not, and there can be considerable avoidable suffering and disability in the interim.

Does asthma cause permanent damage?

The airway obstruction of asthma is generally completely reversible and usually does not cause permanent damage to the lungs, heart, or other organs. However, severe acute episodes of asthma can be associated with life-threatening events and even fatalities. Survival of severe life-threatening events can be associated with damage from lack of oxygen during the severe exacerbation, and lack of oxygen to the brain can cause loss of consciousness and brain damage.

Chronic asthma with ongoing airway inflammation may also be associated with what is called "remodeling" of the airways. This describes permanent changes occurring in the tissues surrounding the airways that results in permanent narrowing of airways. The potential for this emphasizes the importance of monitoring pulmonary function in patients with asthma at regular intervals, particularly those with a chronic pattern of asthma.

What is the goal of asthma treatment?

The primary goal of treatment is the control of asthma.

What does control of asthma mean?

- The ability to deal with acute exacerbations of asthma so that the need for urgent medical care is prevented
- Prevention of hospitalization for asthma
- Tolerating all normal activities up to and including competitive athletics if otherwise able
- The avoidance of symptoms that interfere with sleep
- Normal pulmonary physiology (as measured by pulmonary function equipment)

These goals should be reached safely and with the least interference with a normal life-style. The risks and bother of the treatment must be carefully weighed against the risk and bother of the asthma. The benefit obtained from the treatment must be worth any inconvenience and potential medication risks (and any medication has potential risks) imposed by the treatment.

Basic Facts about Asthma

In other words, it is the goal of treatment to determine the simplest, safest therapeutic measures that minimize disability, normalize lung function, avoid the need for acute medical care of asthma, and permit a normal life.

How are the treatment goals are attained?

Unfortunately, there is no magic bullet for asthma. While treatment can control symptoms safely and effectively for most patients most of the time, it is not a simple matter of the doctor writing a prescription and the patient taking the medication. Successful treatment of asthma is likely to require several steps on the part of physician. These include the following:

- Confirmation of the diagnosis (make sure it's asthma and not some other problem.)
- Characterization of the asthma with regard to:
  - Chronicity (how frequent are the symptoms?)
  - Severity (how bad do the symptoms get?)
  - Identification of triggers (what makes the asthma worse?)
  - Identification of the components of airway obstruction (bronchospasm, inflammation, or both?)
- Development of a plan to identify the least treatment that is safe and effective
- Teach implementation of that plan (what to do and when)

The diagnosis of asthma is suspected when a patient has a history of recurrent or chronic shortness of breath, labored breathing, or cough in the absence of any other obvious reason. The diagnosis is confirmed by obtaining evidence that there is airway obstruction that reverses either spontaneously or as a result of treatment with anti-asthmatic measures. The procedures used to make the diagnosis include a careful history, measurement of pulmonary function (unless not practical, as in young children), and therapeutic trials of medication.

Chronicity refers to the relative persistence of symptoms and signs of asthma. Some patients have only episodic or intermittent asthma; between relatively infrequent episodes of acute symptoms, they are completely asymptomatic. Other patients have extended periods of seasonally recurring symptoms due to seasonal inhalant allergens.

This pattern is classified as seasonal allergic asthma. Yet others have chronic asthma. These patients may also have brief acute exacerbations or recurring seasons of worsened symptoms but differ from intermittent or seasonal allergic asthmatics in that they do not experience extended periods free of symptoms and signs of asthma.

Assessment of severity is independent of chronicity. For any of the classifications, symptoms may range from trivial to life-threatening. Severity of acute symptoms is judged by the degree of medical care needed. Some patients never require an urgent visit to a physician or an emergency room for their asthma while others have required frequent emergency care and hospitalizations. Asthmatic symptoms that have resulted in loss of consciousness or admission to an intensive care unit identifies a particularly dangerous degree of severity.

Severity of chronic symptoms is judged by the degree of disability resulting from the daily or frequently recurring symptoms that occur in the absence of effective medication. Patients may have daily symptoms that cause only minimal discomfort. These patients tolerate activities and sleep undisturbed by their asthma. Others are literally pulmonary cripples with virtually no tolerance of activity and frequent disturbance of sleep by shortness of breath or cough.

Triggers of asthma, those identifiable factors that commonly worsen symptoms, include the following:

- viral respiratory infections (common colds)
- airborne allergens (such as pollens, mold spores, animal dander, and dusts)
- inhaled irritants (such as cigarette smoke, chemical fumes, strong odors, and air pollution)
- cold air
- exertion

Other factors can also worsen asthma on occasion. Hyperventilation, excessively rapid and deep breathing, can worsen asthma. This occurs from anxiety in some patients, particularly when asthma symptoms have begun for some other reason. A vicious cycle then occurs of asthma causing anxiety, which then worsens asthma, thereby causing more anxiety, etc. Ingested substances, such as aspirin, sulfite preservatives, and specific foods can cause acute attacks of asthma in sensitive patients.

Basic Facts about Asthma

The components of airway obstruction in asthma include bronchospasm (constriction of the muscle surrounding the airways) and inflammation. The distinction is important because the responses of each to medical treatment are different. Bronchospasm (constriction of the muscle surrounding the airways) responds to bronchodilators, medication that relaxes the bronchial smooth muscle that causes narrowing of the airway from bronchospasm. Bronchodilator medications, however, have little or no effect on mucosal edema and mucous secretions caused by inflammation. Anti-inflammatory corticosteroids (no relationship to "steroids" used by athletes to build muscle) dramatically, though slowly, reduce the mucosal swelling and mucous secretions but have no direct ability to relax the bronchial smooth muscle and relieve the bronchospasm.

An organized plan should determine specific treatment needs to control the asthma. These include medication needs, environmental alterations, and indications for allergy shots.

Medication requirements can be divided into two categories, intervention measures to relieve acute symptoms and maintenance medication to prevent the rapid return of symptoms once the intervention measures are stopped.

Patients with an intermittent pattern of asthma require only intervention measures.

Patients with sustained periods of asthmatic symptoms or asthma that returns promptly after complete clearing with intervention measures require the use of maintenance medication in addition to intervention measures.

Virtually all patients should be taught to deliver an inhaled bronchodilator to relieve or prevent acute episodes of bronchospasm. This is all that is needed for many patients. The need for corticosteroids as an additional intervention measure should be assessed based on response to bronchodilator and prior history of severity. For those with sustained periods of symptoms, maintenance medication should be selected sequentially until symptoms and signs of asthma are adequately suppressed. The goal is to permit normal sleep and activities without excessively frequent addition of intervention measures (inhaled bronchodilators and short courses of oral corticosteroids) for breakthrough symptoms.

The need for environmental alterations should be individualized as carefully as medication selection. Non-allergic irritants such as cigarette smoke or chemical fumes are usually assumed to be potentially detrimental to asthma. The use of allergy skin testing helps identify potential allergic sensitivity to specific environmental exposures. The use of allergy shots may be indicated when environmental alteration is not practical for treatment of clinically important airborne allergen sensitivity.

The treatment plan can be no more effective than its implementation. Most of the treatment, and certainly the most important aspects of the treatment, are carried out by the patient (or the family for young children). It is the physician's job (with help from other health professionals) to teach, and it is your job to learn how to carry out the treatment plan. This is an interactive and ongoing process. Use each contact, whether in person or by phone, to learn more about managing your (or your child's) asthma.

Chapter 2

Questions and Answers about Asthma

General Information About Asthma

What is asthma?

Asthma is a disease of the airways in the lungs. Its symptoms are caused by inflammation, which makes the airways red, swollen, narrower, and extra-sensitive to irritants. This leads to recurrent attacks of wheezing, breathlessness, chest tightness, and coughing. Mild attacks can settle down without treatment, but treatment usually helps them to resolve more quickly. Appropriate treatment can also reduce the risk of further attacks. If you experience a serious attack you should seek emergency help.

Asthma is a long-term (chronic) disease. Your asthma does not stay the same, but changes over time, and every person with asthma has good and bad days (or longer periods of time).

Asthma is very common. Around one out of every ten people in the Western World develops asthma at some stage in their life.

What is inflammation in the airways?

Inflammation is a reaction to infections and other triggers in the lining of the airways and the underlying tissue.

From "Q&A: What Is Asthma," © Global Initiative for Asthma (http://ginasthma.com); reprinted with permission from the Global Initiative for Asthma.

How does inflammation of the airways affect my asthma?

Inflammation of the airways causes asthma symptoms (wheezing, breathlessness, chest tightness, and coughing) by restricting or limiting the airflow to and from the lungs. It does this by causing the following symptoms:

- swelling of the airways, which makes them narrower
- tightening of the muscles that surround the airways (also called bronchoconstriction), which makes them even narrower
- the production of too much mucus, which can plug up or block the airways
- longer-term damage to the walls of the airways, which prevents them from opening as widely as a normal airway

When the airways have been inflamed for a long time, they become extra-sensitive. This means that they react faster and more strongly to various triggers, such as allergens, viruses, dust, smoke, and stress.

Who gets asthma?

Asthma tends to run in families, which means that you are more likely to develop asthma if someone in your family already has it. Children with eczema or food allergy are more likely than other children to develop asthma.

Allergy to pollen, house dust mites, or pets also increases your chance of developing asthma. Exposure to tobacco smoke, air pollution, or other inhaled irritants can also cause asthma symptoms in those with an underlying tendency to asthma.

At what age does asthma start?

Asthma can start at any age, although about half of all people with asthma have had their first symptoms by the age of 10, and many children with asthma have had their first asthma attack before the age of 6.

Is asthma a chronic disease?

Yes. Asthma is a chronic (long-term) disease that causes inflammation and narrowing of the airways. Some degree of inflammation is usually present, even at times when you are unaware of any symptoms.

Questions and Answers about Asthma

If your asthma is untreated, you will have repeated attacks of asthma symptoms.

Mild attacks can settle down without treatment, but treatment usually helps them to resolve more quickly. Appropriate treatment can also reduce the risk of further attacks. If you experience a serious attack you should seek emergency help.

Your asthma does not stay the same, but changes over time, and every person with asthma has good and bad days (or longer periods of time). However, if asthma is properly treated, you may enjoy long periods without symptoms or attacks.

Causes of Asthma and Trigger Factors

What causes asthma?

The causes of asthma are not fully understood. Its symptoms are caused by inflammation, which makes the airways red, swollen, narrower, and extra-sensitive to irritants. Asthma is probably usually caused by a mixture of hereditary factors (those you are born with) and environmental factors, but how these factors work together is still largely unknown.

Allergens from house dust mites and pets are the most common causes, but many other allergens, such as pollen and molds, can cause asthma. Some people with asthma have no obvious allergies.

What causes asthma symptoms or an asthma attack?

Some causes of symptoms (triggers) are common to all people with asthma, and some are more individual, especially allergens. There are very big differences between people in how easily and how severely they react. The severity of the symptoms or an attack can differ in the same person at different times, and treatment can also be more or less effective.

Your asthma does not stay the same, but changes over time, and every person with asthma has good days and bad days (or longer periods). However, if asthma is properly treated, there can also be long periods without symptoms or attacks.

What are asthma triggers?

Asthma triggers are factors that start asthma symptoms or an asthma attack by irritating the airways or worsening the inflammation in the airways. These triggers can provoke attacks in individuals who already have a tendency to asthma, but they are not necessarily part of the cause of that tendency. The following triggers can cause asthma symptoms or start an asthma attack:

- infections, usually those caused by a virus (for example, colds or flu)
- allergens, most commonly from house dust mites, pets, or pollen
- exercise, especially in cold weather
- emotions, such as excitement, fear, or anger
- irritants, such as air pollution
- smoking—people with asthma and the parents of asthmatic children should avoid smoking
- changes in the weather (for example, a cold spell)
- food additives, such as tartrazine (an artificial food coloring), or food allergens, such as peanuts (sensitized or allergic individuals can have a very severe allergic reaction)
- certain medications—some people may be allergic to some drugs (for example, aspirin)

What are the main asthma triggers?

Different triggers can start an asthma attack and people differ a lot in how easily and how severely they react. Some triggers (also called inciters) only cause tightening of the airways (bronchoconstriction) that lasts for just a short time. These triggers include the following:

- exercise
- cigarette smoke
- changes in air temperature
- laughing
- strong smells

Other triggers (also called inducers) also increase the underlying inflammation of the airways, and may have longer-term effects. Such triggers include the following:

- allergens (for example, pets, house dust mites, and pollen)
- infections (for example, colds, flu)
- certain chemicals

Questions and Answers about Asthma

What chemicals, irritants, or other substances trigger asthma?

Many irritating particles or chemicals in the air can trigger an asthma attack. Here are some examples:

- cigarette smoke
- diesel exhaust
- perfume or other strong scents
- household sprays
- sulfur dioxide
- grain or flour dust
- sawdust

However, there are very big differences between people in how easily and how severely they react. This depends on the severity of the asthma and how well it is treated.

Can medications trigger asthma?

Only a few medications can trigger asthma. Check with your doctor or pharmacist before starting any new medicine. And if your asthma symptoms are worse after starting a new medication, you should see your doctor immediately.

These are the most common medicines that can trigger asthma:

- aspirin (acetylsalicylic acid) and certain other NSAID (non-steroidal anti-inflammatory) drugs, which are used as pain relievers and to treat arthritis and inflammatory conditions
- beta-blockers, which are used to treat high blood pressure, heart conditions, migraine, or anxiety

Not all patients with asthma react to aspirin or NSAIDs, so some people with asthma can use these drugs. However, beta-blockers are more likely to cause symptoms in patients with asthma and should be avoided.

Can weather changes trigger asthma?

Yes, sudden weather changes (for example, cold winds, humidity, and storms) can trigger asthma in some people. Some of these sudden changes can cause the release of allergens, such as pollen, that can make asthma worse in people whose asthma is allergy-related. Cold air can also have a direct irritant effect on inflamed airways.

Can infections trigger asthma?

Yes, viral respiratory infections, such as colds or flu, can trigger asthma symptoms, particularly in children. Try to avoid contact with people if you know they have a respiratory infection.

Can an allergic reaction trigger asthma?

Yes. Once you are sensitized or allergic, both indoor and outdoor allergens can cause asthma symptoms and attacks, as well as other allergic symptoms such as sneezing or a runny nose. It is, therefore, important to consider whether your asthma is caused or worsened by allergens.

Exposure to even small amounts of airborne allergens can cause asthma symptoms. Repeated exposure may not only provoke symptoms, but may also be a cause of long-term (chronic) inflammation in the airways.

Proper advice about which allergens and environments you should avoid can only be given after talking to your doctor and often after you have been tested for allergies.

Why is it sometimes so hard to know what triggers an asthma attack?

People with allergic asthma can often easily identify the most common trigger factor(s) for their asthma (for example, pets or pollen). But many people with untreated or under-treated asthma have an underlying airway inflammation that they are hardly aware of. These people will react easily to many irritants, allergens, and infections, and it can be difficult to identify the most important one.

If your asthma is provoked by more than one trigger at the same time, the reaction can be stronger than if you are only exposed to one trigger. For example, an airway infection may cause you to react to stimuli that you normally would not react to. This is why triggers such as physical exercise, strong smells, plants, chemicals, smoke, weather changes, anxiety, stress, and some medications can sometimes cause an asthma attack and sometimes cause no symptoms.

Questions and Answers about Asthma

Is asthma a psychological (psychosomatic) disease?

No, asthma is not a psychological condition; it is a long-term (chronic) inflammatory disease that leads to extra-sensitive and easily irritated airways, especially when it is not properly treated.

Although asthma is not a psychological condition, emotional stress can trigger the symptoms. For example, financial problems, not enjoying your work, or worrying about your family can all help to trigger symptoms if you already have asthma.

Why does my asthma get worse when I am upset or worried about something?

Not all people with asthma feel worse when they are upset or worried. Those who do may be easily stressed, or may cry or breathe too fast (hyperventilate) easily.

Another reason that your asthma gets worse could be that you are not being treated properly for the inflammation you have in your airways.

Can I get asthma symptoms from a plastic Christmas tree?

Yes, you could if you had asthma symptoms from real Christmas trees in the past (though this is not a common allergy). This phenomenon is called a conditioned reflex. It is the same thing that causes your mouth to water when you see a picture of delicious food.

Asthma Symptoms

What does asthma feel like?

Asthma symptoms typically come and go. You have trouble breathing, your chest feels tight, and you can hear wheezing when you breathe or cough. These symptoms often occur during exercise or during the night.

An asthma attack is when your symptoms rapidly become more severe, usually rather suddenly. During an asthma attack, you have more trouble breathing.

You may get used to the asthma symptoms and not realize that your airflow is impaired and could be improved by treatment.

When your asthma is under good control, the airways are clear and air flows easily in and out.

What happens during an asthma attack?

When asthma is not under control, the airways become inflamed. Inflammation of the airways causes asthma symptoms (wheezing, breathlessness, chest tightness, and coughing) by restricting or limiting the airflow to and from the lungs.

- The airways become red and swollen, which makes them narrower. This can often take several hours or days to develop and may take just as long to reverse after the asthma attack has passed.
- Tightening of the muscles that surround the airways (also called bronchoconstriction) makes them even narrower. This tightening can happen very quickly, depending on the type of trigger and underlying inflammation.
- The airways make more mucus, which can plug up or partly block the airways.
- Attacks can range from mild to severe.

What are the signs of a severe and dangerous asthma attack?

- Symptoms that are rapidly becoming more severe and do not get better even after you take your airway opener (bronchodilator) medication
- Symptoms that do not improve at all, or rapidly return after you have taken your airway opener medication
- Difficulty talking because you are short of breath
- A peak flow reading below 50% of your normal value, which is not improved by the airway opener medication
- A peak flow reading that according to your asthma management plan puts you at risk of an asthma attack

Can a person die from asthma?

Unfortunately, deaths still occur in acute, severe asthma. But this is unusual and can be prevented.

Most asthma deaths occur in people who have not received enough treatment, perhaps because they did not realize or did not want to admit how serious their asthma was, or because they had not received adequate guidance from their doctors and nurses.

The correct use of controlling and preventive medication is the key to preventing these tragedies. People with asthma sometimes forget or choose not to take their anti-inflammatory medication, especially during periods when they are feeling well. When they start to get symptoms of asthma, they increase the dose of airway opener (bronchodilator). However, this will not treat the underlying inflammation, which may lead to severe life-threatening attacks. If you have stopped taking your anti-inflammatory medication, you should re-start it at the first sign of symptoms of asthma, in addition to using an airway opener.

If you are using regular inhaled corticosteroid treatment, you should not stop using this at any time unless you have discussed this with your doctor first.

Why do I lose my breath?

You lose your breath during an asthma attack because the airways become narrow, which restricts or limits the airflow to and from the lungs. The airways become restricted because of the following conditions:

- The lining of the airways becomes inflamed
- The production of mucus (phlegm) increases and may block the airways
- The muscles in the walls of the airways tighten

During an asthma attack, all of these things happen in different degrees.

You can also lose your breath for other reasons than asthma (for example, during physical exercise, especially if you are not in good shape). If you lose your breath without typical asthma symptoms, and if your asthma medication has no effect, you should see your doctor.

How do I know if I am having an asthma attack?

During an asthma attack, you will find it harder to breathe because your airways have become narrower. Your chest feels tight, and you can hear wheezing when you breathe or cough. You may feel as if you are trying to breathe through a straw in your mouth while holding your nose.

If the peak expiratory flow (PEF) value drops to half of the usual level, it's time to seek emergency help.

Can the peak flow meter tell me if I need to see the doctor?

If you take peak flow readings regularly or know the reading you get when your asthma is well controlled then, as a general rule, if the reading falls to less than two-thirds of the usual level, it is time to be cautious and to increase the amount of medication. A reading that is less than half the usual level often indicates the need for immediate help, but this varies from person to person.

It is best if you and your doctor together set a personal peak flow reading that indicates when it is time for you to increase the dose of medication or seek acute help. This should be combined with a written treatment plan for your medications.

It is important to realize that your treatment should not be entirely determined by your peak flow readings. Whenever the usual treatment does not have the effect you wish on the control of your asthma you should discuss this with your doctor, regardless of the peak flow reading.

Can asthma medication help prevent asthma symptoms?

Yes. Asthma medications include very effective airway openers. Even more importantly, they include very effective controllers (inhaled steroids), which can prevent most asthma attacks when used regularly.

Asthma Prognosis

Can my asthma be cured?

No, there is not yet a total cure for asthma.

The causes of asthma are not fully understood. Sometimes children with asthma can grow out of their symptoms, or many years of regular treatment with anti-inflammatory asthma medication may make the disease disappear. However, asthma may recur again later in life in both these groups of patients.

Asthma does not stay the same, but changes over time, and every person with asthma has good days and bad days. It is tempting to think that your asthma has been cured if you have not had symptoms for a long time, but you will usually still have a tendency to asthma if you are exposed to the appropriate triggers in the future.

Allergy treatment using hyposensitization (often called allergy vaccination) can very occasionally achieve a near-cure of asthma in someone with specific reactions to known allergens, but is unhelpful for most people.

Questions and Answers about Asthma

Is there a risk that my asthma will get worse with age?

Yes, that risk cannot be disregarded. Poorly treated asthma gets worse with age, and the lungs of people with untreated asthma function less well than those of non-asthmatic individuals. Modern asthma treatments have not been available for long enough for us to be certain whether or not lung function will still deteriorate more rapidly in patients with treated asthma as they grow older. However, most asthma doctors think that regular, preventive asthma treatment can prevent your asthma from getting worse and help to preserve your lung function.

Can I outgrow my asthma?

Whether you can outgrow your asthma depends on how old you were when it started and how severe it was at the time. Around half the children with mild asthma will have no symptoms by the time they reach their mid-teens. Asthma does, however, often recur in adulthood. Children with more severe asthma are less likely to be free of symptoms when they get older.

Asthma that develops in adulthood can be associated with long-term exposure to specific triggers, such as chemicals or pollution, and can sometimes be greatly improved if the triggers are avoided.

Most asthma can be well controlled with appropriate medication, but as an adult you are unlikely to outgrow it completely.

Is asthma a life-long disease?

Asthma is a long-term (chronic) disease, and the tendency to develop asthma symptoms is probably life-long. In some children, symptoms only appear intermittently. Also, some children with mild asthma will have no symptoms by the time they reach their mid-teens.

Non-Medical Treatment

How can I avoid common triggers?

First, try to discover what triggers your asthma. Common triggers include tobacco smoke, cold air and exercise.

- You should be strict about no smoking inside your home and other places where you spend time. Exposure to tobacco smoke makes asthma worse in most people.

- Cold air triggers symptoms more easily when you are not getting enough treatment for your asthma, and increasing your dose of anti-inflammatory medication will often help.
- Exercise is important and should normally not be discouraged, because asthma symptoms during or following exercise can usually be prevented by good medication.

Some allergens can be avoided. For example, if you are allergic to horses or cats you should keep away from them. Other allergens and environmental triggers, such as house dust mite, pollen, and air pollution, are more difficult to avoid completely.

Remember there is a difference between triggers that cause inflammation (inducers) and those that only cause temporary symptoms. Full advice about which allergens and environments you should avoid can only be given after talking to your doctor and often after you have been tested for allergies.

I'm allergic to pets/furry animals. What can I do?

If you have allergic asthma, it is especially important to avoid or at least reduce your exposure to the relevant allergens. If you are allergic to pets, such as cats and dogs, you should not keep them indoors. You should also reduce your contact with other peoples pets, especially indoors.

Use a vacuum cleaner with a HEPA (high efficiency particulate air) filter and double bags. You may also feel better if you avoid having dust-collecting textiles and furniture.

Should I get a central vacuum cleaner?

It is not scientifically proven that a central vacuum cleaner is more effective than a modern vacuum cleaner with a HEPA (high efficiency particulate air) filter and double bags.

I'm allergic to dust mites. What can I do?

House dust mites and their allergens are difficult to avoid. Try to keep your house, and especially the living area and the bedrooms, dry and well ventilated. Avoid textile floor coverings.

If possible, let someone else do the cleaning. Mop the floors instead of vacuuming them.

It can be a good idea to encase pillows, quilts, and mattresses in airtight covers that do not allow dust mites or their allergens to pass through. Alternatively, wash your pillow, blanket and bedding regularly at 140° F (60° C). Previously, it was recommended that you put your pillow in the freezer regularly to reduce the number of dust mites, but this is unnecessary if you get a cover for your pillow and mattress that does not let the dust mites through. Ask your doctor for advice.

Use a vacuum cleaner with a HEPA (high efficiency particulate air) filter and double bags. You may also feel better if you avoid having dust-collecting textiles and furniture.

Can I reduce my asthma if I get an air purifier?

It is not clear whether using an air purifier in the home is effective. If you have no other way of reducing your exposure to allergens or irritants, it may be worth trying. However, you must use it correctly, which includes keeping doors and windows closed in the room where you are using it.

Can acupuncture help my asthma?

Acupuncture releases the body's own cortisone, among other things, and this can help in some cases. One or two studies have shown a short, temporary effect of acupuncture on asthma, but there are no long-term studies showing any lasting effects.

Asthma Medical Treatment

What are controllers?

Controllers are medicines that prevent asthma attacks from starting. There are two types of controller medicines: anti-inflammatory medicines and airway openers.

Anti-inflammatory medicines work by reducing the inflammation in the airways that occurs in asthma. The most effective and most commonly used anti-inflammatory medicines are inhaled glucocorticosteroids, such as budesonide, beclomethasone, and fluticasone. These medicines help to prevent periods of greater severity of asthma if you take them regularly as instructed by your doctor (usually once or twice every day), and they may relieve you of your symptoms completely for most of the time. If your doctor gives you an inhaled glucocorticosteroid you must take it regularly, even if you are not wheezing.

If the inflammation is not controlled, the airways become red, swollen, narrower, and extra-sensitive. Some degree of inflammation is usually present in your lungs, even when you are unaware of symptoms, and worsening of the inflammation may lead you to feel an attack coming on.

Airway openers, which are also known as bronchodilators, are medicines that help to prevent attacks progressing by quickly opening up the narrowed airways. They do this by relaxing the muscles surrounding the airways. Most airway openers only have a short-term effect and should not be used regularly as controllers. Long-acting airway openers, including formoterol and salmeterol, are effective as controllers when they are used regularly with an inhaled glucocorticosteroid. However, they should not be used regularly on their own as they do not treat the underlying inflammation and their effect on the symptoms of asthma could even hide the fact that it is getting worse.

What are relievers?

Relievers or airway openers are medicines that provide rapid relief from an asthma attack by quickly opening up the narrowed airways (dilating the bronchi). They do this by relaxing the muscles surrounding the airways, and are known to doctors and other asthma professionals as bronchodilators.

There are two types of airway openers: short-acting bronchodilators and long-acting bronchodilators. The most widely used short- and quick-acting airway openers are salbutamol (also known as albuterol) and terbutaline. Salmeterol is a long-acting airway opener that has a slower action, so it is used for longer-term control, but not for the quick relief of symptoms. Formoterol is a long-acting airway opener that is also quick-acting, so it can be used both for the immediate relief of symptoms and for longer-term control.

What are combination medications?

Combination medications contain a reliever and a controller in the same inhaler. So this type of inhaler opens up the airways (preventing the feeling of chest tightening and the worsening of an attack) and also reduces the underlying inflammation that causes asthma. As a result, combination inhalers provide better control of asthma symptoms and reduce the number of inhalers you have to use.

With conventional combination inhalers, you take the same amount of medication all the time. But because every person with asthma has good days and bad days, this means that sometimes you will take a bit more of the medication than you really need, and at other times you will not be getting enough and you may have to use doses from a second inhaler containing an airway opener (bronchodilator).

Recently, a combination inhaler has become available that lets you safely adjust the dosage of your combined medication to match the changes in your asthma. This makes it possible for you to take the right level of medication at the right time and means that you use less medication overall.

What effects do anti-inflammatory medications have?

Asthma is caused by inflammation of the airways, which makes them become red, swollen, narrower, and extra-sensitive to irritants. Anti-inflammatory medicines (controllers) relieve this inflammation so that the swelling goes down and further swelling is prevented. The narrowing due to muscle tightening is reduced, and the airways become less sensitive to asthma triggers.

Anti-inflammatory medications are very effective and can control asthma in most people. The most effective anti-inflammatory medicines are the inhaled glucocorticosteroids, such as budesonide, beclomethasone, and fluticasone.

What effects do airway opener medications have?

Airway openers work by opening up the narrowed airways. They do this by relaxing the muscles surrounding the airways. This makes it easier to get air in and out of the lungs. Most airway openers work quickly and can be used to treat an asthma attack. They are sometimes called relievers or rescue bronchodilators.

What are glucocorticosteroids?

Glucocorticosteroids, which are also known as corticosteroids, are anti-inflammatory medicines. They are used to relieve and prevent inflammation of the airways, which is the cause of asthma. In asthma, glucocorticosteroids are usually inhaled and referred to as inhaled corticosteroids or inhaled steroids. The most effective and commonly used are budesonide, beclomethasone, and fluticasone.

Why are glucocorticosteroid medications inhaled?

In asthma, glucocorticosteroids are usually inhaled so that the medicine goes straight to the lining of the airways affected by inflammation. This also greatly reduces the risk of any possible harmful effects on the rest of the body. The small amount of medicine that goes into the bloodstream is rapidly removed from the body so that normally there are none of the side effects that may occur with other types of steroid treatment. This is exemplified by pregnancy. Long-term treatment with glucocorticosteroid tablets puts both mother and unborn baby at significant risk of various complications. However, the inhaled steroid budesonide has been investigated in large studies of pregnant women, which did not show any increased risk for the mother or unborn baby.

When and why are corticosteroid tablets or injections used?

Corticosteroid tablets (usually prednisolone or prednisone) or injections can be helpful to treat a severe attack of asthma when inhaled corticosteroids have not had enough effect or are not available.

Treatment with corticosteroid tablets or injections for short periods has few side effects. High doses can, however, temporarily affect your mood, either positively or negatively. Long-term treatment with corticosteroid tablets or injections can cause side effects, including osteoporosis, thinning of the skin, weight gain, high blood pressure, and high blood sugar levels. These risks are avoided if you switch back to inhaled corticosteroids as soon as possible (in consultation with your doctor) and avoid the long-term use of corticosteroid tablets or injections.

What is the difference between a corticosteroid and an anabolic steroid?

Both corticosteroids and anabolic steroids are sometimes just called steroids. However, corticosteroids are very different from anabolic steroids. Corticosteroids reduce the swelling in the airways that make breathing difficult and also reduce the amount of mucus produced in the lungs. Anabolic steroids have an effect similar to that of the male hormone testosterone. They are sometimes used illegally by some athletes to increase muscle mass, strength, and endurance. Corticosteroids do not have these effects.

What are inhaled non-steroidal anti-inflammatory medications?

Inhaled non-steroidal anti-inflammatory medications, such as the chromones (sodium cromoglycate, cromolyn, and nedocromil), have weaker anti-inflammatory effects than corticosteroids. If your doctor gives you an inhaled non-steroidal anti-inflammatory medication, you must take it regularly, even if you are not wheezing in the same way as you should take an inhaled corticosteroid. If you are being treated with one of these medications, you will need to take an airway opener from another inhaler to treat any asthma attacks.

Is there an effective alternative to using inhaled corticosteroids?

There are no alternative treatments that control asthma as effectively as inhaled corticosteroids. Inhaled non-steroidal anti-inflammatory medications, such the chromones, are not so effective and do not usually relieve the inflammation completely.

Antileukotrienes are tablets that are taken by mouth and are helpful to some people with asthma. Often they are not an effective alternative to inhaled corticosteroids for the long-term control of asthma and the prevention of attacks, but some patients benefit from their use.

Antihistamine tablets are not helpful in the treatment of asthma. However, patients who also have hay fever may find that their asthma improves when the hay fever is successfully controlled, and antihistamines may be successfully used to treat hay fever.

Some airway openers, such as theophylline, can be taken by mouth in long-acting preparations. To select the safe and effective dose for an individual patient, and thus achieve the best effect, blood levels of the drug may need to be measured and the dose adjusted. In general, long-acting airway openers are not an alternative to inhaled corticosteroids, because these medications do not fully relieve the underlying inflammation of asthma. The inflammation tends to become worse over time, causing more frequent asthma attacks and more severe symptoms. Although some patients find that their asthma can be satisfactorily controlled by the regular use of theophylline tablets or capsules, these treatments have been largely replaced by inhaled medications. If you have been using theophylline for some time, you may want to discuss today's alternative treatments with your doctor.

What are antileukotrienes?

Antileukotrienes are a relatively new type of medication for asthma that are taken as tablets once or twice a day. They work by relieving the part of the airway inflammation caused by chemical substances called leukotrienes, but do not reduce it completely. They may also help to protect against asthma attacks. Often they are not an effective alternative to inhaled corticosteroids for the long-term control of asthma and the prevention of attacks, but some patients benefit from their use.

Inhaled corticosteroids are recommended for treating asthma because they are anti-inflammatory. Aspirin is also anti-inflammatory, but is not recommended for people with asthma. Why?

Corticosteroids and aspirin are both anti-inflammatory, but work in very different ways and relieve different types of inflammation. Aspirin has no effect on the inflammation of the airways that occurs in asthma. More seriously, in some patients with asthma, aspirin may provoke severe attacks of asthma. Any patient who is known to have such aspirin sensitivity should avoid the use of aspirin at all times. Even in other patients, aspirin has no beneficial effects on asthma.

What anti-inflammatory medication can I take for a strained muscle, aching joints, severe back pain, or rheumatism, for example?

If you have asthma and have used aspirin or a similar medicine (often called non-steroidal anti-inflammatory drugs, or NSAIDs) without any worsening of your asthma, you can continue to use it. If, however, you have had asthma symptoms after using aspirin or an NSAID, you should avoid these drugs and use acetaminophen (paracetamol) or another medicine instead. You should discuss appropriate alternatives with your doctor if necessary.

What is hyposensitization (immunotherapy/vaccination)?

Hyposensitization is often referred to as allergy vaccination or immunotherapy. It usually involves having a series of injections of the allergen or allergens that are known to cause your asthma. The dose of the injections is gradually increased, with the aim that the body will learn to handle these allergens better and no longer develop asthma on exposure to them.

Hyposensitization is sometimes suitable for the treatment of asthma provoked by pollen, some animals, or dust mites. It is most likely to be successful if your asthma is caused by only one or a few allergens. If your asthma reacts to many different things, it will not usually get better with this treatment.

Hyposensitization has been used for more than 80 years and is still the only treatment that can potentially reduce your reaction to a specific allergen. The method works for asthma that has been provoked by pollen, furry animals, and dust mites, but not for mold. However, there is a risk of serious reactions to the injections, so they should only be given by a specialist, and usually only in a hospital clinic. The risks of these injections limit their availability in some countries, and the treatment is also relatively expensive.

I'm troubled by my asthma when outdoors in cold weather. What can I do?

First of all, be sure that you are using an effective anti-inflammatory treatment. If cold air causes asthma symptoms, inhaled corticosteroids are probably needed. If you are already taking them, ask your doctor whether you should increase the dose or take additional treatment. A long-acting bronchodilator, such as formoterol, may be the best choice.

A face mask may also help by heating and moisturizing the inhaled air, because cold air dries and irritates the mucus membranes in the airways, especially in people with asthma. Your doctor or pharmacist will be able to advise you.

Asthma Side Effects

Can asthma itself cause side effects?

Many people focus on the side effects of treatment so much that they forget that poorly treated asthma can also cause side effects. Apart from the (fortunately low) risk of dying from asthma, there is also a risk that lung function will deteriorate over the years and that you will become disabled by chronic asthma as you age. Children with poorly treated asthma do not grow properly, and pregnant women with poorly controlled asthma have a higher risk of complications, for example poor growth or death of the unborn baby.

Can tiredness and forgetfulness be caused by my asthma medication?

No, but if you are not sleeping well because you have poorly treated asthma, you can become tired and forgetful.

Theophylline and related medications can also adversely affect your sleep and may therefore make you feel tired indirectly. If you suspect something like this, discuss it with the doctor who treats your asthma.

The older antihistamines can make you feel drowsy. If you use these medications for hay fever or other allergies and feel tired, you should talk to your doctor about possible alternative medications. If you are allergic to pollen, it is also possible that this causes you to feel tired during the pollen season.

Do inhaled corticosteroids cause any long-term side effects?

As with most medications, inhaled corticosteroids may have side effects in some people.

The most common side effect is a fungal infection in the mouth (oral candidiasis). This is easily treated, and can be prevented by rinsing the mouth after inhalation or sometimes by changing your inhalation technique. Inhaled corticosteroids do not cause fungal (or other) infections in the lungs.

Some people find that their voices become husky after using an inhaled corticosteroid. This usually passes when the dose is lowered, but the hoarseness can sometimes prevent further treatment.

Side effects of inhaled corticosteroids elsewhere in the body are very rare, in contrast to the known risks of corticosteroids given by mouth. Occasionally bruising can occur. There is no evidence that the most commonly prescribed doses of inhaled corticosteroids can lead to osteoporosis or to cataracts in the eyes, for example although these are recognized complications of corticosteroid tablets.

Inhaled corticosteroids are a very effective way of treating asthma, and in most people the benefit of this effective treatment is much greater than any risk of side-effects. You should discuss any worries you may have about this with your doctor.

Is it good for me to always use inhaled corticosteroids?

Yes. These anti-inflammatory medications are currently the most effective treatment for asthma, because they treat the causes of asthma instead of just relieving the symptoms. With long-term treatment, the mucus membranes lining the airways return to normal without any harmful effects on the lungs.

Early treatment with inhaled corticosteroids seems to help prevent asthma from getting worse. This may make it less likely that you will have severe attacks and the treatment these require.

Questions and Answers about Asthma

Can I become addicted to the corticosteroids in asthma medications?

No.

Why can I use inhaled corticosteroids for many years, but corticosteroid cream on my skin for only a short period?

The skin and the blood vessels just below the surface of the skin are very sensitive to the effects of corticosteroids. If you apply a corticosteroid cream to the same area of skin for a long time, the skin and the walls of the blood vessels become fragile and break easily, which makes bruising common. Because of this, doctors and scientists have looked very carefully to see whether this could happen in the airways of people treated with corticosteroids over a long period of time. However, no signs of damage to the airways have been seen and it seems that the lining of the airways reacts to corticosteroids in a different way from the skin.

Do I need to rinse out my mouth after using an inhaled corticosteroid?

There is a slight risk of fungal infection in the mouth when using inhaled corticosteroids. Although this affects very few people, it does not hurt to rinse out your mouth after inhaling a corticosteroid, whenever convenient (for example, at home in the morning or evening). If you are out during the day and it is inconvenient to rinse, this is not a problem, as the risk is very small.

If I can't remember whether I actually took my daily maintenance dose of inhaled corticosteroid, is it better to risk taking a double dose or none at all?

There is no risk in taking a double dose on a single occasion, but try not to make a habit of this.

What can I do to prevent osteoporosis?

There is no evidence that inhaled corticosteroids in commonly prescribed doses can cause osteoporosis, but it is reasonable for all patients with asthma (especially older women) to take steps to avoid this, as it is a recognized consequence of increasing age and physical inactivity (and of corticosteroid tablets used in the long-term).

Physical activity will help your skeleton grow stronger and is probably the most important factor in preventing osteoporosis. Inactivity (for example, due to very poor lung function or fear of getting an asthma attack) makes osteoporosis worse. Effective asthma treatment that makes it possible to lead an active life is, therefore, very important. Calcium supplements for middle-aged and older women who are unlikely to get sufficient calcium in their ordinary food may also reduce the risk of osteoporosis, and specific treatments are available for those at special risk. Research in this field will probably lead to further developments in the future.

Asthma and Infections

Do infections cause asthma?

You may remember that your asthma seemed to start in connection with a viral infection, probably when you were a child. However, the infection probably did not cause the asthma; more likely, it only triggered the symptoms. The condition was already there and would have developed sooner or later, with or without the infection. You were probably born with a tendency to develop asthma.

Some children are allergic and have a mild form of asthma (inflammation of the airways) without being aware of it. Then they get a viral infection and the obvious asthma symptoms appear.

Do infections trigger asthma?

Yes, viral respiratory infections, such as the common cold or flu, can trigger attacks in people who have asthma. Try to avoid contact with people if you know they have a respiratory infection.

Viral infections are thought to be more likely to trigger symptoms if the underlying inflammation in asthma is not properly treated.

Why don't antibiotics help against asthmatic inflammation in the airways?

Penicillin and other antibiotics are only effective against bacterial infections. The inflammation in asthma is not caused by bacteria, so antibiotics have no effect. In addition, most infections of the airways are caused by viruses, and would not respond to antibiotic treatment.

People with asthma can get bacterial infections in the lungs (bronchitis or even pneumonia), which may need to be treated with antibiotics. But antibiotics do not have any effect on the long-term, underlying inflammation in asthma. This inflammation needs to be treated with a controller (anti-inflammatory) medication. And since the inflammation usually also causes tightening of the muscles around the airways and narrowing of the airways, it should also be treated with an airway opener or reliever medication (bronchodilator).

Is asthma contagious?

No. Asthma cannot be spread to other people. On the other hand, a person with asthma can catch a respiratory tract infection just as easily as anyone else.

Asthma and Exercise

Is it good for people with asthma to exercise?

Yes. Even though physical exercise is a common trigger of asthma symptoms, it is just as important for people with asthma to exercise as for anyone else. Keep in mind that it takes time to get in shape and you lose fitness quickly when you stop exercising regularly.

With the right medication, most people with asthma will be able to do some kind of physical exercise. Many will feel no restrictions, and some will only react to exercise in combination with other triggers.

Exercise is good for you. So why can it cause asthma symptoms?

The following are common symptoms of exercise-induced asthma:

- wheezing
- abnormal shortness of breath
- tightness in the chest
- coughing

Your may have just one of these symptoms or a combination of them.

Treatment with a airway opener (reliever) medicine, such as a quick-acting bronchodilator, should immediately relieve one or more of the symptoms. If not, you should discuss other possible reasons for the symptoms with your doctor.

How can I avoid exercise-induced asthma?

The best way to avoid exercise-induced asthma is to make sure that your asthma is properly controlled and, if necessary, that you take extra medication before exercising. A good warm-up also reduces the risk of exercise-induced asthma.

Anti-inflammatory treatment, preferably with inhaled corticosteroids, taken regularly will prevent exercise-induced asthma in many people. However, some people still need to take an airway opener (bronchodilator) before exercise. Many people with asthma should have daily treatment with both inhaled corticosteroids and a long-acting airway opener. Combination medications are now available in many countries.

Particular types of exercise, such as running and jogging, are more likely to expose the airways to large volumes of dry air and trigger asthma, while less vigorous activities, like swimming and yoga, are less likely to cause these symptoms.

Are some kind of physical activities more suitable for people with asthma?

Aerobics is an effective activity, which allows you to train in sessions at varying intensities. The purpose of aerobics is to develop your breathing and heart capacity. If you start by warming up with light jogging, you can, for example, increase the intensity for a couple of minutes, slow down again and then increase the speed once more.

Indoor swimming is also thought to be good exercise, because it takes place at a controlled temperature and in a humid environment. You can also try an aerobic approach by increasing and decreasing your swimming speed.

Whatever you do, make sure you warm up first, because this will reduce the likelihood of exercise-induced asthma.

The most important thing is that the exercise you do is fun; otherwise it is easy to skip it. It is important to find the exercise that suits you.

How intensively do I dare to exercise?

Your training program should help you get in better shape gradually. Remember that it takes time to get in shape. As a rule of thumb, you should feel fine after every training session. It is, therefore, important that you do not try to do too much at once. You should not feel totally exhausted for a couple of hours after every training session.

Questions and Answers about Asthma

If you often get asthma symptoms when you exercise intensively, this could be a signal that you are not taking enough medication or that your asthma does not allow such intensive exercise. Talk to your doctor about your treatment to see if anything can be done.

I often feel my asthma when I jog. Do I have to quit jogging?

No. Very often, just preparing yourself for jogging somewhat differently can be enough. There are two things you should remember. First, take your airway opener medication about 15 minutes before you start. Secondly, warm up properly before you go full steam ahead.

What should I do if I get asthma symptoms while exercising?

Make sure that you always carry a quick-relief airway opener medication and use it promptly if necessary.

If exercising often causes asthma symptoms, your may need to take a better preventive medication, or to avoid a particular kind of exercise.

Can I take asthma medications and still take part in competitive sports?

Yes. Most of the commonly prescribed asthma medications are allowed in competitive sports. Generally, the use of inhaled anti-inflammatory medicines and some bronchodilators is allowed, but corticosteroids in tablet, syrup, suppository, or injectable form are banned.

Check with your doctor or the national sports associations (especially if competing internationally) to be sure that your medication does not violate any doping rules. In some cases, you will need a certificate from your doctor about your need for asthma medication.

Asthma and Other Diseases

Is asthma related to other chronic diseases, such as rheumatism and diabetes?

Chronic rheumatism can affect the lungs, but not in the form of asthma. Long-term treatment with corticosteroid tablets (for example, for asthma) can provoke diabetes, but inhaled corticosteroids taken directly into the lungs have not been shown to have this effect. Many people with asthma can experience symptoms from the nose, such as rhinitis, and some also suffer from polyposis. Otherwise, there is no connection between asthma and other chronic diseases.

What is the difference between asthma and COPD (chronic obstructive lung disease)?

COPD is a collective name for chronic bronchitis and emphysema, two diseases that are almost always caused by smoking. Many of the symptoms of COPD are similar to those of asthma (for example, breathlessness, wheezing, production of too much mucus, coughing). COPD is generally a more serious disease than asthma, because the changes in the airways are much more difficult to treat, and it usually has a worse outcome. COPD can cause greater long-term disability and have a greater effect on the heart and other organ systems than asthma.

Is emphysema the same as asthma?

No, emphysema is different from asthma, although some of the symptoms, such as wheezing and difficulty in breathing, may seem similar. Emphysema is a disease in which the cavities in the lungs have been irreversibly damaged by external factors, such as smoking or severe air pollution. Some people are more likely to develop emphysema than others, and there are hereditary forms of the condition.

Asthma is a condition caused by inflammation of the airways leading to the lungs, in which the cavities in the lungs are usually normal. Asthma attacks can be triggered by factors such as exposure to tobacco smoke or cold air or by an allergy to pollens or dust mites.

Both emphysema and asthma involve inflammation, but the type of inflammation and the parts of the airways and lungs that are affected are different. It is possible to have both emphysema and asthma, but this is rare and it is much more common for emphysema to be combined with chronic bronchitis than with asthma.

Lifestyle

What climate is best for a person with asthma?

No specific climate is ideal for all people with asthma, since there are so many triggers for symptoms and these factors differ from person to person. If you move to another area, triggers in the new environment may provoke your asthma symptoms more or less than where you lived before. The levels of many allergens are lower at higher altitudes (for example, in mountainous areas), and this may be beneficial if you have known allergies to pollens or dust mites.

Are relaxing exercises good for my asthma?

Everyone needs to relax sometimes. Learning techniques of relaxation and breathing may help you to avoid feelings of panic during an asthma attack.

Is there a good breathing technique to use when my asthma symptoms get worse?

There are a couple of useful breathing techniques. Sit on a chair, supporting your arms on the back of the chair; or stand up, leaning your arms on a table. Then breathe in and out calmly through slightly closed lips.

Ask your physical therapist or doctor for more specific advice about these techniques.

How does asthma affect my choice of a professional career?

When you decide what type of career interests you, it is important to discuss the alternatives with an asthma specialist. It is probably not a good idea to go for a job which involves spending much time in dusty or smoky environments or in places with potentially irritating smells.

Sometimes people have trouble understanding that I can't cope with perfumes and smoke. What can I do?

Since asthma is invisible, it can be hard for the people around you to understand that you cannot cope with certain things. It is important that you tell them, and remind them whenever necessary, about your condition to help them increase their knowledge and understanding and show the necessary consideration. It is reasonable to ask your friends and relatives not to smoke in your home. A number of brochures and videos with information about asthma are available at your doctor's office, your pharmacy, or on the internet. It could be a good idea to show one of these to your relatives and friends to help them better understand what asthma is all about.

What can I do to improve my home environment in general?

It is important that your home is easy to ventilate and kept clean, particularly the floors. Wood, tile, or linoleum flooring is better than fitted textile carpeting, which tends to collect a lot of dust, dust mites, and allergens.

Do not keep furry animals or birds, even if you are not specifically allergic to them, as they will lead to an increase in the amount of house dust.

Try to avoid strong perfumes, aftershave, deodorants, and fragrant flowers inside the house, as these are all possible triggers of asthma.

Do not allow anyone to smoke indoors (and avoid other smoky environments such as bars).

Can I have pets even though I have asthma?

If you have asthma and are allergic, you should not buy a pet. If you have asthma but no signs of allergy, and do not get any obvious symptoms from your pet, it is probably all right to keep it, but bear in mind that it will contribute to the amount of dust in the house.

When I went to Spain on vacation I felt great. Should I move there?

It is unwise to advise someone to move to another place. Having a vacation is, in itself, a pleasant experience that makes you feel good. Living permanently in location might be quite different. Bear in mind that you will also have been away from allergens in your home and workplace. Consider this: Perhaps your pet or the dust in your home, or allergens at work, are having more of an effect on your asthma than you realized.

My asthma means that I have to miss out on activities that are important to me, such as dancing. This makes me sad and angry. What can I do?

Discuss this with your doctor. One solution is to take extra medication before you go out dancing. An increase in medication may make it possible for you to participate in activities that are important to you.

A chronic disease like asthma can, of course, place limitations on your social life that are hard to accept. You can feel a sense of loss over not being able to participated in certain activities. You may need to work through these feelings so you can move on and find other alternative activities that can be equally pleasant and valuable.

Chapter 3

Can You Prevent Asthma?

The rate of asthma in children is increasing in many parts of the world. It makes sense that if the rate of asthma can go up, modifying the environment children live it should be able to make the rate of asthma go down. This is an area of very active scientific research. This chapter will give some information—based on relatively early research results—on things you can do to prevent your children from developing asthma.

Dust Mites

Dust mite allergy appears to be the most important reason for the increasing rate of asthma in children. As houses become more and more air-tight, amounts of dust mite become higher and higher. Studies from several parts of the world have shown that the larger the amount of dust mite in the home (especially the child's bedroom), the higher the risk of dust mite allergy in children, and the greater the risk of developing asthma.

Things you can do to reduce the amount of dust mites in your home (and especially your child's bedroom) include:

- Plastic-covered mattresses (the kinds used for cribs and toddler's beds) are ideal for reducing dust mite in your child's crib or bed—the most important source of dust mite for small

---

"Can You Prevent Asthma?" © 2000 Children's Hospital of Eastern Ontario (http://www.cheo.on.ca); reprinted with permission. Reviewed by David A. Cooke, M.D., January 2006.

children. You should remove the bedsheets weekly, damp wipe the plastic mattress, and wash the bedsheets. Blankets should be washed monthly.

- When your child moves to a regular mattress, if you can afford it, encase it in dust mite-proof covers from a medical supply store.
- Have a hard wood floor in the child's bedroom.
- Avoid excess clutter (excess toys, books, etc.) in the child's bedroom.
- Keep the household humidity level at 50% or less.

Cigarette Smoke

Cigarette smoke is probably the second most important factor for risking asthma rates in children. You should not allow your child to be exposed to cigarette smoke. If you smoke, you should quit—if at all possible—for the sake of your health, your spouse's health, and your children's health. Your doctor can advise you of techniques available to help you quit smoking—including counseling, community support groups, and medications. If someone in your house cannot quit, they should smoke completely outside—not in the basement, bathroom, etc. Smoke re-circulates in air-tight houses.

Breastfeeding

One Canadian study has suggested that breastfeeding for at least the first four months of age reduces the risk of asthma. In this study, a hydrolyzed formula (Carnation Good Start®) reduced the risk of asthma similarly, although formulas do not contain live cells to fight infections and other important factors found in breast milk.

Pets

Some very early Canadian research suggests that adults regularly exposed to a furry animal are more likely to develop asthma. It is possible that this may also be true for children. In families where allergic diseases (asthma, hay fever, eczema, allergies) are common, it may be prudent to avoid buying pets.

Dirt?

Recent research from several countries suggests that if the immune system of infants under six months of age is very busy fighting off

Can You Prevent Asthma?

infections, "it may be too preoccupied" to develop the kinds of cells and chemicals needed to develop allergic reactions. There is some evidence that children who are exposed to more "germs"—such as children with several older siblings, children in day care before six months of age, and children who live on farms are less likely to develop allergies and allergic-type diseases, such as asthma. These children may have more viral infections, possibly leading to more wheezing episodes when they're very small, but they may be less likely to develop more long-lasting asthma associated with allergies.

Chapter 4

What Happens during an Asthma Attack?

An Asthma Attack

Doctors are not exactly certain how you get asthma. But they do know that once you have it, your lungs react to things that can start an asthma attack.

For instance, when you have asthma, you might get an asthma attack when you have a cold (or some other kind of respiratory infection). Or, you might get an attack when you breathe something that bothers your lungs (such as cigarette smoke, dust or feathers).

When this happens, three changes take place in your lungs:

- Cells in your air tubes make more mucus than normal. This mucus is very thick and sticky. It tends to clog up the tubes.
- The air tubes tend to swell, just as skin swells when you get a scrape.
- The muscles in your air tubes tighten.

These changes cause the air tubes to narrow. This makes it hard to breathe.

Asthma attacks may start suddenly. Or they may take a long time, even days, to develop. Attacks can be severe, moderate or mild.

Reprinted with permission from "Asthma Attacks." © 2005 American Lung Association. For more information about the American Lung Association or to support the work it does, call 1-800-LUNG-USA (1-800-586-4872) or log on to www.lungusa.org.

Severe Attacks

When these happen, you may become breathless. As you're less and less able to breathe, you may have trouble talking. Your neck muscles may become tight as you breathe. Your lips and fingernails might have a grayish or bluish color. The skin around the ribs of your chest might be sucked in. This happens most often in children. If you are using a peak flow meter you will drop below 50% of your personal best.

In the case of a severe asthma attack:

- Take your asthma medicine and get emergency medical help right away.
- You can get into trouble if you wait too long to get help. This is how people die from asthma.
- Go quickly to your doctor's office or an emergency room. The sooner you see doctor, the faster you get the help you need.

Moderate and Mild Attacks

These attacks are more common. You may start to feel tight in your chest. You might start coughing or spit up mucus. You may feel restless or have trouble sleeping. You might make a wheezing or whistling sound when you breathe. This can happen as you breathe air in and out of your narrowed air tubes.

What should you do in the case of a moderate or mild asthma attack? Take your asthma medicine. Usually then the air tubes in your lungs open up in minutes. Sometimes, though, it can take several hours. Ask your doctor how long it takes for the medicine to work.

If your medicine does not work in the time it is supposed to, call your doctor.

The Second Wave

In some cases, your asthma attack may seem to ease up. But, changes may take place in your air tubes that cause another attack or second wave. This can be more severe and more dangerous than the first attack.

In the second wave, the air tubes continue to swell. This may happen even when you're not having asthma symptoms. At this time, you might find it harder to breathe.

What Happens during an Asthma Attack?

The second wave may last for days or even weeks after the first attack. Your lungs become more sensitive to other irritants. This can trigger more attacks.

During the second wave, you may have to be admitted to a hospital. Doctors need to take care of your asthma and give you medicines that will reduce the swelling in your air tubes and relax the tightened muscles.

In any kind of asthma attack:

- Don't take cough medicine. This will not help your asthma.
- Take only the asthma medicines that the doctor gives you.

Chapter 5

How to Identify an Asthma Emergency

Most asthma attacks start out slowly (over hours or days), building gradually before symptoms reach emergency status. But sometimes sudden attacks occur. Asthma symptoms can become life threatening, requiring immediate medical attention. Contact your doctor or go directly to the emergency department of the nearest hospital if you experience these symptoms:

- Coughing, wheezing, shortness of breath, or tightness in the chest that does not respond to inhaled or oral medications
- Difficulty talking
- Rapid or shallow breathing
- Flared and enlarged nostrils
- Tightly pulled skin in the neck area and/or around the rib cage with each breath

---

This chapter begins with text from "How to Identify an Asthma Emergency," "What to Expect When Calling 9-1-1," and "What to Do Until Paramedics Arrive," © Allergy and Asthma Network Mothers of Asthmatics (http://www.aanma.org). Reprinted courtesy of Allergy & Asthma Network Mothers of Asthmatics (AANMA), 800-878-4403, www.breatherville.org. The chapter concludes with "Dealing with Anxiety, Fear, and Panic during an Acute Exacerbation of Asthma," which is from "Managing Asthma for Patients and Families" by Miles Weinberger, MD, September 2004. This copyright protected material used with permission of the author and the University of Iowa's Virtual Hospital, www.vh.org.

- A gray, dusky, or bluish skin color, beginning around the mouth or under the fingernails
- A peak expiratory flow rate (PEFR) that falls 50 percent below your target PEFR or that falls into the danger zone as determined by your physician

Work with your doctor to develop a personalized asthma management plan that explains what to do when asthma symptoms worsen and learn to recognize the early signs of an attack. The sooner medications are started, the easier it is to reverse an episode.

What to Expect when Calling 9-1-1

Calling 9-1-1 is an important step when seeking emergency medical treatment. Knowing ahead of time what to expect when summoning help is one way to alleviate anxiety during emergency situations.

When calling 9-1-1, it's important to keep calm. Although you may be frightened, take a moment to compose yourself so you can provide emergency dispatchers with vital information.

Once you have a dispatcher on the line, you'll be asked to do the following:

- Describe the problem
- Give the age of the patient (and weight if it is a child)
- Give the location where emergency personnel can find you
- Describe the condition of the patient:
  - Is the patient active or lethargic?
  - Is the patient's skin pale, blanched, dusky, or bluish?
  - Is the patient struggling to breathe?
  - Is the patient breathing rapidly, slowly, or shallowly?
- If known, list any medications the patient is currently taking

In some states, the address where the phone call originates flashes on a screen at the 9-1-1 dispatch center. You may be asked to confirm this address or provide the address where you are calling from for the dispatcher.

Finally, do not hang up the phone until instructed to do so by the emergency dispatcher. Dispatchers are specially trained to assist you while waiting for an ambulance and may stay on the phone with you

How to Identify an Asthma Emergency

until emergency personnel arrive. By staying on the line, they can continue to gather information and monitor the situation as it develops.

What to Do until Paramedics Arrive

So you've called 9-1-1 . . . now what?

- First, remain calm. Stay with the patient, offering support and encouragement that help is on the way.
- Follow the asthma management plan as prescribed by your physician (such as using a nebulizer or metered-dose inhaler in case of an emergency).
- If it is nighttime, turn on an outside light to help guide emergency personnel to your door.
- Have a written copy of the patient's asthma management plan available, as well as a list of all medications currently being taken.
- If younger siblings are at home, make arrangements to have them stay with a neighbor or friend if necessary.
- Take a deep breath and try to stay calm.

Dealing with Anxiety, Fear, and Panic during an Acute Exacerbation of Asthma

It is frightening and anxiety-producing to be unable to breathe comfortably. For some, anxiety interferes with treatment of acute asthmatic symptoms. If you (or your child) fail to respond to an inhaled bronchodilator but then rapidly respond to similar medication given by inhalation or injection at a doctor's office or emergency room, a likely explanation is that anxiety was interfering with the proper technique needed for delivery of the aerosol to the airways. This occurs because anxiety causes more rapid and often shallower breathing that can both aggravate the asthma further and decrease delivery of an inhaled medication. It is, therefore, medically essential that anxiety be controlled at least sufficiently to permit effective use of the inhaled bronchodilator.

How do I control anxiety?

Just saying "Relax" will not do the job. For children, it is essential that parents (or babysitters) keep their cool. It is difficult for visibly panicky parents to deal effectively with anxiety in a child. For children or adults, anxiety is often controlled by focusing on some specific behavior, such as rate of breathing.

Two techniques are used to slow respiration increased by anxiety:

- slow drinking of any liquid
- breathing exercises

Sitting down with a glass of liquid (ranging from water to any flavored beverage) imposes a degree of relaxation by distracting patients from their discomfort. Additionally, breathing must slow down in order to drink. Once breathing is slowed, use of the inhaled bronchodilator is likely to be more effective.

Breathing exercises are a method of gaining control of respirations by "overriding" the anxiety-producing ventilatory drive. The technique is as follows:

1. Sit down

2. Take a long slow deep breath while pushing on your upper abdomen with folded hands.

3. Let the air out slowly through "pursed" lips (that is, the lips should be kept almost completely closed, sufficient to cause considerable resistance.)

4. Repeat the slow inhalation with abdominal compression and "pursed" lip expiration at least 2 more times.

5. Try the prescribed inhaled bronchodilator again concentrating on the proper technique.

6. Repeat procedures 1 through 5 if needed.

If difficulty breathing is so severe and sudden in onset that the above relaxation technique does not permit effective delivery of inhaled medication, a self-injecting adrenalin syringe (EpiPen or AnaGuard) provides a useful though rarely needed emergency measure for temporary relief. This can then permit the above procedure to be used. Discuss this with your doctor if you feel that your situation justifies this measure.

Chapter 6

Asthma in Infants

What is asthma?

Asthma is a disease in which the airways become blocked or narrowed. These effects are usually temporary, but they cause shortness of breath, breathing trouble, and other symptoms. If an asthma attack is severe, a person may need emergency treatment to restore normal breathing.

About 15 million Americans have asthma, including nearly five million children under age 18. This health problem is the reason for nearly half-a-million hospital stays each year. People with asthma can be of any race, age, or sex. Its treatment costs billions of dollars each year.

Despite the far-reaching effects of asthma, much remains to be learned about what causes it and how to prevent it. Although asthma can cause severe health problems, in most cases treatment can control it and allow a person to live a normal and active life.

What causes asthma attacks?

Things in the environment trigger an asthma attack. These triggers vary from person to person, but common ones include cold air, exercise, allergens (things that cause allergies)—such as dust mites, mold, pollen, animal dander, or cockroach debris—and some types of viral infections.

"Asthma in Infants," reprinted with permission from the Asthma and Allergy Foundation of America, © 2005. All rights reserved. For additional information about asthma and related topics visit the AAFA website at http://www.aafa.org.

When you breathe in, air travels through your nose and/or mouth through a tube called the trachea (sometimes referred to as the "windpipe"). From the trachea, it enters a series of smaller tubes that branch off from the trachea. These branched tubes are the bronchi, and they divide further into smaller tubes called the bronchioles. It is in the bronchi and bronchioles that asthma has its main effects.

This is how the process occurs: When the airways come into contact with an allergen, the tissue inside the bronchi and bronchioles becomes inflamed (inflammation). At the same time, the muscles on the outside of the airways tighten up (constriction), causing them to narrow. A thick fluid (mucus) enters the airways, which become swollen. The breathing passages are narrowed still more, and breathing is hampered.

Why are some infants and toddlers more susceptible to getting asthma?

The process just described can be normal, up to a point. Everyone's airways constrict somewhat in response to irritating substances like dust and mold. But in a person with asthma, the airways are hyperreactive. This means that their airways overreact to things that would just be minor irritants in people without asthma.

To describe the effects of asthma, some doctors use the term "twitchy airways." This is a good description of how the airways of people with asthma are different from those without the disease. Not all patients with hyperreactive airways have symptoms of asthma, though.

We still do not know what causes some people to develop asthma. Research shows that a family history of asthma or allergies, a specific allergy in the child, or cigarette smoking during pregnancy may increase the likelihood that a person will develop asthma early in life.

One of the most common causes of asthma symptoms in children five years old and younger is a respiratory virus. Although both adults and children experience respiratory infections, children have more of them and some preschool children are plagued with viral infections. At least half of children with asthma show some sign of it before the age of five. Viruses are the most common cause of acute asthma episodes in infants six months old or younger.

How is asthma in very young children different than adult asthma?

Infants and toddlers have much smaller bronchial tubes than older children and adults. In fact, these airways are so small that even small

Asthma in Infants

blockages caused by viral infections, tightened airways, or mucous can make breathing extremely difficult for the child.

Is it asthma?

Asthma symptoms can look like symptoms of other illnesses or diseases. Croup, bronchitis, epiglottis, cystic fibrosis, pneumonia, bronchiectasis, upper respiratory tract viruses, gastroesophageal reflux, congenital abnormalities, or even a foreign body inhaled by the child—all have some of the same symptoms of asthma.

Signs of asthma in a baby or toddler include:

- Noisy breathing or breathing increased 50 percent above normal. Normal respiration rates are as follows:
  - newborns 30–60 breaths/minute
  - 1st year 20–40 breaths/minute
  - 2nd year 20–30 breaths/minute
- Wheezing or panting with normal activities
- Lethargy, disinterest in normal or favorite activities
- Difficulty sucking or eating
- Crying sounds softer, different

Parents may not be aware that asthma symptoms are becoming serious, possibly leading to a medical emergency. If your child demonstrates any of the symptoms listed below, seek medical help immediately:

- Breathing increased 50 percent or more above normal
- Difficulty with sucking or eating that leads to a refusal to eat altogether
- Cyanosis—very pale or blue coloring in face, lips, fingernails
- Rapid movement of nostrils
- Ribs or stomach moving in and out deeply and rapidly
- Expanded chest that does not deflate when child exhales
- Failure to respond to or recognize parents

How is asthma diagnosed in babies and toddlers?

Diagnosing asthma in very young children is difficult. Since they are not able to communicate, they cannot describe how they are feeling. A baby's fussy behavior could mean many things; however, toddlers and preschoolers often continue to be fairly active in spite of increasing chest tightness or difficulty with breathing.

To help the pediatrician make a correct diagnosis, parents must provide information about family history of asthma or allergies, the child's overall behavior, breathing patterns, and responses to foods or possible allergy triggers. Lung function tests—often used to make a definitive asthma diagnosis—are very hard to do with young children. Instead, the physician may see how the child responds to medications to improve breathing. Blood tests, allergy testing, and x-rays may be done to gather additional information.

Using all this information, the doctor then can make the best diagnosis. Parents may be referred to a pediatric allergist or pulmonologist (lung specialist) for specialized testing or treatment.

How is asthma treated in very young children?

Babies or toddlers can use most medications used for older children and adults. The dosage, of course, is lower, and the way the medication is given is different. Inhaled medications are preferred because they generally act more rapidly to reduce symptoms and produce fewer side effects.

Medications to treat asthma symptoms in infants and toddlers are usually given in a tasty liquid form or with a nebulizer. A nebulizer (sometimes referred to as a "breathing machine") is a small machine that uses forced air to create a "medication mist" for the baby to breath through a small face mask. Nebulizer treatments take about 10 minutes and are given several times each day until symptoms decrease. Although a nebulizer treatment is gentle, babies and young children often are frightened by the mask and fight the treatment at first.

Some toddlers are able to use an inhaler containing asthma medication with a spacer and mask attachment. A spacer is a small tube, or "AeroChamber," which holds the medication released by the inhaler fitted into it. The inhaler/spacer device allows children to breathe in the medication at their own speed.

Various medications are used to treat asthma. Bronchodilators (for example, Proventil or Ventolin) are "quick relief" medications, opening up airways immediately to make breathing easier. "Long-term control" medications, such as corticosteroids (for example, Prelone or Pediapred) or cromolyn sodium (for example, Intal), help keep asthma symptoms at a minimum. Most people with asthma, including very

Asthma in Infants

young children, use a combination of medications depending on the severity and frequency of symptoms. You will need to work with your child's health care providers to develop an asthma care management plan.

What can be done to reduce asthma symptoms?

You can reduce asthma symptoms by controlling allergy triggers in your child's environment. Concentrate on the bedroom, where very young children spend as much as 12–18 hours each day. Cover the pillows, mattress, and box springs in allergen-proof casings. Wash bed linens weekly in hot water (130° F). Use washable area carpets. Buy only washable stuffed animals. Vacuum weekly or more. Don't allow pets in the bedroom (or house). Restrict smoking in the house. (Even if someone smokes in the basement of a multi-storied house, smoke filters through the vents to all parts of the house). For children sensitive to animal dander, use air cleaners with a high efficiency particulate air (HEPA) filter if there is an animal in the home.

There is some evidence that breast-feeding helps prevent children from developing eczema and food allergies, but it probably does not reduce asthma. Also, if there is a history of allergies in your family or if you think your baby may have allergies, slowly introduce new foods in his/her diet so you can monitor responses. Be especially careful of the foods known to cause an allergic response in many people: nut-based foods (like peanut butter), dairy products, soy, fish, shellfish, wheat products, and eggs. Watch for hidden ingredients in packaged foods.

Can a child "outgrow" asthma?

Approximately 50 percent of children with asthma appear to outgrow asthma when they reach adolescence. Once someone develops sensitive airways, they remain that way for life, although asthma symptoms can vary through the years. As a child's airways mature, they are able to handle airway inflammation and irritants better, so their asthma symptoms may notably decrease. About half of those children find their asthma symptoms reappear in varying degrees when they reach their late thirties or early forties. There is no way to predict which children may experience greatly reduced symptoms as they get older. New triggers may set off symptoms at any time in people who have asthma. If your child has asthma, keep "quick relief" medications on hand (and up-to-date), even if symptoms are rare.

Tips for Parents

When a very young child has a chronic illness, parents can feel stretched to their limits as they try to manage. Consider these tips for coping:

- Learn the warning signs for increasing asthma in infants and toddlers. Know your child's particular asthma symptom "pattern."

- Develop an asthma care management plan with your child's physician. Make sure the plan provides guidelines to follow if asthma symptoms get worse. Understand when your child's symptoms require emergency care.

- Follow your asthma care plan every day. Don't alter from the plan until you consult your healthcare provider. Even if your child's symptoms are gone, stick with the plan until you discuss changes with the doctor.

- Get regular check-ups to help reduce your anxiety.

- Teach your toddler or preschooler to tell you when they are not feeling well.

- Work out an emergency plan of action to follow if your child has a serious asthma episode. What hospital will you use? (Be sure your doctor uses that hospital and it is in your health care plan.) Who will take care of your other children? How does your medical coverage provide for emergency care?

Above all, don't let your child's asthma become the focus of your relationship. If you use good health care practices to manage your baby or toddler's asthma, you'll be able to think less about asthma and enjoy your child more.

Chapter 7

Childhood Asthma

Asthma is the most common chronic disease of childhood, and yet many parents know little about it. In the United States, it is estimated that nearly 5 million youngsters under age 18 have this disease. In 1993 alone, asthma was the reason for almost 200,000 hospital stays and about 340 deaths among persons under age 25.

The numbers of young people and children with asthma is rising. In children ages 5–14 years, the rate of death from asthma almost doubled between 1980 and 1993. The disease is more common in Blacks and in city-dwellers than in Whites and those who reside in suburban and rural areas. A government survey of young people with asthma (those aged 15–24 years) showed that more Blacks than Whites died of the disease from 1980 to 1993. Among children aged 0–4 years in 1993, Blacks were six times more likely to die from asthma than Whites. Among children aged 5–14, Blacks were four times more likely than Whites to die of the illness.

Although asthma can occur in people of any age, even in infants, most children with the illness developed it by about age five. Asthma seems to be more common in boys than in girls in early childhood. The survey mentioned above showed that in 1993, boys aged 0–4 were 1.4 times more likely than girls the same age to die from asthma. This increased risk remained in boys aged 5–14, who were 1.3 times more

---

"Childhood Asthma," reprinted with permission from the Asthma and Allergy Foundation of America, © 2005. All rights reserved. For additional information about asthma and related topics visit the AAFA website at http://www.aafa.org.

likely to die from asthma than girls in that age group. By the teen years, the risk seems to even out between girls and boys.

These numbers can be cause for alarm, but the best defense against childhood asthma begins with knowledge of the disease. This is the best way to ensure that, if your child does develop asthma, you and your doctor can work together to control the illness.

What is asthma?

Asthma is a chronic (long-term) illness in which the airways become blocked or narrowed. This is usually temporary, but it causes shortness of breath, trouble breathing, and other symptoms. If asthma becomes severe, the person may need emergency treatment to restore normal breathing.

When you breathe in, air travels through your nose and/or mouth through a tube called the trachea (sometimes referred to as the "windpipe"). From there, it enters a series of smaller tubes that branch off from the trachea. These branched tubes are the bronchi, and they divide further into smaller tubes called the bronchioles. It is in the bronchi and bronchioles that asthma has its main effects.

The symptoms of asthma are triggered by things in the environment. These vary from person to person, but common triggers include cold air, exercise, allergens (things that cause allergies)—such as dust mites, mold, pollen, animal dander, or cockroach debris—and some types of viral infections.

This is how the process occurs: When the airways come into contact with one of these triggers, the tissue inside the bronchi and bronchioles becomes inflamed (inflammation). At the same time, the muscles on the outside of the airways tighten up (constriction), causing them to narrow. Then the fluid (mucus) is released into the bronchioles, which also become swollen. The breathing passages are narrowed still more, and breathing becomes very difficult.

This process can be normal, up to a point. Everyone's airways constrict somewhat in response to irritating substances. But in a person with asthma, the airways are hyperreactive. This means that their airways overreact to things that would just be minor irritants in people without asthma.

To describe the effects of asthma, some doctors use the term "twitchy airways." This is a good description of how the airways of people with asthma are different from those without the disease. (Not all patients with hyperreactive airways have symptoms of asthma, though).

Childhood Asthma

In mild cases of asthma, the symptoms usually subside on their own. Most people with asthma, though, need medication to control or prevent the episodes. The need for medication is based on how often asthma attacks occur and how severe they are. With the treatments available today, most children with asthma can do almost everything that children without the disease can do.

Who gets asthma and what triggers it?

Some traits make it more likely that a child will develop asthma. These risk factors can alert you to watch for signs of the disease so that your child can be treated promptly.

Heredity: To some extent, asthma seems to run in families. Children whose brothers, sisters, or parents have asthma are more likely to develop the illness themselves. If both parents have asthma, the risk is greater than if only one parent has it. For some reason, the risk appears to be greater if the mother has asthma than if the father does.

Atopy: Certain types of allergies can increase a child's risk of developing asthma. A person is said to have atopy (or to be atopic) when he or she is prone to have allergies. This tendency is passed on from the person's parents. It is not the same as inheriting a specific type of allergy. Rather, it is merely the tendency to develop allergies. In other words, both the child and the parent might be allergic to something, but not necessarily to the same thing.

Substances in the environment that cause allergies—things like dust mites, mold, or pollen—are known as allergens. Atopy causes the body to respond to allergens by producing immunoglobulin E (IgE) antibodies. Antibodies are proteins that form in response to foreign substances in the body. One way to test a person for allergies is to perform skin tests with extracts of the allergens or do blood tests for IgE antibodies to these allergens.

What are some asthma triggers?

It is important to be aware of the things in your environment that tend to make asthma worse. These factors vary from person to person. Some of the more common factors or triggers are described here.

Allergens: Some allergens (substances that cause allergies) are more likely to trigger an asthma attack. For instance, babies in particular may have food allergies that can bring on asthma symptoms. Some of the foods to which American children are commonly allergic include eggs, cow's milk, wheat, soybean products, tree nuts, and peanuts.

A baby with a food allergy may have diarrhea and vomiting. He or she is also likely to have a runny nose, a wet cough, and itchy, flaky skin. In toddlers, common allergens that trigger asthma include house dust mites, molds, and animal hair. In older children, pollen may be a trigger, but indoor allergens and molds are more likely to be a cause of asthma.

Viral infections: Some types of viral infections can also trigger asthma. Two of the most likely culprits are respiratory syncytial virus (RSV) and parainfluenza virus. The latter affects the respiratory tract in children, sometimes causing bronchitis (inflammation of the bronchi) or pneumonia (inflammation of the lining inside the lungs). RSV can cause diseases of the bronchial system known as bronchopneumonia and bronchiolitis. A young child who has wheezing with bronchiolitis is likely to develop asthma later in life.

Tobacco smoke: Today most people are aware that smoking can lead to cancer and heart disease. What you may not be aware of, though, is that smoking is also a risk factor for asthma in children and a common trigger of asthma for all ages.

It may seem obvious that people with asthma should not smoke, but they should also avoid the smoke from others' cigarettes. This "secondhand" smoke, or "passive smoking," can trigger asthma symptoms in people with the disease. Studies have shown a clear link between secondhand smoke and asthma in young people. Passive smoking worsens asthma in children and teens and may cause up to 26,000 new cases of asthma each year.

Other irritants in the environment can also bring on an asthma attack. These irritants may include paint fumes, smog, aerosol sprays, and even perfume.

Exercise: Exercise—especially in cold air—is a frequent asthma trigger. A form of asthma called exercise-induced asthma is triggered by physical activity. Symptoms of this kind of asthma may not appear until several minutes of sustained exercise. (When symptoms appear sooner than this, it usually means that the person needs to adjust his or her treatment). The kind of physical activities that can bring on asthma symptoms include not only exercise, but also laughing, crying, holding one's breath, and hyperventilating (rapid, shallow breathing).

Childhood Asthma

The symptoms of exercise-induced asthma usually go away within a few hours. With proper treatment, a child with exercise-induced asthma does not need to limit his or her overall physical activity.

Other triggers: Cold air, wind, rain, and sudden changes in the weather can sometimes bring on an asthma attack.

The ways in which children react to asthma triggers vary. Some children react to only a few triggers, others too many. Some children get asthma symptoms only when more than one trigger occurs at the same time. Others have more severe attacks in response to multiple triggers.

In addition, asthma attacks do not always occur right after exposure to a trigger. Depending on the type of trigger and how sensitive the child is to it, asthma attacks may be delayed.

Each case of asthma is unique to that particular child. It is important to keep track of the factors or triggers that you know to provoke asthma attacks in your child. Because the symptoms do not always occur right after exposure, this may take a bit of detective work.

What are the symptoms of asthma?

Common symptoms of asthma include the following:

Wheezing is a high-pitched, whistling sound that your child may make during an asthma attack. If you hear this sound as your child breathes, be sure to let your doctor know. Not all people who wheeze have asthma, and not all those who have asthma wheeze. In fact, if asthma is really severe, there may not be enough movement of air through a person's airways to produce this sound.

- **Chronic cough,** especially at night and after exercise or exposure to cold air, can be a symptom of asthma.

- **Shortness of breath,** especially during exercise, is another possible sign. All children get out of breath when they're running and jumping, but most resume normal breathing very quickly afterward. If your child doesn't, a visit to your doctor is in order.

- **Tightness in the chest** is a symptom that you may have to ask your child about. If you notice any of the signs just described, it's a good idea to ask your child whether he or she feels a tight, uncomfortable feeling in the chest.

What is the treatment for asthma?

Because each case of asthma is different, treatment needs to be tailored for each child. One general rule that does apply, though, is removing those things in the child's environment that you know act as triggers for asthma symptoms. When possible, keeping down levels of dust mites, mold, animal dander, and cockroach debris in the house—especially in the child's bedroom—can be helpful. When these measures are not enough, it may be time to try one of the many medications that are available to control symptoms.

New guidelines from the National Institutes of Health advise treating asthma with a "stepwise" approach. This means using the lowest dose of medication that is effective, "stepping up" the dose and the frequency with which it is taken if the asthma gets worse. When the asthma gets under control, the medicines are then "stepped down."

Asthma medications may be either inhaled or in pill form. These medications are divided into two types—quick relief and long-term control. The first group (quick relief) is used to relieve the immediate symptoms of an asthma attack. The second group (long-term control) does not provide relief right away, but over time these medications help to lessen the frequency and severity of attacks.

Like any medication, asthma treatments often have side effects. Be sure to ask your doctor about the side effects of the medications your child is prescribed and what warning signs should prompt you to contact your doctor.

Quick-relief medications: Medications that provide immediate relief of asthma symptoms relax the muscles around the airways, making breathing easier. They begin to work within minutes after they are used, and their effects may last for up to six hours.

Most of the quick-relief medications are inhaled through a pocket-sized device that your child can easily learn to use when he or she feels symptoms coming on. These medications can also be used before exercise to help ward off asthma symptoms. Commonly used quick-relief treatments for asthma include albuterol, bitolterol, metaproterenol, pirbuterol, and terbutaline. In addition, ipratropium is an inhaled asthma medication that works more slowly than the above medications. It is not effective for exercise-induced asthma, but it is helpful in people who cannot tolerate the side effects of the medications listed above, such as older adults.

Other quick-relief medications are methylprednisolone, prednisolone, and prednisone. These oral corticosteroids are taken by mouth in short bursts to establish initial control or to control symptoms during a period of gradual deterioration.

Long-term control medications: The long list of long-term control medications for asthma include both oral and inhaled medications. Unlike the quick-relief medications, long-term medicines do not provide quick relief in the midst of an asthma episode. Rather, they work over the long term to reduce the frequency and severity of attacks. Most of these medications take several weeks of regular use to achieve their full effect, and all work only when they are taken consistently.

The long-term control medications can be divided into four broad categories:

- Inhaled anti-inflammatory agents
- Oral corticosteroids
- Long-acting bronchodilators
- Oral leukotriene modifiers

Anti-inflammatory agents prevent and reduce airway inflammation. They also make airways less sensitive to asthma triggers.

Corticosteroids are the most potent and consistently effective long-term control medications. Children with moderate to severe persistent asthma take inhaled corticosteroids daily, while those with mild persistent asthma may take an inhaled corticosteroids or inhaled non-steroids such as cromolyn sodium or nedocromil.

Inhaled anti-inflammatory medications are taken through a metered-dose inhaler (MDI). This is a device that delivers a measured amount of medication each time it is used. Most can also be inhaled through a nebulizer. With this device, medication is turned into a vapor that is inhaled deeply into the lungs.

The non-steroids have very few mild side effects. Potential side effects of inhaled steroids are cough, hoarseness, oral thrush, and perhaps a slowing of the rate of growth. Thrush is a type of yeast infection in the mouth. To decrease the chance of thrush and other systemic reactions, patients are advised to rinse out the mouth with water after each use of an MDI and to use a spacer or holding chamber attached to the MDI. Ask your doctor about potential side effects in relationship to the goal of adequately controlling asthma.

Long-term oral corticosteroids can have total body (systemic) side effects. Talk with your doctor about how to minimize these while maintaining adequate control of your child's asthma.

Oral corticosteroids may be given in liquid or tablet form and begin to work within a few hours. They are given for a short period of time, such as a few days, to control severe asthma episodes and to speed recovery. These medications may be given for longer periods in patients who have very severe and recurrent asthma attacks. Patients taking corticosteroids must never stop using these medications all at once because this can cause side effects. Rather, their use must be tapered off. It is especially important to take these medications exactly as prescribed by your doctor.

Long-acting bronchodilators relax the muscles around the airways, making breathing easier. Their effects last up to 12 hours, and like the inhaled anti-inflammatory agents, they continue to work only if they are taken regularly. These medications can be taken either through a metered-dose inhaler or by mouth, in tablet, capsule, or liquid form. Their side effects may include nervousness, dry mouth, or rapid heartbeat. As with any medications, talk with your doctor about potential side effects.

Leukotriene modifiers are the latest class of medications used to treat asthma. These medications prevent and reduce airway inflammation and constriction of the airway muscles. They also make airways less sensitive to asthma triggers and can reduce the need for short-acting reliever medications. Leukotriene modifiers seem to have fewer side effects than other asthma treatments. Depending on what type of leukotriene modifier is used, side effects may include upset stomach, diarrhea, and changes in liver function tests. As with any new type of medication, frequent, clear communication between you and your doctor is required.

Sometimes asthma medications are combined to provide better treatment than any one used alone can offer. The goals of asthma treatment are to allow restful nighttime sleep, avoid the need for hospital stays, and allow your child to engage in normal play and school activities—in other words, to give him or her a normal life. Many treatment options exist to achieve this goal. The choice of treatment depends on the details of your child's own case.

Be Involved in Your Child's Care

Asthma is an illness that is best understood, rather than feared. If your child has asthma, learn all you can about the disease and work with your child's doctor. This will afford your child the best chance of controlling asthma and allowing him or her to lead a normal, healthy and happy life.

Chapter 8

Asthma and Teenagers

Asthma affects about one in seven teenagers. The teenage years are difficult for some, and having asthma can be seen as just one more thing to worry about. However, effective management of asthma can reduce the impact that it can have on study, sport and social activities.

Coping with Change

The teenage or adolescent years are a time of great physical and emotional change. Most teenagers survive these years without many problems, but some find it hard to cope with the changes. Having asthma can add to these difficulties and dealing with the condition can become a low priority. Teenagers need the help and support of parents and family.

The Importance of Self-Management

Teenagers should be aware that, although their parents are there to help, they can successfully and responsibly manage their own condition by:

© 2004 Better Health Channel, Victoria, Australia. This information was provided by the Better Health Channel. Material on the Better Health Channel regularly updated. For the latest version of this information please visit: www.betterhealth.vic.gov.au.

- Taking medication regularly.
- Understanding their own asthma trigger factors and avoiding these where possible.
- Being aware of any limitations that their condition may have on social or physical activities.

How Teenagers Can Help Themselves

Some helpful hints for the teenager with asthma include:

- Spend time learning about your own condition, including familiarizing yourself about medication and how to use your medication devices correctly.
- Visit your doctor every six months or more often if you have a severe attack.
- Ask your doctor to develop an asthma action plan that you can clearly understand.
- Learn how you can manage your asthma so you can participate in sport and social activities.

Risk-Taking Behaviors

During the adolescent years teenagers become independent and want to spend more time with their friends. Taking risks and experimenting with alcohol and smoking are a normal part of growing up. Teenagers need to be aware of the risks associated with these behaviors, so they can make informed choices to mange their asthma and to care for their health in general.

Effects of Steroid Medication

Some teenagers tend to avoid taking medication because they are worried about the long term or physical side effects of steroid medications. Steroids used in asthma are very different from steroids used in sport and they do not affect the body in the same way. These steroids are called corticosteroids and, for most people, the standard inhaled doses have no side effects. These drugs—usually present in preventative asthma medications—are very effective in allowing people with asthma to lead normal lives.

Exercise and Sport

Exercise can sometimes trigger asthma. However, we also know exercise is important because it keeps you fit and it is a great way of managing your asthma. Teenagers with managed asthma can play almost any sports (scuba diving should be avoided). These tips should be followed if you do exercise or sport:

- Always warm up before exercise, 15 to 20 minutes of light exercise and stretching is recommended.
- Check with your parents or your doctor which puffer to use before sport and use it five to 10 minutes before you warm up.
- Remember to carry your blue reliever puffer at all times.
- Always cool down after exercise.

Things to Remember

- The adolescent years are a time of great physical and emotional change.
- Having an asthma management plan is very important.
- With support teenagers should be able to manage their own asthma.
- The steroids in asthma medication are safe and effective.

Chapter 9

Adult Onset Asthma

What is asthma?

Asthma is a common disease that affects the lungs. About 15 million Americans have asthma. People who have asthma may experience wheezing, coughing, increased mucous production, and difficulty breathing. These symptoms are caused by inflammation and/or obstruction of the airways, which transport air from the nose and mouth to the lungs.

People with asthma may have allergies "triggered" by various allergens. Allergens are substances found in our everyday environment.

What is adult onset asthma?

Many people develop asthma in childhood. However, asthma symptoms can appear at any time in life. Individuals who develop asthma as adults are said to have adult onset asthma. It is possible to first develop asthma at age 50, 60, or even later in life.

Adult onset asthma may or may not be caused by allergies. Some individuals who had allergies as children or young adults with no asthma symptoms could develop asthma as older adults. Other times,

---

"Adult Onset of Asthma," reprinted with permission from the Asthma and Allergy Foundation of America, © 2005. All rights reserved. For additional information about asthma and related topics visit the AAFA website at http://www.aafa.org.

adults become sensitized to everyday substances found in their homes or food and suddenly begin to experience asthma symptoms.

Who gets adult onset asthma?

We do not know what causes asthma. There is evidence that asthma and allergy are in part determined by heredity.

Several factors may make a person more likely to get adult onset asthma. Women are more likely to develop asthma after age 20. For others, obesity appears to significantly increase the risk of developing asthma as an adult.

At least 30 percent of adult asthma cases are triggered by allergies. People allergic to cats may have an increased risk for developing adult onset asthma. Exposure to cigarette smoke, mold, dust, feather bedding, perfume, or other substances commonly found in the person's environment may trigger the first asthma symptoms. Prolonged exposure to certain workplace materials may set off asthma symptoms in adults.

Hormonal fluctuations and changes in women may play a role in adult onset asthma. Some women first develop asthma symptoms during or after a pregnancy. Women going through menopause can develop asthma symptoms for the first time. An ongoing Harvard Nurses Health Study found that women who take estrogen supplements after menopause for ten years or more are 50 percent more likely to develop asthma than women who never used estrogen.

Different illnesses, viruses, or infections can be a factor in adult onset asthma. Many adults first experience asthma symptoms after a bad cold or a bout with the flu.

Adult onset asthma is not caused by smoking. However, if you smoke or are exposed to cigarette smoke (secondhand smoke), it may provoke asthma symptoms.

What are the signs and symptoms of adult onset asthma?

Asthma symptoms can include the following:

- dry cough, especially at night or in response to specific "triggers"
- tightness or pressure in the chest
- difficulty breathing
- wheezing—a whistling sound—when exhaling

- shortness of breath after exercise
- colds that go to the chest or "hang on" for ten days or more

How does adult onset asthma compare with childhood asthma?

Unlike children who often experience intermittent asthma symptoms in response to allergy triggers or respiratory infections, adults with newly diagnosed asthma generally have persistent symptoms. Daily medications may be required to keep asthma under control.

After middle age, most adults experience a decrease in their lung capacity. These changes in lung function may lead some physicians to overlook asthma as a possible diagnosis. Untreated asthma can contribute to even greater loss of lung function.

How is adult onset asthma diagnosed?

Asthma symptoms can mimic other illnesses or diseases—especially in older adults. Hiatal hernia, stomach problems, or rheumatoid arthritis can create asthma-like symptoms. Chronic obstructive pulmonary disease (COPD) has many of the same symptoms as asthma. COPD, which includes emphysema and chronic bronchitis, is very common in older adults, especially those who are or have been smokers.

To diagnose asthma, your physician will question you about your symptoms, do a physical exam, and conduct lung function tests. In addition, you may be tested for allergies. Your primary care physician may refer you to a pulmonologist (lung specialist) or an allergist for specialized testing or treatment.

If you have any asthma symptoms, don't ignore them or try to treat them yourself. Get a definitive diagnosis from your health care provider.

How can adult onset asthma be managed?

There are four key steps to successfully managing asthma:

- Learn about asthma and stay up-to-date on new developments.
- Take prescribed medications. Don't make any changes until you check with your doctor. Don't use over-the-counter medications unless prescribed by your doctor. Check your lungs daily at home with a peak flow meter.

- You often can detect changes in your lungs with a flow meter before you actually feel your symptoms increasing. Visit your doctor regularly for further in-office tests. These lung tests are painless and provide valuable data that help your physician make adjustments in your medications.
- Make an asthma management plan with your health care provider. A plan establishes guidelines that tell you what to do if your asthma symptoms get worse.

How can asthma symptoms be controlled or reduced?

If your asthma symptoms are caused by allergies, take steps to control known or potential triggers in your environment. Allergy-proof your house for dust, mold, cockroaches, and other common indoor allergens to which you are allergic. Reduce your outdoor activities when pollen counts or ozone levels are high. Choose foods that don't contribute to your asthma or allergy symptoms. Evaluate your workplace for possible allergens and take the necessary steps to reduce your exposure to them.

Can asthma reappear in adults after disappearing years ago?

Asthma is usually diagnosed in childhood. In many patients, however, the symptoms will disappear or be significantly reduced after puberty. Around age 20, symptoms may begin to reappear. Researchers have tracked this tendency for reappearing asthma and found that people with childhood asthma tend to experience reappearing symptoms through their 30s and 40s at various levels of severity. Regardless of whether your asthma is active, continue to avoid your known triggers and keep your rescue medications or prescriptions up-to-date and handy in case you need them.

Are there any special considerations for adults with asthma?

Many adults take several medications and/or use over-the counter medications, such as ibuprofen or aspirin, regularly. Work with your doctor to simplify your medication program as much as possible. Explore the possibility of combining medications or using alternate ones that will have the same desired effect. Be sure to discuss potential drug interactions with anything you take, including vitamins.

Adult Onset Asthma

Some asthma medications increase heart rate. If you have a heart condition, discuss those side affects with your health care provider. Older "first generation" antihistamines can cause men with enlarged prostates to retain urine. Oral steroids can make symptoms of glaucoma, cataracts, and osteoporosis worse.

Adults with arthritis may need special inhalers that are easier to operate. Anyone with asthma should consider getting an annual flu shot. Older adults also should talk with their doctor about getting a pneumonia vaccination. People with multiple medical conditions need to be aware of how their illnesses may affect one another.

Chapter 10

Asthma and Older People

Can I get asthma at my age?

Yes. Many people who develop asthma as adults remember that they had breathing problems as children. Asthma is a breathing problem that can affect people at any age.

Sometimes people have asthma when they are very young and it goes away as they grow up. It may come back later in life. Sometimes people get asthma for the first time when they are older.

Asthma can develop at any age. Over 20.3 million Americans have asthma including 2 million people over age 65. In 2001, over 860,000 people over 65 had an asthma attack or episode.

What is asthma?

Asthma is a breathing problem that makes it more difficult for you to get air in and out of your lungs. When you breathe in (inhale), fresh air comes in through your nose. It passes down through tubes (called bronchi) to your lungs. When you breathe out (exhale), stale air from your lungs is breathed out through the same tubes.

When a person has asthma, the breathing tubes are sensitive. They may react to smoke, pollen, dust, air pollution, allergies, or other

---

Reprinted with permission. © 2005 American Lung Association. For more information about the American Lung Association or to support the work it does, call 1-800-LUNG-USA (1-800-586-4872) or log on to www.lungusa.org.

triggers. In a person with asthma, the breathing tubes may tighten, becoming inflamed and swollen.

When the breathing tubes react, or when they get inflamed, they become narrow. That makes it harder for you to breathe fresh air in and stale air out.

Your difficulty in breathing may change. Sometimes you will feel fine. Other times you may have breathing problems.

Is asthma common among older people?

Yes. Some older people had asthma when they were children or young adults, and now the problem has come back. Other older people may get asthma as adults.

Asthma and symptoms like asthma are very common among adults. More than a quarter of the people over 65 included in two studies had some form of wheezing, a common symptom of asthma. They may wheeze with or without colds, or may have attacks of shortness of breath with wheeze. You can have asthma even if you don't wheeze.

In older people, it is sometimes difficult for the doctor to decide whether the problem is asthma or another lung disease. Other lung diseases that cause similar problems are bronchitis and emphysema, particularly in people who smoke.

In some adults, bronchitis and emphysema may seem like asthma. Or asthma may seem like bronchitis and emphysema. Heart disease may also cause breathing problems. And a person can have heart and lung disease at the same time.

What are the symptoms of asthma?

The symptoms of asthma can be confusing, but the most common symptoms are:

- **A wheezing sound when you breathe:** Sometimes this happens only when you have a cold.

- **Cough:** You may cough up mucus. The cough often comes back and it may last more than a week.

- **Shortness of breath:** You may have difficulty breathing only now and then, or you may have problems quite often. It feels as if you can't get enough air into your lungs.

- **Chest tightness:** Your chest may feel tight in cold weather or during exercise. Chest tightness may be one of the first signs that your asthma is getting worse.

Asthma and Older People

Is asthma serious?

Yes. Asthma is a serious health problem. And it is a continuing problem. But the good news is that it can be successfully treated.

People with asthma can live normal, productive lives. They need regular medical care from an experienced doctor. However, without proper treatment, asthma can be extremely dangerous, even fatal.

What causes asthma?

Scientists are not sure why some people have asthma and others don't. For many people, a tendency to asthma may be inherited. Other factors may also be involved. The basic problem is inflammation of the airways. Among the things that scientists know are involved are:

Smoking: Smoking cigarettes, cigars, pipes, or anything else, increases your risk of developing asthma symptoms. If you smoke at home, your child has a greater chance of developing asthma. It's smart to avoid smoke and people who smoke.

In the family: Asthma can "run in the family." It can be inherited. It may be more common in Hispanic people, especially those who come from Puerto Rico. If you have a blood relative with asthma or allergies (father, mother, sister, brother, son, daughter), you may be at higher risk of getting asthma.

Allergies: People who are allergic to pollen, pets, or dust are at higher risk of developing asthma.

Medications: Some medications may cause asthma symptoms or make asthma worse. Make sure your doctor and your pharmacist know all the medications you are taking. Keep an up-to-date list of all medications you use, both prescription and over-the-counter medicines.

Is asthma "psychosomatic"? Is it all in the head?

No. People used to think asthma was a psychological problem. It is not. Asthma is a real medical problem, but too much stress can make asthma worse.

Can asthma be treated?

Yes. The good news is that most people with asthma can be treated very successfully. The treatment may mean medication that you inhale (breathe in from an inhaler or puffer) or pills.

Successful treatment of asthma is a partnership. It takes cooperation between the patient and the doctor. You and your doctor will work out an asthma treatment plan. The treatment plan will tell you what to do for your asthma when you're feeling well, and when you're sick.

Your treatment plan will help you know when to take your medications. You will understand what the medications should do. You will know when to call your doctor, especially if your asthma is getting worse.

What are the keys to a good asthma treatment plan?

If you have asthma, you have to know your own body well so you can notice when changes happen. Asthma gives early warning signs of trouble. You also have to work closely with a doctor.

You need to know what the best treatments are for you. You need to know the signs of trouble and when to call your doctor. You need a doctor who will talk to you and answer all your questions. You need a pharmacist who can give you information about any medicine you use.

Many good treatments for asthma are available today. The treatments will relax the air tubes in your lungs and help you breathe easier. The treatments reduce the swelling and inflammation in the air tubes.

It's important to follow your doctor's advice about your treatment. Some medicines help prevent asthma. You need to take these medicines all the time, even when you feel well.

Other medicines may be needed if your asthma starts to get worse. If your asthma is getting worse, it's important to start treatment early, as soon as your symptoms begin.

Remember that asthma is a problem that does not go away. It is a chronic disease, like diabetes or heart problems. You need a doctor who knows how to treat asthma.

Regular care is part of your treatment plan. Don't wait until you have problems to see the doctor.

You have to keep on top of asthma, working with the help of your doctor. Your doctor will teach you how to use medications and tell you the signs of serious problems. Be sure you understand. Don't just smile and say "OK."

If you don't understand what your doctor said, ask questions until you do understand. Your doctor will tell you:

- what medications you should take;
- when you should take them;

- what your medications are supposed to do;
- what the signs of problems are;
- when to call your doctor for advice;
- when to go to an emergency room.

Are there special tools that help people with asthma?

There are several different devices that may help you control your asthma and use your asthma medicine better. Ask your doctor about a peak flow meter and a spacer or holding chamber.

There's even a special device to help people with arthritis use their medication inhaler more easily.

Should I try those drugstore remedies?

No. They may help a little. But everyone is an individual and needs their own asthma treatment plan. If you have asthma, you need an experienced doctor.

Good treatment for your asthma means working with your doctor on a regular basis, not buying drugstore remedies that may be expensive and may not treat the problem.

If I have asthma, are there medications I should avoid?

Maybe. Some drugs may cause problems for people with asthma. Tell your doctor what medications you are taking for other conditions. Some asthma drugs may cause irregular heart beats (cardiac arrhythmias). Tell your doctor if this happens to you.

As a reminder, here are some drugs that may interact with asthma medications:

Blood pressure and heart drugs: Some people with asthma find that their asthma gets worse when they take certain blood pressure drugs. Some of these drugs are called beta-adrenergic blockers (such as propranolol, nadolol, timolol). Others are called ACE inhibitors.

Aspirin: Some people with asthma may have problems if they take aspirin or drugs related to aspirin. Such drugs include many drugstore cold remedies and pain remedies.

Sleeping pills and tranquilizers: Sleeping pills, tranquilizers and other sedative drugs may also cause problems for older people with asthma. These drugs make you breath more slowly and less deeply. That can be dangerous if you have lung problems such as asthma.

Remind your doctor about your asthma every time you are given a new prescription.

If I am having problems with my asthma, what should I do?

Act now: The best control of asthma starts with an asthma treatment plan and early treatment for asthma problems. Serious problems from asthma may result if you delay treatment.

Don't wait: If you are having severe breathing problems or if your medication is not working, Call your doctor. Follow your doctor's advice. If you cannot reach your doctor, go to the nearest hospital emergency room.

Call your doctor right away, even if you are worried about bothering your doctor. Do not wait to see if you feel better. Asthma can be serious. It's better to be safe than sorry.

Are there special problems about asthma in older people?

Yes and no. Treatment of asthma means recognizing asthma triggers, understanding your asthma treatment, knowing your asthma's early warning signs, and talking with your doctor. Those rules are the same for young people and older people.

Older people are more likely to have other health problems. They have high blood pressure or heart problems. They may take medication for these problems. Sometimes a drug that is good for one health problem is bad for another.

Your doctor should know about all your health problems and medications. Your doctor should know all the drugs you are taking.

If you have more than one doctor, remember to tell each doctor what your problems are and what drugs you are taking. If you have a problem, ask the doctor whether one drug might be interacting with another to cause your problem.

Keep an up-to-date list of all the medicines you take. Carry the list with you.

Many older people still smoke. Smoking makes asthma and other lung problems worse. Tell your doctor if you smoke or if someone in your household smokes. You may be at high risk for lung problems.

Asthma and Older People

Other people in your home may also be at high risk for lung problems.

What is the good news?

You can control your asthma. Good treatment is a partnership between you and your doctor.

- You need an asthma treatment plan.
- You have to talk to your doctor.
- Your doctor has to talk to you.
- Young and old people can control asthma.

Chapter 11

Asthma and Pregnancy

Maintaining adequate control of asthma during pregnancy is important for the health and well-being of both the mother and her baby. Asthma has been reported to affect 3.7 to 8.4 percent of pregnant women, making it potentially the most common serious medical problem to complicate pregnancy. The largest and most recent studies suggest that maternal asthma increases the risk of perinatal mortality, preeclampsia, preterm birth, and low birth weight infants. More severe asthma is associated with increased risks, while better-controlled asthma is associated with decreased risks.

New Treatment Guidelines for Pregnant Women with Asthma

In January 2005, the National Asthma Education and Prevention Program (NAEPP) issued the first new guidelines in more than a decade for managing asthma during pregnancy. The report reflects new

---

This chapter includes excerpts from "Quick Reference from the Working Group Report on Managing Asthma During Pregnancy: Recommendations for Pharmacologic Treatment," National Asthma Education and Prevention Program, National Heart, Lung, and Blood Institute (NHLBI), NIH Pub. 05-5246, January 2005 (full text available online at http://www.nhlbi.nih.gov/health/prof/lung/asthma/astpreg/astpreg_qr.pdf); and excerpts from "New Treatment Guidelines for Pregnant Women with Asthma," an NHLBI press release dated January 11, 2005 (full text available online at http://www.nih.gov/news/pr/jan2005/nhlbi-11.htm)

medications that have emerged, and it updates treatment recommendations for pregnant women with asthma based on a systematic review of data on the safety of asthma medications during pregnancy.

The guidelines emphasize that controlling asthma during pregnancy is important for the health and well-being of the mother as well as for the healthy development of the fetus. A stepwise approach to asthma care similar to that used in the NAEPP general asthma treatment guidelines for children and nonpregnant adults is recommended. Under this approach, medication is stepped up in intensity if needed, and stepped down when possible, depending on asthma severity. Because asthma severity changes during pregnancy for most women, the guidelines also recommend that clinicians who provide obstetric care monitor asthma severity during prenatal visits of their patients who have asthma.

"The guidelines review the evidence on asthma medications used by pregnant patients," said Barbara Alving, M.D., acting director of the National Heart, Lung, and Blood Institute (NHLBI), which administers the NAEPP. "The evidence is reassuring, and suggests that it is safer to take medications than to have asthma exacerbations."

"Simply put, when a pregnant patient has trouble breathing, her fetus also has trouble getting the oxygen it needs," added William W. Busse, M.D., professor of medicine at the University of Wisconsin Medical School, and chair of the NAEPP multidisciplinary expert panel that developed the guidelines. "There are many ways we can help pregnant women control their asthma, and it is imperative that providers and their patients work together to do so."

Asthma worsens in approximately 30 percent of women who have mild asthma at the beginning of their pregnancy, according to a recent study by the National Institute of Child Health and Human Development Maternal-Fetal Medicine Units Network and cofunded by NHLBI. The study also found that, conversely, asthma improved in 23 percent of the women who initially had moderate or severe asthma.

"We cannot predict who will worsen during pregnancy, so the new guidelines recommend that pregnant patients with persistent asthma have their asthma checked at least monthly by a healthcare provider," explained Mitchell Dombrowski, M.D., chief of obstetrics and gynecology for St. John Hospital in Detroit, and a member of the NAEPP expert panel. "Clinicians who provide obstetric care should be part of the patient's asthma management team, working with the patient and her asthma care provider to adjust her medications if needed to keep her asthma under control and to lower the risk of complications from asthma for her and her baby."

The following are key recommendations from the guidelines regarding medications:

- Albuterol, a short-acting inhaled beta2-agonist, should be used as a quick-relief medication to treat asthma symptoms. Pregnant women with asthma should have this medication available at all times.

- Women who have symptoms at least two days a week or two nights a month have persistent asthma and need daily medication for long-term care of their asthma and to prevent exacerbations. Inhaled corticosteroids are the preferred medication to control the underlying inflammation in pregnant women with persistent asthma.

- For patients whose persistent asthma is not well controlled on low doses of inhaled corticosteroids alone, the guidelines recommend either increasing the dose of inhaled corticosteroid or adding another medication—a long-acting beta agonist.

- Oral corticosteroids may be required for the treatment of severe asthma.

"Several studies have shown that taking inhaled corticosteroids improves lung function during pregnancy and reduces asthma exacerbations—and other large, prospective studies found no relation between taking inhaled corticosteroids and congenital abnormalities or other adverse pregnancy outcomes," said Michael Schatz, M.D., M.S., chief of the Department of Allergy for Kaiser Permanente San Diego Medical Center. Schatz is also a member of the NAEPP expert panel on asthma during pregnancy and author of an editorial accompanying the guidelines report.

The guidelines highlight other important aspects of asthma management during pregnancy, such as identifying and limiting exposure to asthma triggers. Similarly, women with other conditions that can worsen asthma, such as allergic rhinitis, sinusitis, and gastroesophageal reflux, should have those conditions treated as well. Such conditions often become more troublesome during pregnancy.

"As important as medications are for controlling asthma, a pregnant woman can reduce how much medication is needed by identifying and avoiding the factors that make her asthma worse, such as tobacco smoke or allergens like dust mites," added Dr. Schatz.

Recommendations for Managing Asthma during Pregnancy

The treatment goal for the pregnant asthma patient is to provide optimal therapy to maintain control of asthma for maternal health and quality of life as well as for normal fetal maturation. Asthma control is defined as:

- minimal or no chronic symptoms day or night;
- minimal or no exacerbations;
- no limitations on activities;
- maintenance of (near) normal pulmonary function;
- minimal use of short-acting inhaled beta2-agonist;
- minimal or no adverse effects from medications.

It is safer for pregnant women with asthma to be treated with asthma medications than for them to have asthma symptoms and exacerbations. Monitoring and making appropriate adjustments in therapy may be required maintain lung function and, hence, blood oxygenation that ensures oxygen supply to the fetus. Inadequate control of asthma is a greater risk to the fetus than are asthma medications. Proper control of asthma should enable a woman with asthma to maintain a normal pregnancy with little or no risk to her or her fetus.

The obstetrical care provider should be involved in asthma care, including monitoring of asthma status during prenatal visits. A team approach is helpful if more than one clinician is managing a pregnant woman with asthma.

Asthma treatment is organized around four components of management:

- **Assessment and monitoring of asthma, including objective measures of pulmonary function:** Because the course of asthma changes for about two-thirds of women during pregnancy, monthly evaluations of asthma history and pulmonary function are recommended.
- **Control of factors contributing to asthma severity:** Identifying and controlling or avoiding such factors as allergens and irritants, particularly tobacco smoke, that contribute to asthma severity can lead to improved maternal well-being with less need for medications.

Asthma and Pregnancy

- **Patient education:** Asthma control is enhanced by ensuring access to education about asthma and about the skills necessary to manage it—such as self-monitoring, correct use of inhalers, and following a plan for managing asthma long term and for promptly handling signs of worsening asthma.

- **A stepwise approach to pharmacologic therapy:** In this approach to achieving and maintaining asthma control, the dose and number of medications and the frequency of administration are increased as necessary, based on the severity of the patient's asthma, and are decreased when possible.

Stepwise Approach for Managing Asthma

- **Step 1: Mild Intermittent Asthma:** Short-acting bronchodilators, particularly short-acting inhaled beta2-agonists, are recommended as quick-relief medication for treating symptoms as needed in patients with intermittent asthma. Albuterol is the preferred short-acting inhaled beta2-agonist because it has an excellent safety profile and the greatest amount of data related to safety during pregnancy of any currently available inhaled beta2-agonist.

- **Step 2: Mild Persistent Asthma:** The preferred treatment for long-term-control medication in Step 2 is daily low-dose inhaled corticosteroid. This preference is based on the strong effectiveness data in nonpregnant women as well as effectiveness and safety data in pregnant women that show no increased risk of adverse perinatal outcomes. Budesonide is the preferred inhaled corticosteroid because more data are available on using budesonide in pregnant women than are available on other inhaled corticosteroids, and the data are reassuring. It is important to note that there are no data indicating that the other inhaled corticosteroid preparations are unsafe during pregnancy. Therefore, inhaled corticosteroids other than budesonide may be continued in patients who were well controlled by these agents prior to pregnancy, especially if it is thought that changing formulations may jeopardize asthma control.

- **Step 3: Moderate Persistent Asthma:** Two preferred treatment options are noted: either a combination of low-dose inhaled corticosteroid and a long-acting inhaled beta2-agonist, or increasing the dose of inhaled corticosteroid to the medium dose range. No data from studies during pregnancy clearly delineate that one option is recommended over the other.

- **Step 4: Severe Persistent Asthma:** If additional medication is required after carefully assessing patient technique and adherence with using Step 3 medication, then the inhaled corticosteroid dose should be increased within the high-dose range, and the use of budesonide is preferred. If this is insufficient to manage asthma symptoms, then the addition of systemic corticosteroid is warranted. Although the data are uncertain about some risks of oral corticosteroids during pregnancy, severe uncontrolled asthma poses a definite risk to the mother and fetus.

Management of Acute Exacerbations

Asthma exacerbations have the potential to lead to severe problems for the fetus. Therefore, asthma exacerbations during pregnancy should be managed aggressively.

Pharmacologic Management of Allergic Rhinitis

Rhinitis, sinusitis, and gastroesophageal reflux are conditions that are often associated with asthma, are frequently more troublesome during pregnancy, and may exacerbate coexisting asthma. If these conditions are present, appropriate treatment is an integral part of asthma management.

Part Two

Understanding Types of Asthma and Common Co-Occurring Conditions

Chapter 12

What Causes Asthma?

Introduction

The word asthma originates from an ancient Greek word meaning panting. Essentially, asthma is an inability to breathe properly. When any person inhales, the air travels through the following structures:

- Air passes into the lungs and flows through progressively smaller airways called bronchioles. The lungs contain millions of these airways.
- All bronchioles lead to alveoli, which are microscopic sacs where oxygen and carbon dioxide are exchanged.

The major features of the lungs include the bronchi, the bronchioles and the alveoli. The alveoli are the microscopic blood vessel-lined sacks in which oxygen and carbon dioxide gas are exchanged.

Asthma is a chronic condition in which these airways undergo changes when stimulated by allergens or other environmental triggers. Such changes appear to be two specific responses:

- The hyperreactive response (also called hyperresponsiveness)
- The inflammatory response

Excerpted from "Asthma in Adults," © 2005 A.D.A.M., Inc. Reprinted with permission.

These actions in the airway cause patients to cough, wheeze, and experience shortness of breath (dyspnea), the classic symptoms of asthma.

Hyperreactive Response

In the hyperreactive response, smooth muscles in the airways constrict and narrow excessively in response to inhaled allergens or other irritants. It should be noted that the airways in everyone's lungs respond by constricting when exposed to allergens or irritants. There are major differences, however, in the hyperreactive response that occurs in people with asthma:

- When people without asthma breathe in and out deeply, the airways relax and open in order to rid the lungs of the irritant.
- When people with asthma try to take those same deep breaths, their airways do not relax but instead narrow and the patients pant for breath. Smooth muscles in the airways of people with asthma may have a defect, perhaps a deficiency in a critical chemical that prevents the muscles from relaxing.

Inflammatory Response

The hyperreactive stage is followed by the inflammatory response, which generally contributes to asthma in the following way:

- The immune system responds to allergens or other environmental triggers by delivering white blood cells and other immune factors to the airways.
- These so-called inflammatory factors cause the airways to swell, to fill with fluid, and to produce a thick sticky mucus.
- This combination of events results in wheezing, breathlessness, inability to exhale properly, and a phlegm-producing cough.

Inflammation appears to be present in the lungs of all patients with asthma, even those with mild cases, and plays a key role in all forms of the disease.

Causes

Asthma has dramatically risen worldwide over the past decades, particularly in developed countries, and experts are puzzled over the

What Causes Asthma?

cause of this increase. The mechanisms that cause asthma are complex and vary among population groups and even from individual to individual. Many asthma sufferers have allergies, and some researchers are targeting common factors in both these conditions. Not all people with allergies have asthma, however, and not all cases of asthma can be explained by allergic response. Other contributing causes need to be studied.

Asthma is most likely to be caused by a convergence of factors that can include genes (probably several) and various environmental and biologic triggers (for example, infections, dietary patterns, hormonal changes in women, and allergens).

The Allergic Response

Nearly half of adults with asthma have an allergy-related condition, which, in most cases developed first in childhood. (In patients who first develop asthma during adulthood, the allergic response usually does not play a strong causal role, although it may be increasing.) Important irritants or allergens included the following:

- Dust mites, specifically mite feces, which are coated with enzymes that contain a powerful allergen: These are the primary allergens in the home.
- Animal dander
- Pollen: An asthma attack from an allergic response to pollen is more likely to occur during extreme air changes, such as thunderstorms. Major weather changes, such as El Niño, can affect the timing of allergy seasons. For example, in 1998, when the effects of El Niño were very strong, allergy and asthma attacks were markedly increased and maximum tree pollen counts occurred two to four weeks earlier and mold counts two to three months earlier than in 1997.
- Molds: A 2002 study suggested that molds might produce a worse asthma attack in adults than other allergens.
- Fungi
- Cockroaches: Cockroaches are major asthma triggers and may reduce lung function even in people without a history of asthma.
- Fossil Fuels. Certain chemicals may trigger allergic rhinitis. Of particular note, some experts believe that refined fossil fuels, such as diesel fuel and particularly kerosene, may be important

triggers for allergic rhinitis. And, in people who already have allergies or asthma, exposure to such fossil fuels may worsen symptoms.

The Allergic Process. The allergic process, called atopy, and its connection to asthma is not completely understood. It involves various airborne allergens or other triggers that set off a cascade of events in the immune system leading to inflammation and hyperreactivity in the airways. One description is as follows:

- The conductor in an orchestra of immune factors that contribute to allergies and asthma appears to be a category of white blood cells known as helper T-cells, in particular a subgroup called TH2-cells.
- TH2-cells overproduce interleukins (ILs), immune factors that are molecular members of a family called cytokines, powerful agents of the inflammatory process.
- Interleukins 4, 9, and 13, for example, may be responsible for a first-phase asthma attack. These interleukins stimulate the production and release of antibody groups known as immunoglobulin E (IgE). (People with both asthma and allergies appear to have a genetic predisposition for overproducing IgE.)
- During an allergic attack, these IgE antibodies can bind to special cells in the immune system called mast cells, which are generally concentrated in the lungs, skin, and mucous membranes. This bond triggers the release of a number of active chemicals, importantly potent molecules known as leukotrienes. These chemicals cause airway spasms, over-produce mucus, and activate nerve endings in the airway lining.
- Another cytokine, interleukin 5, appears to contribute to a late-phase inflammatory response. This interleukin attracts white blood cells known as eosinophils. These cells accumulate and remain in the airways after the first attack. They persist for weeks and mediate the release of other damaging particles that remain in the airways.

Remodeling and Causes of Persistent Asthma

Over the course of years the repetition of the inflammatory events involved in asthma can cause irreversible structural and functional changes in the airways, a process called remodeling. The remodeled

What Causes Asthma?

airways are persistently narrow and can cause chronic asthma. Researchers are trying to determine how this process occurs:

Interleukins: Some researchers are looking at potent immune factors, including interleukins 11 and 13. They have been linked to a number of processes possibly involved in remodeling, including overgrowth of cells in the smooth muscles that line the airways and scarring in the airways.

Growth Factors: Compounds known as vascular endothelial growth factor (VEGF) have been observed in the airways of asthma patients. VEGF is a powerful promoter of cell growth in blood vessel linings and some researchers believe it may be major factor in remodeling.

Genetic Factors

About one-third of all persons with asthma share this condition with another member of their immediate family. Asthma may be more likely to be passed to children from the mother than from the father. Both allergies and asthma are strongly associated with hereditary factors and they share certain genetic markers, but they are not always inherited together.

Research, then, on the genetics of these conditions is confusing and difficult. Of some significant promise, researchers have identified a gene (*ADAM33*), which has been linked to asthma. The gene regulates one of the enzymes called metalloproteases, which are involved with the smooth muscle in the airway. A mutation of this gene, then, could play a role in airway changes that occur after inflammation.

Female Hormones

Hormones or changes in hormone levels appear to play a role in the severity of asthma in women.

Menstrual-Related Asthma: Between 30% and 40% of women with asthma experience fluctuations in severity that are associated with their menstrual cycle. One study indicated that women with menstrually associated asthma tended to have the following characteristics:

- were older
- had asthma for a long time

- had severe asthma attacks that were likely to occur three days before and four days into the menstrual period

Oral contraceptives (OCs) theoretically should help asthma sufferers by leveling out hormonal changes, but they do not appear to have much effect. (There have been a few reports of asthma exacerbation with OCs, but these are uncommon events.)

Asthma during Pregnancy: During pregnancy, one-third of asthmatic women suffer more from the condition, one-third suffer less, and the other third experience no difference in severity. One interesting but unsubstantiated study suggests that expectant asthmatic mothers carrying a female baby tend to have more severe symptoms than do those who are bearing a male.

Menopause and Asthma: Around the time of menopause (called perimenopause) when estrogen declines, the risk for hospitalization in women with asthma increases fourfold compared to previous years. Although it should then follow that hormone replacement therapy (HRT), which contains estrogen, should benefit postmenopausal women studies are inconsistent. As with OCs, if there is an effect one way or the other, it is likely to be weak.

NSAIDs and Acetaminophen

About 10% of asthmatic adults and some fewer children have aspirin-induced asthma (AIA). With this condition, asthma gets worse when patients take aspirin. Aspirin is one of the drugs known as nonsteroidal anti-inflammatory drugs (NSAIDs). Although aspirin is used to reduce inflammation in other disorders, it appears to have the opposite effect in many asthma cases. It is not wholly known why this occurs. AIA often develops after a viral infection. It is a particularly severe asthmatic condition and is associated with up to 25% of asthma-related hospitalizations. In about 5% of cases, aspirin is responsible for a syndrome that involves multiple attacks of asthma, sinusitis, and nasal congestion. Such patients also often have polyps (small benign growths) in the nasal passages.

Patients with aspirin-induced asthma (AIA) should avoid aspirin and most likely other NSAIDs, including ibuprofen (Advil) and naproxen (Aleve).

Acetaminophen (for example, Tylenol) has been the traditional alternative for relief of minor pain for patients who are aspirin-sensitive.

What Causes Asthma?

Unfortunately, recent evidence has muddied these recommendations. In fact, some asthmatic episodes have been linked to high consumption of acetaminophen among adults.

Experts hope that the new NSAIDs COX-2 inhibitors, which include celecoxib (Celebrex) and rofecoxib (Vioxx), may be safe for AIA. To date, studies are promising but more research is needed to confirm their safety in people with this condition.

Exercise-Induced Asthma

Exercise-induced asthma (EIA) is a limited form of asthma in which exercise triggers coughing, wheezing, or shortness of breath.

Nocturnal Asthma

Asthma occurs primarily at night (called nocturnal asthma) in as many as 75% of asthma patients. Attacks often occur between 2 and 4 A.M. Factors that might play role in nocturnal asthma may include one or more of the following:

- chemical and temperature changes in the body during the night that increase inflammation and narrowing of the airways
- delayed allergic responses from exposure to allergens during the day
- the wearing off of inhaled medications toward the early morning
- an increase in acid reflux (back up of stomach acid) that causes airways to narrow
- postnasal drip that occurs during sleep
- conditions relating to sleep, such as sleep apnea or sleeping on one's back, which may worsen any asthma attack that occurs at night

Some experts believe that nocturnal asthma may actually be a unique form of asthma with its own specific biologic mechanisms that occur only at night and which reduce natural steroid hormones (which block inflammation).

Contributing Medical Conditions

Infections: The role of infections in asthma is complicated. Respiratory infections may play a role in some cases of adult-onset asthma, but may be protective against asthma in small children. (In both children and adults with existing allergic asthma, however, an upper respiratory tract infection often worsens an attack.)

Researchers are particularly interested in the organisms *Chlamydia pneumoniae* and *Mycoplasma pneumoniae*. They are major causes of both mild and serious respiratory infections and are becoming important suspects in many cases of severe adult asthma. (If such respiratory infections occur in young children, they are unlikely to have any affect on adult-onset asthma.)

In one study, patients whose asthma was initiated after infections had more severe conditions than those whose asthma was due to other causes. The infection-initiated asthma, however, lasted only 5.6 years compared to 13.3 years in the non-infection group.

In any age group, respiratory infections worsen existing asthma in people who have it already. Rhinovirus (the common cold virus) has been reported to be the most common infectious agent associated with asthma attacks. In one study, it was associated with 61% of asthma exacerbations in children and 44% in adults. Some research suggests that colds promote allergic inflammation and increase the intensity of airway responsiveness for weeks.

GERD: At least half of asthmatic patients have gastroesophageal reflux disease (GERD), the cause of heartburn. It is not entirely clear which condition causes the other or whether they are both due to common factors.

Heartburn is a condition where the acidic stomach contents back up into the esophagus causing pain in the chest area. This reflux usually occurs because the sphincter muscle between the esophagus and stomach is weakened. Standing or sitting after a meal can help reduce the reflux which causes heartburn. Continuous irritation of the esophagus lining as in gastroesophageal reflux disease is a risk factor for the development of adenocarcinoma.

Some theories for the causal connection between GERD and asthma are as follows:

- Acid leaking from the lower esophagus in GERD stimulates the vagus nerve which runs through the gastrointestinal tract. This stimulated nerve triggers the nearby airways in the lung to constrict, which causes asthma symptoms.
- Acid backup that reaches the mouth may be inhaled into the airways (aspirated). Here, the acid triggers a reaction in the airways that cause asthma symptoms.

What Causes Asthma?

GERD is sometimes hard to detect and might be suspected as a contributor in the following asthmatic patients:

- Those who do not respond to asthma treatments
- Those whose asthma attacks follow episodes of heartburn
- Those whose attacks are worse after eating or exercise
- Those whose coughs follow episodes of acid reflux: One study found that GERD was associated with about half of the episodes of coughs and wheezes in asthmatic patients.

Treating GERD symptoms with anti-acid agents may resolve asthma in some (but not all) patients who share both conditions. A small 2005 small observational study found that while GERD was common in asthma patients, treatment of GERD had no effect on asthma symptoms.

Sinusitis: Almost half of children and adults with allergic asthma have sinus abnormalities, and in various studies, between 17% and 30% of asthmatic patients develop true sinusitis. The presence of sinusitis, however, does not appear to increase the severity of asthma.

Chapter 13

Recognizing and Diagnosing Asthma

Symptoms

Asthma symptoms vary in severity from occasional mild bouts of breathlessness to daily wheezing that persists despite taking large doses of medication. After exposure to asthma triggers, symptoms rarely develop abruptly but progress over a period of hours or days. In some cases, the airways have become seriously obstructed by the time the patient even calls the doctor.

The classic symptoms of an asthma attack are the following:

- Wheezing when breathing out is nearly always present during an attack. Usually the attack begins with wheezing and rapid breathing, and, as it becomes more severe, all breathing muscles become visibly active.

- Shortness of breath (dyspnea): Shortness of breath is a major source of distress in asthma patients. It should be noted, however, that the severity of this symptom does not always reflect the degree to which lung function is impaired. In fact, according to one study, a quarter of patients are not aware that they are experiencing shortness of breath (referred to as "a blunted perception of dyspnea"). Such patients are at particular risk for very serious and even life-threatening asthma attacks, since they are less conscious of symptoms. Those at highest risk for this effect

---

Excerpted from "Asthma in Adults," © 2005 A.D.A.M., Inc. Reprinted with permission.

tend to be older, female, and to have the disease for a longer period of time.

- Coughing: In some people the first symptom of asthma is a nonproductive cough. In fact, in a 2001 survey, 12% of asthma patients reported coughing as a significant problem. Patients surveyed tended to feel that daytime cough was even more distressing than wheezing or sleep disturbances.
- Chest tightness or pain: Initial chest tightness without any other symptoms may be an early indicator of a serious attack.
- The neck muscles may tighten, and talking may become difficult or impossible.
- Rapid heart rate
- Sweating
- Chest pain occurs in about three-quarters of patients. It can be very severe, although its intensity is not necessarily related to the severity of the asthma attack itself.

The end of an attack is often marked by a cough that produces a thick, stringy mucus. After an initial acute attack, inflammation persists for days to weeks, often without symptoms. (The inflammation itself must still be treated, however, because it usually causes relapse.)

Diagnosis

When asthma is suspected, the patient should describe for the physician any pattern related to the symptoms and possible precipitating factors, including the following:

- whether symptoms are more frequent during the spring or fall (allergy seasons)
- whether exercise, a respiratory infection, or exposure to cold air has ever triggered an attack
- any family history of asthma or allergic disorders, such as eczema, hives, or hay fever
- any occupational or long-term exposure to chemicals: Early detection of occupational asthma is very important. If symptoms improve on weekends and vacation and are worse at work, the job is likely to be the source of the asthma, although this is not

always the case. Asthma is common, and exacerbation at work may be coincidental.

Ruling Out Other Diseases

A number of disorders may cause some or all of the symptoms of asthma:

- Asthma and chronic obstructive lung diseases (chronic bronchitis and emphysema) affect the lungs in similar ways and, in fact, may all be present in the same person. Unlike the other chronic lung conditions, asthma usually first appears in patients less than 30 years old and with chest x-rays that are normal. Still, it may be difficult to distinguish these disorders in some adults with late onset asthma.
- Panic disorder can coincide with asthma or be confused with it.
- Gastroesophageal reflux disorder (GERD) is a common companion in asthma and may affect treatment.
- Other diseases that must be considered during diagnosis are pneumonia, bronchitis, severe allergic reactions, pulmonary embolism, cancer, heart failure, tumors, psychosomatic illnesses, and certain rare disorders (such as tapeworm and trichomoniasis).

Pulmonary Function Tests

If symptoms and a patient's history are indicative of asthma, the physician will usually perform tests known as pulmonary function tests to confirm the diagnosis and determine the severity of the disease.

Using a spirometer, an instrument that measures the air taken into and exhaled from the lungs, the physician will determine several values:

1. vital capacity (VC), which is the maximum volume of air that can be inhaled or exhaled

2. peak expiratory flow rate (PEFR), commonly called the peak flow rate, which is the maximum flow rate that can be generated during a forced exhalation

3. forced expiratory volume (FEV1), which is the maximum volume of air expired in one second

Spirometry is a painless study of air volume and flow rate within the lungs. Spirometry is frequently used to evaluate lung function in people with obstructive or restrictive lung diseases such as asthma or cystic fibrosis.

If the airways are obstructed, then these measurements will fall. Depending on the results, the physician will take the following steps:

- If measurements fall, then the physician typically asks the patient to inhale a bronchodilator. This is a drug that is used in asthma to open the air passages. The measurements are taken again. If the measurements are more normal, than the drug has most likely cleared the airways and a diagnosis of asthma is strongly suspected.

- If measurement results fail to show airway obstruction, but the doctor still suspects asthma, he or she may perform a challenge test. In this case a specific drug (histamine or methacholine) is administered that usually increases airway resistance only when asthma is present. The challenge test may be quite useful in ruling out occupational asthma. It is not always accurate, particularly in asthmatic patients whose only symptom is persistent coughing.

Another method for inducing airway resistance is to administer cold air. This test is very accurate for ruling out asthma, but it is not sensitive enough to accurately identify adults who actually are asthmatic.

Allergy Tests

The patient may be given skin or blood allergy tests, particularly if a specific allergen or occupational agent is suspected and available for testing. Allergy skin tests may be the best predictive test for allergic asthma, although they are not recommended for people with year-round asthma.

Other Tests

Tests that either rule out other diseases or obtain more information about the causes of asthma include the following:

- a complete blood count
- chest and sinus x-rays

Recognizing and Diagnosing Asthma

- computed tomography (CT) scans: CT scans may be helpful in certain cases, such as for determining wall thickness in airways in patients who are difficult to treat, which could signify a higher risk for lung damage.

- examination of the patient's sputum for eosinophils (white blood cells that in high levels are associated with severe allergic asthma): One 2002 study suggested that asthma might be effectively managed by using treatment goals based on achieving a normal eosinophil counts.

- investigative measurements of certain chemicals in sputum or exhaled air that indicate airway inflammation: Such chemical markers include nitric oxide and hydrogen peroxide. For example, high levels of nitric oxide in exhaled air is proving to be a simple and noninvasive way of diagnosing asthma.

If aspirin-induced asthma (AIA) is suspected, an investigative noninvasive test called acoustic rhinometry may be useful. A solution of lysine acetylsalicylic acid (L-ASA) is instilled into the patient's nostril. Patients who experience symptoms such as sneezing, itching, congestion, and secretion are likely to have AIA.

Chapter 14

Allergic Asthma

Allergic (extrinsic) asthma is characterized by symptoms that are triggered by an allergic reaction. Allergic asthma is airway obstruction and inflammation that is partially reversible with medication. Allergic asthma is the most common form of asthma. Many of the symptoms of allergic and non-allergic asthma are the same (coughing, wheezing, shortness of breath or rapid breathing, and chest tightness). However, allergic asthma is triggered by inhaled allergens such as dust mite allergen, pet dander, pollen, mold, etc. resulting in asthma symptoms.

Questions about Allergic Asthma

What is allergic asthma?

Allergic asthma is how doctors describe a particular type of asthma. In people with this common condition, certain types of allergens can trigger asthma attacks and symptoms such as coughing, wheezing, and shortness of breath.

How common is it?

The National Institutes of Health estimates that 60% of the people in the United States with asthma have allergic asthma.

This chapter includes "Allergic Asthma," "Allergic Asthma FAQs," and "Allergic Asthma A-to-Z," reprinted with permission from the Asthma and Allergy Foundation of America, © 2005. All rights reserved. For additional information about asthma and related topics visit the AAFA website at http://www.aafa.org.

What triggers allergic asthma?

You are probably aware of many things that can trigger your asthma. Mold, dust mites, cockroaches, and pet dander are common examples of year-round allergens. What you may not know is how something as simple as visiting a friend who has a pet can lead to an asthma attack. The reason, in part, is a substance produced by the body called IgE.

What is IgE?

IgE is short for immunoglobulin E. This substance, which occurs naturally in your body in small amounts, plays an important role in allergic asthma. If you have allergic asthma, your body makes more IgE when you breathe an allergen. This can cause a series of chemical reactions known as the allergic-inflammatory process in allergic asthma. It can result in two things:

1. The muscles that surround the airways in your lungs begin to tighten (this is known as constriction of the airways).
2. Your airways become irritated and swell up (this is known as inflammation of the airways).

Together, constriction and inflammation of the airways make it harder for you to breathe. This can lead to an asthma attack.

How can I tell if I have allergic asthma?

Only a doctor can confirm a diagnosis of allergic asthma. This is typically done using a skin or blood test to see if your asthma is triggered by year-round allergens in the air.

Allergic Asthma A-to-Z

Are you taking a proactive role in managing your allergic asthma? Knowing the terminology is the first step to helping you better communicate with your healthcare provider to keep your allergic asthma under control. Here are some of the most common terms:

Allergic asthma is a disease of the lungs in which an allergic reaction to inhaled allergens causes your asthma symptoms to appear. Common inhaled allergens include dust mite allergen, pet dander, pollen, and mold spores.

Allergic Asthma

Blood tests done by your doctor can help determine if you have allergic asthma. Knowing if you have allergic asthma or non-allergic asthma is very important to help your doctor develop the right management and treatment plan for you.

Cascade, often called the "allergic cascade," is the name for the series of reactions your immune system goes through after you've been exposure to an allergen. At the end of this "cascade," your allergy or asthma symptoms appear. That's why it's important to know what things trigger your personal "allergic cascade" so you can avoid and prevent the cascade from ever starting.

Diagnosis of allergic asthma begins with a discussion with your doctor about your medical history, a physical exam that includes a lung function test, and, in some cases, a chest or sinus x-ray.

Extrinsic asthma is just another name for "allergic asthma," the most common form of asthma affecting over 10 million people in the U.S.

Family history of asthma or allergies is something that doctors look at to help determine if you might have allergic asthma. This disease tends to be more common among people who have a family history of allergies or asthma.

Genetics play a role in asthma. People whose brothers, sisters, or parents have asthma are more likely to develop the illness themselves. If only one parent has asthma, chances are one in three that each child will have asthma. If both parents have asthma, chances are seven in ten that their children will also.

Home environment is a critical factor in managing your allergic asthma. If pet dander, smoke, mold, or other triggers are all over your house, your asthma symptoms are likely to be much worse than if you eliminated these from your home environment.

Immunoglobulin E (IgE) is the name of the antibody that plays a major role in allergic diseases. Your body produces the IgE antibody when it detects an allergen and causes the "allergic cascade" to begin. New advances in treatment for certain people with allergic asthma include "anti-IgE therapy," such as Xolair, which blocks IgE and helps to prevent the allergic cascade from staring.

Just because you haven't used your rescue inhaler lately doesn't mean your asthma is under control. Talk to your doctor to learn more about what it means to be in control of your asthma.

Keeping track of your asthma symptoms can help determine your triggers and prevent future attacks. Create an "asthma management plan" with your doctor.

Long-term control medicines, or anti-inflammatory drugs, make airways less sensitive. These important medicines help reduce coughing and wheezing and allow you to live an active "life without limits."

Mortality rates (death rates) among African Americans who have asthma are three times higher than others. If you're in this high-risk group, talk to your doctor about more ways to recognize and prevent asthma symptoms so you don't become a statistic.

Non-allergic asthma (also called intrinsic asthma) is triggered by irritants, not allergens. Many of the symptoms of allergic and non-allergic asthma are the same (coughing, wheezing, shortness of breath or rapid breathing, and chest tightness), but, with non-allergic asthma, symptoms are not caused by an allergic reaction.

Occupational asthma is when asthma symptoms are triggered by things related to conditions at your workplace. Symptoms are the same as other types of asthma, but some of the irritants that cause symptoms may be unique to your workplace, such as exposure to certain chemicals, dirt or dust, vapors, etc. People who work in factories, manufacturing plants, and even bakers who are exposed to airborne flour may show symptoms of asthma.

Peak flow meter is a diagnostic tool to measure how well your lungs are able to expel air. During an asthma flare up, the large airways in the lungs slowly begin to narrow. A peak flow meter will show the speed of air leaving the lungs to measure the peak expiratory flow (PEF).

Quick reliever medications should only be used in emergency situations, such as during an asthma attack. If you are taking long-term controller medications properly, you should almost never need these emergency medicines.

Rhinitis—sneezing, runny nose—may be caused by irritants or allergens, and, if not treated, it can lead to difficulty breathing. Nearly half of all those who have asthma also have "allergic rhinitis," so make sure you talk with your doctor about avoidance of rhinitis triggers and prevention of symptoms.

Sinusitis is sinus inflammation caused by a bacterial or viral infection, or an allergic reaction. More than 50 percent of people with moderate to severe asthma also have chronic sinusitis.

Allergic Asthma

Triggers are different substances that can cause your asthma to act up. Allergic triggers can cause a series of chemical reactions resulting in the constriction and inflammation of the airways in your lungs. Common allergic triggers include pollen, dust mites, mold spores, and pet dander.

Understanding your asthma triggers is a key to controlling your condition. Knowing your triggers can help your healthcare professional make better prevention and treatment recommendations.

Viral respiratory infections—such as head or chest colds—are common among people with asthma; in fact, it's the number one asthma trigger among kids. Studies show that viral respiratory infections can make asthma symptoms worse for kids and adults. That's why it's important to get a flu shot and to protect against cold and flu every year.

Weather changes, cold air, or dry wind can sometimes trigger asthma symptoms. During the hot weather season, outdoor ground-level ozone can be a problem, and people with asthma and allergies should drink plenty of fluids.

Xolair is a new breakthrough treatment for people with moderate to severe allergic asthma. Instead of treating symptoms, Xolair treats the underlying cause—it stops the allergic cascade—by blocking immunoglobulin E (IgE). Learn more at www.xolair.com.

You're in control. Don't let asthma control you. With proper prevention, treatment and management of your asthma you can live "life without limits."

Zoom! Traveling with asthma just means that you have to put a little extra thought and preparation into your trip.

Chapter 15

Exercise-Induced Asthma

Do you or your child:

- Become short of breath with physical activity?
- Usually cough during or after running?
- Experience chest pain with exercise?
- Have trouble keeping up with others during sports?
- Have a family history of asthma?

If you answered "Yes" to any of these questions, exercise-induced asthma may be the culprit. Exercise-induced asthma, or EIA, is a common ailment that affects many of the more than 17 million individuals who have asthma as well as those with no clinical evidence of asthma. Both adults and children can be affected resulting in various degrees of reduced exercise tolerance. The good news is that EIA is treatable.

Questions about Exercise-Induced Asthma

What is exercise-induced asthma?

Asthma is a lung disease that causes the airways of the lung to become narrowed and inflamed. This narrowing is called bronchoconstriction. The inflamed airway also produces an overabundance of

---

Reprinted with permission from Children's Asthma Respiratory & Exercise Specialists, Glenview, IL, http://www.wecare4lungs.com, © 2005. All rights reserved.

mucus narrowing the airways even further. The result of these events is the feeling of chest tightness and difficulty in moving air into and out of the lungs.

Many "triggers" are responsible for bronchoconstriction in the lungs. Exercise is one of the more common triggers. Bronchoconstriction during exercise is called exercise-induced asthma. In most cases of EIA, bronchoconstriction occurs 4–8 minutes into the exercise and peaks about 10 minutes after stopping. Often this condition results in decreased performance. The airways usually return to a normal state within 30–60 minutes after the activity has ceased.

What happens during exercise-induced asthma?

It is believed that people with asthma have airways that are highly sensitive to various conditions and environments. The airways of some people may be more sensitive to dust in the air while others have trouble breathing when the temperature outside is very cold. Those who have difficulty breathing when they exercise may have EIA. EIA is thought to be caused by very rapid cooling and drying of airways.

As you exercise, you breathe faster moving large amounts of cool, dry air into your lungs. This cool, dry air must be warmed. As we breathe faster and faster, the process of warming the air becomes increasingly difficult. This rapid change in temperature is thought to be one of the causes of airway narrowing.

Certain conditions, such as the environment and level of exertion, may put a person at risk of having an attack. These conditions are likely to increase the magnitude of stress on the airways of someone with EIA.

What might trigger exercise-induced asthma?

Effort Level

- Extreme exertion
- High effort
- Examples: Running, soccer, cycling, rowing

Environment

- Cold, dry air
- Dusty or polluted area
- Examples: Cross-country skiing, winter running, or hockey

Exercise-Induced Asthma

What might lessen symptoms of exercise-induced asthma?

Effort Level

- Intermittent exertion
- Low to moderate effort
- Examples: Baseball, weight lifting, gymnastics

Environment

- Warm, humid air
- Little to no pollutants
- Examples: Swimming, climate controlled work-outs in a gym

How is exercise-induced asthma diagnosed?

When the classic symptoms of EIA are present, your family physician may readily diagnose and treat asthma symptoms. If treatment is unsuccessful, consultation with an asthma specialist, such as a pulmonologist, may be necessary.

Classic Symptoms

- Chest tightness
- Shortness of breath
- Wheezing
- Feeling out of shape
- Other lung problems
- Coughing

If test results do not support EIA, a physician may need to consider these diagnoses:

- Gastroesophageal reflux
- Vocal cord paresis or dysfunction
- Deconditioning
- Anxiety
- Cardiac dysfunction
- Sinusitis

How is exercise-induced asthma treated?

The most common way to treat EIA is through medications prescribed by your physician. These medications work in a variety of ways and their therapeutic benefit is usually based on symptoms. However effective the prescribed medications prove to be, the alternate treatments described below can further assist an athlete in dealing with EIA.

Nasal Breathing: By breathing in through the nose and out through the mouth, one can humidify the air breathed to nearly 100%, while warming the air to body temperature. The use of a mask or scarf may also help to warm the air. (Comment: May not be comfortable for some.)

Refractory Period: This is the time after an asthma attack when the individual is at decreased risk of developing a second attack. By inducing a mild asthma attack prior to competing, you may protect yourself from an attack during the competition. (Comment: May not benefit athletes in sprint-like activities.)

Relaxation Techniques: By reducing the anxiety level of an individual, breathing rates remain controlled. The psychological benefits of relaxation may also help enhance performance. (Comment: May be difficult for some individuals with extreme anxiety.)

What medications are used to treat exercise-induced asthma?

Table 15.1. lists commonly used medications. It is to serve only as an information tool and is not all inclusive. The medical protocol which works best for you or your child's symptoms may include one or more of the medications listed. By working in conjunction with your physician and/or asthma care specialist, treatment strategies for management of your EIA can be designed. For further information regarding each of the drugs listed, consult your physician.

Does being in better shape help reduce the risk of having an asthma attack?

It appears that those individuals who keep themselves in better physical condition are less likely to have an attack, especially at intensities below a level of peak exertion. This may be due to the body's

Exercise-Induced Asthma

Table 15.1. Medications Commonly Used to Treat Exercise-Induced Asthma

	Beta agonist	Ipratropium Bromide	Mast Cell Stabilizer	Corticosteroids	Theophylline
Trade Names	Ventolin Proventil Serevent	Atrovent	Intal Nedocromil	Prednisone Beclovent Flovent Vanceril AeroBid Pulmicort	Slo-bid Slo-Phyllin Theo-Dur
How It Works	Bronchodilator (B-agonist)	Bronchodilator (Anti-Cholinergic)	Anti-inflammatory, prevents mast cell release of histamine	Anti-inflammatory	Bronchodilators (Xanthine derivatives)
How Effective	90–100%	uncertain	70–80%	Highly effective	65–80%
How Taken	Inhaled, Capsule	Inhaled	Inhaled	Inhaled, Tablet	Capsule, Tablet, Syrup
Side Effects	Increased heart rate Nervousness	Palpitations Nervousness	Dizziness (rare) Nausea (rare) Coughing	Behavior changes, monitor long-term growth	Palpitations Insomnia Nausea
Comments	Most commonly used	Not a first line medication	Unclear mechanism for prevention of EIA	Oral form banned by U.S. Olympic Committee	Very rarely used for EIA

123

adaptive response to chronic exercise. This adaptation allows the body to handle increasing intensities without increasing the breathing rate. However, during the maximal exertion there seems to be little protective effect of fitness level.

Questions about Children with EIA and Sports

Will my child outgrow exercise-induced asthma?

While your child may not completely outgrow EIA, his/her symptoms may improve or worsen based on the season, the environmental conditions, or even the current level of activity.

The thing to remember is that through awareness, exercise strategies, and proven treatments, your child can achieve the highest levels of competition, no matter what the sport.

Will having EIA affect my child's relationship with his/her coaches or teachers?

Coaches and/or teachers should be informed of your child's condition. Educate them about treatment strategies and routines that will enable your child to perform at his/her peak level. Through a team effort with your physician, family, and coach, one can achieve success at every level.

My child is a swimmer who suffers from EIA like symptoms, should he/she consider a different sport?

Swimming, with its warm and moist environmental conditions, is actually one of the best activities individuals with asthma can participate in. If the symptoms persist, your physician should be able to help your child deal with the breathing difficulties while they continue to develop within the sport.

My child would like to play sports in college and has concerns about his eligibility and the use of his asthma drugs. What are the rules regarding such issues?

The NCAA (National Collegiate Athletic Association) and USOC (United States Olympic Committee) both have a list of banned substances which may affect your child. This list is updated annually. Consult your physician or asthma specialist for up to date information.

Exercise-Induced Asthma

Taking Control

Taking control of the symptoms of exercise-induced asthma is as simple as following the prescribed treatment plan. Don't "tough it out." Never hesitate to ask your doctor or asthma care specialist about any concerns you or your child have and remember to comply with the treatment measures and medications. This will ensure that you or your child will be able to enjoy activities like exercising, playing sports, running, dancing, or whatever it is you like to do. Exercise-induced asthma should not be viewed as a roadblock to achieving your goals and following your dreams.

Chapter 16

Occupational Asthma

What is occupational asthma?

Occupational asthma, one form of asthma, is a lung disease in which the airways overreact to dusts, vapors, gases, or fumes that exist in the workplace. When these irritants are inhaled:

- airway inflammation begins;
- muscles in the airways tighten;
- the airway tissue swells;
- too much mucus is produced.
- These changes all make breathing difficult.

Occupational asthma is usually reversible, but permanent lung damage can occur if exposure to the substance that causes the disease continues. In highly sensitive persons, even very low levels of exposure may provoke an episode.

What are its symptoms?

The symptoms of occupational asthma include:

- wheezing;

Reprinted with permission © 2005 American Lung Association. For more information about the American Lung Association or to support the work it does, call 1-800-LUNG-USA (1-800-586-4872) or log on to www.lungusa.org.

- a tight feeling in the chest;
- coughing;
- shortness of breath.

Sometimes the worker will only have a cough or any one of the other symptoms. Symptoms usually occur while the worker is exposed to a particular substance at work.

In some cases, symptoms may develop several hours after the person leaves work, and then subside before the worker returns to the job the next day.

In the early stages of the disease, symptoms usually decrease or disappear during weekends or vacations, only to recur upon return to work. In later stages of the disease, symptoms may occur away from work after exposure to common lung irritants.

Once the airways have a pattern of overreacting, many common substances such as cigarette smoke, house dust, or cold air may produce asthma-like symptoms.

Who gets occupational asthma?

Workers in hundreds of occupations are exposed to substances in the air that may cause occupational asthma in susceptible people. Many of these substances are very common and not ordinarily considered hazardous.

Only a small proportion of exposed workers develop occupational asthma.

Workers most likely to develop the disease are those with a personal or family history of allergies or asthma and frequent exposure to highly sensitizing substances. But the disease also can develop in persons with no known allergies.

Occupational asthma may be suspected whenever a worker begins to develop respiratory symptoms. It may take several years to develop.

A thorough physical examination and medical history for a worker with asthma symptoms should include a detailed listing of his or her work history and workplace conditions.

What causes occupational asthma?

New processes and substances that can cause occupational asthma are being identified continually. The following list includes some of the airborne substances and some related occupations known to be associated with the disease:

Occupational Asthma

- Chemical dusts or vapors from plasticizers, polyurethane paints, insulation, foam mattresses and upholstery, and packaging materials used in manufacturing and processing operations. Among specific chemicals known to cause asthma are the isocyanates, trimellitic anhydride, and phthalic anhydride.

- Animal substances such as hair, dander, mites, small insects, bacterial or protein dusts. Exposed workers at special risk include farmers, animal handlers, shepherds, grooms, jockeys, veterinarians, and kennel workers.

- Organic dusts such as flour, cereals, grains, coffee and tea dust, papain dust from meat tenderizer. These substances can cause asthma in millers, bakers, and other food processors.

- Cotton, flax, and hemp dust inhaled by workers in cotton processing and textile industries.

- Metals such as platinum, chromium, nickel sulfate, and soldering fumes. Workers are exposed in refining and manufacturing operations.

How is occupational asthma diagnosed?

A careful, detailed history is essential to relate the occurrence of symptoms to work exposure. A physical examination of the chest is often normal if done several hours after exposure has taken place but is useful in ruling out other causes of shortness of breath.

Pulmonary function tests given before and after the work shift may detect narrowing of the airways. Laboratory tests on blood and sputum may be useful.

Special studies can sometimes confirm the diagnosis, but inhalation of a suspected agent (challenge test) may be necessary. A chest x-ray is essential to exclude other lung disorders, but has no direct role in the diagnosis of occupational asthma.

Is occupational asthma preventable?

In trades and industries in which there is a known risk to workers, steps can be taken to eliminate or at least reduce the number of workers who will be affected.

A change in the manufacturing process or use of modern industrial hygiene techniques, engineering controls, and changed work practices can diminish or eliminate pollutant concentration in the workplace air.

Persons at increased risk because of a family or personal history of allergy or asthma should be aware of the potential problems involved in entering trades with obvious hazards and seek advice.

Periodic medical surveillance may allow early identification of affected workers before they have any permanent lung damage.

If a worker begins to have asthma symptoms due to occupational exposure, the disease usually can be reversed and permanent lung damage prevented by changing jobs. Sometimes, a transfer to a different location within the same plant is helpful.

Because changing jobs may cause a severe financial hardship, such a recommendation should be made only after careful medical evaluation.

What else can be done to treat occupational asthma?

The best "treatment" is to completely avoid the substance causing the asthma. In some circumstances, where exposure is unavoidable or intermittent, drug treatment may be recommended.

In advanced cases of occupational asthma with complications resulting in severely damaged airways, combined medical treatment including drugs, physical therapy, and breathing aids may be needed.

Persons with occupational asthma should avoid exposure to gases such as sulfur dioxide, chlorine, or nitrogen dioxide. Breathing these irritating gases can make asthma symptoms worse.

How does smoking affect occupational asthma?

Smoking may make the disease more severe. Smoking also increases the chances of getting other complicating lung diseases, such as emphysema, chronic bronchitis, or lung cancer.

Workers with occupational asthma who change their job environment and quit smoking are more likely to recover fully than a worker who changes jobs but continues to smoke.

Secondhand smoke from other smokers may also increase the symptoms of the worker with occupational asthma.

Chapter 17

Steroid-Resistant Asthma

Airway inflammation and immune activation plays an important role in chronic asthma. Current guidelines of asthma therapy have, therefore, focused on the use of anti-inflammatory therapy, particularly inhaled glucocorticoids (GCs). While the majority of patients respond to regular inhaled GC therapy, a subset of patients are poorly responsive even when treated with high doses of oral prednisone. This review will examine the mechanisms underlying steroid resistant (SR) asthma.

Definition of Steroid Resistant Asthma

At present there is no universally accepted definition of steroid resistant asthma. It is frequently defined by the failure to improve baseline A.M. (morning) pre-bronchodilator FEV1 (forced expiratory volume in one second) by greater than 15% predicted following 7–14 days of 20 mg twice daily oral prednisone. Although most patients do not have an absolute resistance, but rather a glucocorticoid insensitivity, and some patients might respond to higher doses of prednisone or its equivalent given for longer periods of time, such doses would be undesirable because they are associated with marked adverse effects. Importantly, the diagnosis of steroid resistant asthma should

---

"Steroid Resistant Asthma: Definition and Mechanisms," by Donald Y.M. Leung, M.D., Ph.D., © Copyright 2005 National Jewish Medical and Research Center. All rights reserved. For additional information, visit http://asthma.national jewish.org/ or call 1-800-222 LUNG.

only be made after an extensive evaluation to rule out other potential causes of wheezing or factors that contribute to the severity of asthma. Patients with steroid resistant asthma should fulfill the American Thoracic Society (ATS) criteria for diagnosis of asthma and have a bronchodilator response of greater than 15% improvement in FEV1.

Immune Responses to Glucocorticoids in Steroid Resistant Asthma

One of the major mechanisms by which glucocorticoids act in asthma is by reducing airway inflammation and immune activation. However, patients with steroid resistant asthma have higher levels of immune activation in their airways than do patients with steroid sensitive (SS) asthma. Furthermore, glucocorticoids do not reduce the eosinophilia [a condition often seen in the presence of infections or allergens in which there is an increased number of eosinophils—a type of while blood cell—in the blood] or T cell activation found in steroid resistant asthmatics. This persistent immune activation is associated with high levels of IL [interleukin]-2, IL-4 and IL-5 in the airways of these patients [interleukins are substances produced by the body to help regulate the immune system].

Glucocorticoid Receptor (GCR) Abnormalities in Steroid Resistant Asthma

Two types of steroid resistant asthma have been described. One group with acquired steroid resistance (Type 1) and a second with primary steroid resistance (Type II).

Patients with acquired steroid resistance have poor glucocorticoid receptor binding affinity for steroids and the DNA sites recognized by the glucocorticoid receptor. Clinically they present as patients with steroid resistant asthma who develop severe side effects including adrenal gland suppression from chronic treatment with systemic steroids. Their defect is localized to the immune system, reversible in vitro, and can be induced in their T cells by the combination of IL-2 and IL-4.

In contrast, the primary form (Type II) of steroid resistant asthma is not associated with the development of steroid-induced side effects, and the glucocorticoid receptor defect involves decreased GCR numbers. It may be analogous to patients with primary cortisol resistance, which has a genetic basis, as Type II steroid resistant asthma has an irreversible glucocorticoid receptor defect that involves all cell types.

Steroid-Resistant Asthma

It should be noted that most patients who have a provisional diagnosis of primary steroid resistant asthma are simply NOT taking their medications. As a result, they develop no side effects after being prescribed oral prednisone and they obviously derive no therapeutic effects from the steroids. When patients present with a history of primary steroid resistant asthma, it is important to confirm they are taking the oral steroid under strict supervision by checking their A.M. serum cortisol after a course of steroid therapy. The acquired form (Type I) accounts for more than 95% of steroid resistant asthma. Therefore any patient presenting with primary steroid resistant asthma, should be suspected of poor adherence to therapy until proven otherwise.

Chapter 18

Status Asthmaticus

A Case Study

I first met Susan in the emergency room. She was a 25-year-old graphic designer and had been suffering from severe asthma since she was a teenager. Her symptoms had worsened over the previous three days, after she'd caught a cold. Now she was using her inhaled bronchodilator (drug that expands the airway) every hour with no relief. She delayed calling her primary doctor's office in the hope that her symptoms would get better.

Susan frequently suffered from cough, wheezing, and chest tightness. These symptoms were usually exacerbated by various environmental allergens, cold air, exercise, or respiratory infections. She awakened with night-time symptoms two to three times per week and had taken oral steroids several times over the last year for worsening symptoms. She was using high-dose inhaled steroids daily to decrease airway inflammation and also using inhaled albuterol, a beta adrenergic medication, which relaxes the airway smooth muscle (muscle that controls airway diameter). She had a history of multiple hospitalizations for asthma, including one admission to the intensive care unit two years earlier. At that time, she had required mechanical ventilation (machine-assisted breathing) for several days.

Susan was markedly short of breath and could only speak in short sentences. She had a fever of 101 degrees, was breathing rapidly, and

---

"Status Asthmaticus," by Maritza Groth, MD, © 2004 Healthology, Inc. All rights reserved. Additional information is available at www.heathology.com.

her heart rate was 150/minute. Her air passages were so constricted that she was no longer wheezing, and I could barely hear any breath sounds at all. Her lips were a little blue and I measured her oxygen saturation to be only 84% (normally this value is greater than 90%). She was too short of breath for me to measure her peak flows (maximum force of air at outset of exhalation).

Over the next two hours she required multiple nebulized albuterol treatments (aerosolized asthma medications administered by face mask), oxygen by nasal cannula, and high doses of intravenous steroids. To my dismay, she did not improve. She was becoming visibly tired, laboring with each breath. Blood was drawn from the radial artery in her wrist in order to measure its carbon dioxide and oxygen levels. I became concerned because her carbon dioxide level was elevated. This is an ominous sign in asthmatic patients, and often indicates the need for mechanical ventilation.

Status Asthmaticus

I admitted Susan to the medical intensive care unit with a diagnosis of status asthmaticus. Status asthmaticus means that an asthma attack is so severe that the patient doesn't respond to high doses of inhaled bronchodilators and steroids. This resistance to treatment is probably the result of three things:

- bronchospasm: intense spasm of the airways
- edema: swelling of the lining of the airways
- thick mucus secretions in the airways

These three factors make it very difficult to get air in and out of the lungs.

How Asthmatics Breathe

When we breathe in, our airways are pulled open as the chest wall gets larger, but when we breathe out, the airways tend to collapse, trapping air in the chest. If you are an asthmatic, emptying the lungs takes a long time because your airways are narrowed. You cannot completely empty the lungs before you have to take another breath. The more short of breath you are, the faster you try to breathe and the less time there is to exhale. The result of this is that the lungs retain, or "trap," a lot of air. This is called air-trapping, or hyperinflation. This process makes it harder to take another breath in, and your

Status Asthmaticus

breathing muscles have to work harder to take in any air. A young or otherwise healthy asthmatic can usually overcome this difficulty, but at the cost of significant strain on the breathing muscles. If this demand is sustained too long, for example as a result of resistance to medication, your breathing muscles can fatigue and you will develop respiratory failure.

Respiratory Failure

Respiratory failure is characterized by either a reduced oxygen level or an elevated carbon dioxide level in arterial blood. In asthmatic attacks, the decrease in oxygen is usually not too severe, but may cause breathlessness, rapid breathing, and blue lips. In less severe asthmatic attacks, the respiratory rate rises and the carbon dioxide levels are usually lower than normal; this is called hyperventilation. If the carbon dioxide level is high (or even normal) during an asthma attack, it suggests that the respiratory muscles are fatigued and heralds respiratory failure. As the carbon dioxide level rises, you can become confused, sleepy, and possibly comatose. The acidity of the blood is also altered, so that many vital organs cannot function normally. The reduced oxygen level in status asthmaticus is easily corrected with nasal, or face mask oxygen. The treatment of an elevated carbon dioxide level, however, usually requires mechanical ventilation.

Mechanical Ventilation

A mechanical ventilator takes over the work of breathing during status asthmaticus, but it does nothing to reverse bronchospasm and airway inflammation. Its major function is to maintain breathing for the fatigued muscles until various medications become effective. In order to receive mechanical ventilation, Susan needed an endotracheal tube. This is a plastic tube that is inserted through the mouth or nose into the windpipe (trachea) and is connected to the ventilator. Susan also had to be sedated with fentanyl (an opioid-like morphine) and medically paralyzed in order to allow the ventilator to work effectively and to make her comfortable.

Treatment

I prescribed continuous nebulization of albuterol for the first eighteen hours after Susan's admission to the Intensive Care Unit and then switched to intermittent albuterol every two hours. I added inhaled ipratropium every six hours. Ipratropium is an anticholinergic bronchodilator, and it decreases bronchoconstriction by a different mechanism. Susan continued to be treated with a high dose of intravenous corticosteroids. I also gave her antibiotics, because she had a fever, increased cough and mucus, and a high white blood cell count, suggesting that she had an infection.

I considered adding theophylline by intravenous drip, but decided against it, because Susan's heart was beating rapidly (tachycardia). The use of theophylline in acute asthma has fallen into disfavor, as the data suggest little or no benefit and significant additional toxicity, which includes tachycardia, arrhythmias (irregular heartbeat), nausea, and vomiting.

I was relieved when she finally started to improve, and I could hear wheezing, indicating more airflow. I had very few additional treatments to offer if she hadn't gotten better.

Some of the treatments of last resort used in status asthmaticus include providing general anesthesia with inhalational anesthetics, which are very potent bronchodilators. However, we would need the help of an anesthesiologist to provide this type of treatment. Intravenous anesthetics, such as ketamine, can also be helpful. We have occasionally used intravenous magnesium for some patients with severe status asthmaticus, but the benefits of this treatment are not clearly documented in clinical studies.

The next day, Susan was clearly much better. She was now getting albuterol every 4 hours. She needed less oxygen, and I could hear better breath sounds and less wheezing.

Risk for the Development of Status Asthmaticus

Although patients with mild asthma will occasionally have episodes of status, this dangerous condition occurs mostly in patients with very severe disease and in those who have had previous severe attacks. Susan had required mechanical ventilation once before for her asthma and this identified her as a patient at risk for repeat episodes of status. As a result, I take a cautious approach with patients like Susan. I prescribe more frequent bronchodilator treatments, monitor breathing and overall medical condition in an intensive care setting, and initiate larger doses of intravenous corticosteroids.

The best way to decrease the possibility of having a severe asthma attack is to take your medications regularly as prescribed. My patients know never to stop taking their inhaled steroids or leukotriene modifiers ("controller" asthma drugs) unless instructed to do so. When they develop increasing symptoms or their peak flow drops, they initiate an action plan that includes treatment with higher dose of inhaled steroids or oral corticosteroids. I tell my patients to call me when they are experiencing any of the following:

- increasing breathlessness
- increased wheezing
- falling peak flows
- more frequent use of inhaled bronchodilators

Many patients worry about taking oral corticosteroids because of the multiple side effects, such as hypertension, weight gain, leg edema, glucose intolerance, cataracts, and osteoporosis. However, if you are at risk for developing status asthmaticus, taking oral corticosteroids can prevent a serious attack, and possibly save your life.

How to Keep Your Asthma Under Control

Although there are many new medicines to treat asthma, asthma mortality is actually rising. To minimize your chances of having a severe attack, I suggest the following:

- Recognize and control your asthma triggers.
- Take your medications as prescribed—non-compliance is one of the most common causes of severe attacks.
- Don't be afraid to take oral corticosteroids when prescribed by your physician—they are the most effective therapy for severe asthma.
- If your symptoms worsen, contact your healthcare provider immediately to step up your medications.
- If your asthma is not responding to medication as quickly as it usually does, take immediate action: call your physician or go to the nearest emergency room.

Chapter 19

Heart Disease and Asthma: A Complex Combination

The symptoms are easy to recognize: wheezing (especially wheezing that worsens at night), shortness of breath, and difficulty breathing. Time to reach for your inhaler, right? Maybe, maybe not. It depends on whether this is asthma or something else.

When most people say "asthma," they are discussing bronchial asthma, an increasingly common medical condition in which the patient experiences periods of breathing difficulties such as wheezing, chest tightness, and coughing. But there is another condition with very similar symptoms that can be easily confused with bronchial asthma: it is called cardiac asthma.

Cardiac Asthma

Cardiovascular disease contributes to a reduction in lung capacity and functioning. It can cause chest tightness, shortness of breath, wheezing, elevated blood pressure, and an increased heart rate. This condition, called "cardiac asthma," may be perceived by the patient as bronchial asthma. Yet for many individuals, especially those over the age of 55, these symptoms may be an indication of serious cardiovascular diseases, such as congestive heart failure and coronary heart disease.

"Heart Disease and Asthma: A Complex Combination," by Gretchen W. Cook, from *Asthma Magazine*, March/April 2003. Reprinted by permission from Elsevier.

J. McLean Trotter, MD, University of Mississippi Medical Center, works with many patients who show signs of cardiac asthma. "It's increasingly common as people age, particularly with current or past smokers," says Trotter. "As the population as a whole ages, we expect we'll see more and more heart disease and more cardiac asthma."

According to Philip Corsello, MD, medical director of disease management programs, National Jewish Medical and Research Center in Denver, Colorado, there are very real problems associated with not distinguishing the underlying cause of symptoms. "Cardiac asthma is wheezing associated with congestive heart failure," says Corsello. "In that regard it's not really asthma—it's just a response of the airways to the heart failure that mimics asthma. The danger is, if you treat this kind of wheezing as bronchial asthma, you're treating the wrong disease. If a person has cardiac asthma and you're treating them with asthma drugs, you are not diagnosing and treating the congestive heart failure."

Need for Cardiac Evaluation

Even if a person has been diagnosed with asthma, there may be a real need for a cardiac evaluation to ensure there are not other problems as well—especially with older patients who have other risk factors for heart disease. "Heart disease of any type can be particularly tricky to diagnose and treat when the patient has what we call co-morbid conditions—other serious health problems along with the heart disease," says Trotter. "Asthma is one common condition we see along with heart disease older patients. On the other hand, if there is diagnosed heart disease and a suspicion of asthma, I'd recommend a thorough pulmonary evaluation from a qualified allergy specialist or pulmonologist."

"A person known to have or suspected to have both heart disease and asthma should first be treated optimally for the asthma," says Corsello. "Then the patient should be evaluated by a cardiologist. If the person has asthma and is known to have heart disease and the treatment of the asthma has them symptom free, then the need for a cardiology consultation is not so urgent. But if you treat the asthma optimally and the patient still has shortness of breath, then it is imperative that the person promptly see a cardiologist."

Medicine Matters

When a person has both asthma and heart disease, it is important that he or she be treated by qualified specialists. One reason for this

Heart Disease and Asthma: A Complex Combination

is that the medicines used to treat each of these conditions have the potential to cause adverse reactions that may aggravate the other condition. Many of the drugs used to treat cardiovascular problems may interfere with asthma medications or cause asthma exacerbations. Furthermore, some asthma medicines contribute to side effects, such as a rapid or irregular heart beat, tremors, or chest pain, and may not be not appropriate for individuals with cardiovascular disease.

Table 19.1. Potential Drug Reactions/Interactions for Patients with Heart Disease and Asthma

Drug	Possible Side Effect
Asthma/Allergy Medications	
Oral corticosteroids	Cardiovascular or metabolic disturbances
Theophylline	Cardiac arrhythmias
Inhaled beta2-agonists (albuterol)*	Increased heart rate and increased blood pressure
Oral beta2-agonists	Increased heart rate and increased blood pressure
Non-sedating anti-histamine	Heart arrhythmias, particularly if patient is using a diuretic or a beta2-agonist
Heart Disease Medications	
Non-specific beta-blocker	Acute bronchospasm (Not recommended for patients with asthma)
Selective beta-blocker	Bronchospasm (May be used with caution for patients with asthma)
Diuretics	Some diuretics, when combined with beta2-agonists (albuterol) can increase the risk of cardiac arrhythmias
ACE inhibitors (angiotensin-converting-enzyme, a high blood pressure medicine)	Cough that can be mistakenly attributed to asthma and kidney problems

Note: When seeing more than one doctor, be sure to make each doctor aware of all medications you take to help guard against adverse reactions or drug interactions.

*Ipratropium bromide is recommended as a substitute for inhaled beta-2 agonists for those experiencing side effects as long as the patient's responsiveness to it is established.

Two drugs that have the potential to cause problems sound remarkably similar, but are in fact very different. These are beta-blockers and beta-agonists.

Beta-blockers improve the heart's functioning or pumping ability and can also reduce the heart rate. Beta-blockers are frequently prescribed for people with heart failure, high blood pressure, irregular heartbeat, or angina. They can, however, cause side effects, including triggering asthma symptoms. "In those individuals who have asthma, the use of beta-blockers [to treat heart disease] should be avoided because a significant number of them will have a worsening of their asthma when they use a beta-blocker," says Corsello.

Beta-agonists are perhaps best known as the active ingredient in rescue inhalers used by people with asthma. They quickly reduce chest tightness or wheezing by relaxing the muscles around the airways during an asthma episode. While they are very effective at treating an asthma episode, these drugs can affect the functioning of the heart.

The problem lies in the way beta-blockers and beta-agonists work. "There are two types of beta-receptors in the body," says Corsello. "Beta-1 receptors are primarily in the heart, while beta-2 receptors are primarily in the airways." To treat an asthma exacerbation it is common to use a beta-2 "stimulator," such as albuterol. To treat heart problems, very often a beta "blocker" is used. But the operative word is primarily. "When we say receptors in the heart are primarily beta-1, that might be 90%," explains Corsello. "There will be a small percentage of beta-2 receptors in the heart, and these may respond to the beta-agonist, such as albuterol."

Therefore, if you are taking a beta-blocker, such a propanolol, one commonly prescribed for heart disease, it may also affect the beta-receptors in the airways. "In this case, propanolol is a non-specific beta-blocker," Corsello explains. "It affects both beta-1 and beta-2 receptors. When you use it as a heart drug, it will address the beta-1 receptors in the heart, but it will also block the beta-2 receptors in the lungs, which is not good for patients with asthma. There is another beta-blocker called Metoprolol. It will primarily block the beta-receptors in the heart because it is a fairly specific beta-1 blocker."

"A cardiologist has the training and experience to determine the best combination of drugs to treat the heart without exacerbating the asthma," says Corsello. It is important to note that not everyone reacts to these drugs in the same way. Some people with asthma may tolerate a beta-blocker with no problems, while others may experience a dramatic worsening of asthma symptoms.

Heart Disease and Asthma: A Complex Combination

Communication

In many instances, patients see more than one doctor. This is especially true within the elderly population. Unfortunately, it often falls to the patient to take an active role in communicating to each doctor the various medications he or she is taking, diagnoses that have been made, or treatment plans that have been prescribed by other health care providers. "In instances where there are multiple health conditions, the patient must absolutely become his own advocate," says Trotter.

Trotter suggests the following three techniques to facilitate this communication:

1. "Take each of your prescription and over-the-counter medicines with you to every doctor or emergency room visit. This is the most effective way to let the doctor know what [medications] you take."

2. Educate yourself about your medical conditions and ask questions during doctor's visits. "Write up a list in advance, if necessary. And do not hesitate to double check the doctor's instructions. Both doctors and patients make mistakes."

3. Take notes. "Ask your questions and take notes of the answers. A lot is going on during an office consultation, and it's easy to forget things."

When the Patient Is Overwhelmed

Sometimes, because of age or health problems, a person can simply be overwhelmed and unable to adequately communicate with the attending physicians. If this is the case, it is imperative that family members or friends go along to provide assistance and act as an advocate.

"In elderly patients, it's not uncommon to see someone on 10 different medications," explains Trotter. "It's easy to get confused. In these cases, it takes a dedicated caregiver to assist."

For many people living with asthma coupled with heart problems, managing this complex combination is a daily challenge. "With careful attention to the symptoms and medications, asthma in the heart patient can be well controlled," says Trotter. "With clear communication between doctor and patient and a proactive approach, even these complex health issues can be addressed effectively to allow the patient a full and rewarding life."

Chapter 20

Asthma and Chronic Obstructive Pulmonary Disease (COPD)

What does the term COPD mean? It stands for chronic obstructive pulmonary disease and refers to a problem with breathing air out from your lungs. If you have difficulty breathing "used" air out of your lungs, not enough space is left for oxygen-rich air to enter your lungs.

Until recently, most people who had COPD were grouped together and considered to have one disease. We now know that several different diseases cause this difficulty in releasing air from the lungs. Asthmatic bronchitis, chronic bronchitis, and emphysema are three of the major diseases that are grouped together as COPD.

Asthmatic and Chronic Bronchitis

Both asthmatic and chronic bronchitis occur when the large airways or bronchi are inflamed and swollen. Imaging what happens to your skin when you've gotten an insect bite and it becomes swollen, red, and painful. This same idea can be applied to the swelling that occurs with bronchitis. The lining of the air tubes becomes swollen and produces large amounts of mucus. Because mucus clogs the airways, it complicates the problem, much like pus infects and irritates a wound and delays healing.

"Lung—COPD and Asthma," © 2004 National Lung Health Education Program. Reprinted with permission. For additional information, visit http://www.nlhep.org/.

The muscles that surround the airways may tighten when they should not, causing bronchospasm. These narrowed airways prevent all the "used" air from leaving the lungs. Bronchospasm, inflammation, and swelling all make the space inside the airways smaller. This reduces the amount of air that can flow in and out of the lungs.

The first symptom of chronic bronchitis is a persistent cough that brings up mucus. This is often followed by wheezing, shortness of breath, and frequent chest infections. The symptoms of bronchitis can usually be relieved or improved with treatment.

Emphysema

Emphysema develops when many of the small air sacs, or alveoli, in the lungs are destroyed. This reduces their elasticity and decreases their ability to pass oxygen into the blood and remove carbon dioxide from the blood.

Shortness of breath is the major symptom of emphysema. At first, this difficulty in breathing may occur only with heavy exercise. Later it happens with light exercise and, still later, even when walking or engaging in other everyday activities. Many people who have emphysema also have chronic bronchitis. The mucus produced by these inflamed airways makes breathing even more difficult.

In most cases, a person's lungs can take a lot of abuse. It may be 20 or more years before someone who has emphysema notices a change in his or her health. However, when emphysema is diagnosed early, more can be done to treat it. By stopping smoking and using appropriate treatments or medication, persons with emphysema can generally lead a comfortable life.

Causes of COPD

Asthmatic bronchitis, chronic bronchitis, and emphysema develop as a result of one or more of these factors:

- cigarette smoking
- family susceptibility
- inhaling large amounts of dust at work or at home

Conditions that can make these diseases worse are frequent colds or infections in the nose, sinus, throat, or chest.

It is also known that emphysema can be hereditary. In some families this might be due to a lack of normal lung "defenses" that fight

Asthma and Chronic Obstructive Pulmonary Disease (COPD)

damage within the lung. It may also be because certain habits are passed along to other family members. For example, if parents smoke, there is a good chance that their children will smoke. Since smoking is the main cause of COPD, persons with family members who smoke are at greater risk of getting these diseases.

Chapter 21

Rhinitis and Its Impact on Asthma

Summary

Allergic rhinitis is a major chronic respiratory disease due to its prevalence, impact on quality of life, impact on work/school performance and productivity, economic burden, and links with asthma. In addition, allergic rhinitis is associated with sinusitis and other co-morbidities (co-occurring disorders) such as conjunctivitis.

Allergic rhinitis should be considered as a risk factor for asthma along with other known risk factors. A new subdivision of allergic rhinitis has been proposed: intermittent and persistent. The severity of allergic rhinitis has been classified as "mild" or "moderate/severe" depending on the severity of symptoms and quality of life outcomes. Depending on the subdivision and severity of allergic rhinitis, a stepwise therapeutic approach has been proposed.

The treatment of allergic rhinitis combines allergen avoidance (when possible), pharmacotherapy (medications), and immunotherapy (allergy shots). The environmental and social factors should be optimized to allow the patient to lead a normal life.

Patients with persistent allergic rhinitis should be evaluated for asthma by history, chest examination and, if possible and when necessary, the assessment of airflow obstruction before and after bronchodilator.

Excerpted from National Guideline Clearinghouse (NGC). Guideline summary: Allergic Rhinitis and its Impact on Asthma. In: National Guideline Clearinghouse (NGC) http://www.guideline.gov. Rockville (MD): [cited 2005 Sept 01]. Available: http://www.guideline.gov.

Patients with asthma should be appropriately evaluated (history and physical examination) for rhinitis. A combined strategy should ideally be used to treat co-existent upper and lower airway diseases in terms of efficacy and safety.

Specific Recommendations

Diagnosis and Assessment of Severity

History: History should take into account some associated symptoms common in patients with rhinitis. They include:

- loss of smell (hyposmia or anosmia);
- snoring, sleep problems;
- post nasal drip or chronic cough, in particular if sinusitis is present;
- sedation, which may be caused by rhinitis;
- questions on asthma and conjunctivitis.

The history includes a full-length questionnaire:

- The frequency, severity, duration, persistence or intermittence and seasonality of symptoms should be determined.
- It is important to assess their impact on the patients' quality of life in terms of impairment of school/work performance, interference with leisure activities and any sleep disturbances.
- Potential allergic triggers should be documented including exposure in the home, workplace and school. Any hobbies which may provoke symptoms should also be noted.
- An occupational history should be obtained.
- The effects of previous allergen avoidance measures should be noted, bearing in mind that up to 3–6 months of vigorous cleaning may be needed to eradicate mites, cat dander, and other relevant allergens from the home.
- Response to pharmacological treatment and previous immunotherapy should be recorded in terms of improvement and side effects.
- Compliance with treatment and patients' fears about treatment should be explored, particularly if the response to treatment has been below that expected.

- Drugs affect skin tests, and it is always necessary to ask patients about the drugs they have taken.

Examination of the Nose

In patients with mild intermittent allergic rhinitis, a nasal examination is optimal. All patients with persistent allergic rhinitis need a nasal examination. Nasal examination should describe:

- the anatomical situation in the nose (for example, the septum, the size of the inferior turbinate and if possible the structures in the middle meatus);
- the color of the mucosa;
- the amount and aspect of the mucus.

Anterior rhinoscopy, using a speculum and mirror, gives information which is sometimes limited, but it remains an appropriate method for studying the major modifications observed in most cases of allergic rhinitis.

Nasal endoscopy can find nasal and sinus pathology that might easily be missed with routine speculum and nasopharyngeal examination. Ear, nose, and throat (ENT) examination in the clinic is now considerably facilitated by the use of rigid Hopkins rods or flexible fibre-optic endoscopes.

The administration of intranasal anesthesia is recommended at initial assessment. Specific attention is paid to abnormality within the middle meatus and nasopharynx.

Allergy Diagnosis

Skin Tests

- Immediate hypersensitivity skin tests are widely used to demonstrate an IgE-mediated allergic reaction of the skin and represent a major diagnostic tool in the field of allergy. If properly performed, they yield useful confirmatory evidence for a diagnosis of specific allergy. As there are many complexities for their performance and interpretation, it is recommended that they should be carried out by trained health professionals. Delayed hypersensitivity tests provide little information.

- Scratch tests should not be used any longer because of poor reproducibility and possible systemic reactions.

- Prick and puncture tests (SPT) are usually recommended for the diagnosis of immediate type allergy. Skin prick tests should be 2 cm apart.

IgE

- The measurement of total serum IgE is barely predictive for allergy screening in rhinitis and should no longer be used as a diagnostic tool.
- In contrast to the low predictive value of total serum IgE measurements in the diagnosis of immediate type allergy, the measurement of allergen-specific IgE in serum is of importance.

Nasal Challenge

Indications for nasal challenge tests:

- Allergen provocations
    - When discrepancies between history of allergic rhinitis and tests or between tests are present (for example, in cases of diagnostic doubt)
    - For diagnosis of occupational allergic rhinitis
    - Before immunotherapy for allergic rhinitis. Although it is still not very common to use nasal provocation before starting immunotherapy, it has been considered that a laborious long-lasting therapy is justified by a proper diagnosis. This holds true particularly in the case of perennial allergic rhinitis.
    - For research
- Lysine-aspirin: Nasal provocation is recommended as a substitute for oral provocation in aspirin intolerance. Whenever such a nasal provocation is negative, an oral test is still required.
- To test non-specific hyperreactivity: nasal provocation with non-specific stimuli (histamine, methacholine, cold dry air, etc.) is not relevant for daily clinical practice and diagnosis but can be used in research.

Assessment of the nasal response: Symptom scores are combined with objective measures.

- Counting sneezes or attacks of sneezes

Rhinitis and Its Impact on Asthma

- Measuring volume or weight of nasal secretion
- Changes of nasal patency, airflow or airflow resistance

Diagnosis of Asthma

The diagnosis of asthma may be difficult due to the transient nature of the disease and the reversibility of the airflow obstruction spontaneously or after treatment. Key indicators for diagnosing asthma are presented below.

Consider asthma if any of the following are present:

- Wheezing: high-pitched whistling sounds when breathing out—especially in children. (A normal chest examination does not exclude asthma.)
- History of any of the following:
    - Cough, worse particularly at night
    - Recurrent wheezing
    - Recurrent difficult breathing
    - Recurrent chest tightness

Note: Eczema, hay fever, or family history of asthma or atopic diseases are often associated with asthma, but they are not key indicators.

- Symptoms occur or worsen at night, awakening the patient.
- Symptoms occur or worsen in the presence of:
    - Exercise
    - Viral infection (common cold)
    - Animals with fur
    - Domestic dust mites (in mattresses, pillows, upholstered furniture, carpets)
    - Smoke (tobacco, wood)
    - Pollen
    - Changes in temperature
    - Strong emotional expression (laughing or crying hard)
    - Aerosol chemicals
    - Drugs (aspirin, beta blockers)

- Reversible and variable airflow limitation as measured by using a peak expiratory flow (PEF) meter or forced expiratory volume in 1 second (FEV1) in any of the following ways:
  - PEF or FEV1 increases more than 12% 15 to 20 minutes after inhalation of a short-acting beta2-agonist, or
  - PEF or FEV1 varies more than 20% from morning measurement upon arising to measurement 12 hours later in patients taking a bronchodilator (more than 10% in patients who are not taking a bronchodilator), or
  - PEF or FEV1 decreases more than 15% after 6 minutes of running or exercise.

Assessment of Severity of Rhinitis

For rhinitis, there is no accepted measure of nasal obstruction. The nasal inspiratory peak flow (NIPF) has been extensively studied but results are not consistent among the different studies. Moreover, the correlation between the objective measurement of nasal resistance and subjective reports of nasal airflow sensation is usually poor.

Management Recommendations

Allergen Avoidance: Allergen avoidance, including house dust mites, should be an integral part of a management strategy.

Medication

Oral H1 antihistamines: Because of their more favorable risk/benefit ratio and enhanced pharmacokinetics, new H1-antihistamines should be considered as a first-choice treatment for allergic rhinitis when they are available and affordable. The anti-allergenic activities exerted by some drugs would suggest that long-term use is preferable to an "on demand" regimen, especially in persistent disease. In perennial allergic rhinitis, when obstruction is the predominant symptom, intranasal glucocorticosteroids should either be added to a H1-antihistamine or used as a first choice drug.

Intranasal or intraocular (topical) H1 antihistamines: Topical H1-antihistamines have a rapid onset of action (less than 15 minutes) at low drug dosage, but they act only on the treated organ. Topical H1-antihistamines usually require twice-a-day administrations to maintain a satisfactory clinical effect. Their use may therefore be recommended for mild organ-limited disease, as an "on demand" medication in conjunction with a continuous one.

Intranasal corticosteroids: A recent meta-analysis has demonstrated that intranasal glucocorticoids are more efficacious in reducing the symptoms of allergic rhinitis than antihistamines. The advantage was most obvious for nasal blockage. However, in clinical practice, compliance, drug preference, drug availability and potential side effects should be considered.

Because intranasal glucocorticosteroids are more effective in moderate to severe rhinitis and can suppress many stages of the allergic inflammatory disease, the therapeutic risk/benefit ratio has to be considered. Generally, the groups of patients with persistent allergic rhinitis who usually suffer from nasal blockage are better managed with intranasal glucocorticosteroids. When symptoms are mild or only intermittent, an H1-antihistamine is a good choice. The balance between intranasal glucocorticosteroids and H1-antihistamines has to be individualized.

In conclusion, intranasal glucocorticosteroids should be regarded as a highly effective first-line treatment for patients suffering from allergic and non-allergic rhinitis with moderate to severe and/or persistent symptoms. Even though intranasal glucocorticosteroids may be less effective in non-allergic rhinitis, they are worth trying.

Systemic glucocorticosteroids: Systemic glucocorticosteroids are never the first line of treatment for allergic rhinitis. They can be used as a last resort of treatment when other treatments are ineffective. Oral glucocorticoids have the advantage over depot injections that treatment adjustments can follow the pollen count. Systemic glucocorticoids, in contrast to intranasal treatment, reach all parts of the nose and paranasal sinuses, therefore short courses in patients with severe perennial rhinitis or nasal polyposis can be helpful.

Systemic glucocorticosteroids should be avoided in children, pregnant women and patients with known contraindications.

Intranasal or intraocular chromones: In placebo-controlled trials, disodium cromoglycate (DSCG) four times daily has been shown to be effective in allergic rhinitis and conjunctivitis, although less effective than H1-antihistamines or intranasal glucocorticosteroids.

Nedocromil sodium has also been shown to be effective in allergic rhinitis and conjunctivitis and has the advantage of a twice-a-day dosing regimen.

In adults, chromones are not a major therapeutic option in the treatment of allergic rhinitis, although they maintain a valued place for the treatment of allergic conjunctivitis.

Decongestants: In general, because of the risk of rhinitis medicamentosa, the use of intranasal decongestants should be limited to a duration of less than 10 days. Short courses of intranasal decongestants can be useful to promptly reduce severe nasal blockage while co-administering other drugs.

Decongestants should be used with care in children under one year of age because of the narrow range between therapeutic and toxic doses. Furthermore, it is advised not to prescribe pseudoephedrine to patients over 60 years of age, to pregnant women and, in general, to patients suffering from hypertension, cardiopathy, hyperthyroidism, prostatic hypertrophy, glaucoma, and psychiatric disorders as well as to those taking beta-blockers or monoamine oxidase (MAO) inhibitors.

Topical anti-cholinergics: Studies performed in perennial allergic rhinitis demonstrated that ipratropium bromide only improves nasal hyper-secretion. (No data are available for seasonal rhinitis.) Since patients with perennial rhinitis usually suffer also from nasal congestion, itching, and sneezing, other drugs are preferable as first-line agents to ipratropium in the vast majority of cases of allergic rhinitis. However, the ipratropium bromide nasal spray alone should be considered in patients for whom rhinorrhea (runny nose) is the primary symptom. Its use in combination with an intranasal glucocorticosteroid or an H1-antihistamine may be considered in patients where rhinorrhea is the predominant symptom, or in patients with rhinorrhea who are not fully responsive to other therapies. Moreover, ipratropium may be used in patients with or without allergic rhinitis who suffer from rhinorrhea when in contact with cold air. In elderly patients, ipratropium may be of interest in the treatment of isolated rhinorrhea.

Antileukotrienes: In seasonal allergic rhinitis, the combination of a CysLT (cysteinyl leukotriene) receptor antagonist, montelukast, and loratadine showed that symptoms of rhinitis and conjunctivitis were more effectively treated with the combination of these drugs as opposed to any one of them alone or with the placebo.

Treatments with a lack of demonstrable efficacy (homeopathy, acupuncture, chiropractic, traditional medicine and phytotherapy, other alternative therapies): None of the methods used in alternative medicine can be supported scientifically to be clinically effective. The public should be warned against methods of diagnosis and treatment which may be costly and which have not been validated. Properly designed randomized clinical trials are required to assess the value of these forms of treatment.

Antibiotics: In non-complicated rhinitis, antibiotics are not a recommended treatment.

Nasal douching: Nasal douching with a traditional alkaline nasal douche or a sterile seawater spray was shown to improve symptoms of rhinitis.

Surgery: Indications for surgical intervention are:

- drug-resistant inferior turbinate hypertrophy;
- anatomical variations of the septum with functional relevance;
- anatomical variations of the bony pyramid with functional/aesthetic relevance;
- secondary or independently developing chronic sinusitis;
- different forms of nasal unilateral polyposis (choanal polyp, solitary polyp, allergic fungal sinusitis) or therapy-resistant bilateral nasal polyposis;
- fungal sinus disease (mycetoma, invasive forms) or other pathologies unrelated to allergy (cerebrospinal fluid leak, inverted papilloma, benign and malignant tumours, Wegener's disease, etc.).

Aspirin Intolerance

In order to prevent life-threatening reactions, patients with aspirin-intolerant rhinitis/asthma should avoid aspirin, all products containing aspirin and other analgesics that inhibit cyclooxygenase (COX). The education of physicians and patients regarding this matter is extremely important.

The patient should obtain a list of drugs that are contraindicated, preferably with both the generic and trade names. If necessary, these patients can take acetaminophen or paracetamol; it is safer not to exceed a dose of 1000 mg. Sodium salicylate, benzydamine, azapropazone, and dextropropoxyphene can be administered.

Specific Immunotherapy (SIT)

In order to make the patient as symptom-free as possible, immunotherapy is indicated as a supplement to allergen avoidance and as a drug treatment in patients with rhinitis predominantly induced by dominating allergens.

Immunotherapy should be initiated early in the disease process to reduce the risk of side effects and to prevent the further development of severe disease. Arguments for specific immunotherapy are:

- insufficient response to conventional pharmacotherapy;
- side effects from drugs;
- rejection of drug treatment.

Injection (subcutaneous) specific immunotherapy may be used in severe or prolonged allergic rhinitis (eventually associated with asthma). Local (intranasal and sublingual-swallow) specific immunotherapy may be considered in selected patients with systemic side effects and with refusal to injection treatment.

Contraindications: Specific immunotherapy is contraindicated in patients with: serious immunopathological and immunodeficiency diseases, malignancy, severe psychological disorders, treatment with beta-blockers, even when administered topically, poor compliance, severe asthma uncontrolled by pharmacotherapy, and/or patients with irreversible airways obstruction (FEV1 is consistently under 70% of predicted values after adequate pharmacological treatment), significant cardiovascular diseases which increase the risk of side effects from epinephrine, and children under 5 years of age unless there are specific indications.

Education

It is important to educate both the patient and relevant family members regarding the nature of the disease and available treatments. This should include general information regarding the symptoms, causes and mechanisms of rhinitis.

In addition, education about means of avoidance, immunotherapy, and drug therapy must be provided. It is vital that patients understand the potential side effects of therapy, especially drug side effects, in order to insure that they do not abruptly discontinue beneficial therapy but rather communicate adverse events to their physician so they can deal with them in a manner best for the patient.

It is also important to provide patients with education about the complications of rhinitis, including sinusitis and otitis media, and about comorbid conditions such as nasal polyps. They should be aware of how such complications are recognized and how they are treated.

Patients need to be aware of the potential negative impact of rhinitis on the quality of life and potential benefits of complying with therapeutic recommendations.

Patients must also have realistic expectations for the results of therapy and should understand that complete cures do not usually occur in the treatment of any chronic disease, including rhinitis.

Chapter 22

Sinusitis and Asthma

Introduction

Background: In the United States, 35 million persons have sinus problems and 15 million persons have asthma. Clinically, physicians know that a sinus infection can contribute significantly to the frequency and severity of asthma attacks. The purpose of this chapter is to outline the factors common to both conditions and to note how best to improve these conditions.

Asthma and sinusitis both have been recognized in ancient literature. In the 1940s and 1950s, considerable sinus surgery was performed to help people with asthma. Purulent diseased tissue was removed, the nasal airway was opened, and excellent results were achieved for some of these patients. Then, in the 1960s, the improvements following sinus surgery were thought to be related more to the stress reaction than to the surgical technique; therefore, sinus surgery became less popular as a principle of asthma management.

With the introduction of the CT scanning technique in the 1970s, accurately pinpointing the location and extent of the sinus pathology became possible. A return to corrective surgery for individuals with sinusitis and individuals with asthma has occurred. Then, in the 1980s,

---

Excerpted and reprinted with permission from "Asthma and Sinusitis," by Murray Grossan, MD, Consulting Staff, Department of Otolaryngology, Cedars Sinai Hospital of Los Angeles, June 8, 2004, © 2004 eMedicine.com, Inc. The complete text of this document may be viewed online at http://www.emedicine.com.

functional endoscopic sinus surgery (FESS) and the ability to physiologically improve sinus function became available.

In the 1990s, as CT scanning enhanced the view of the sinus and as endoscopic surgery, especially with the computer-assisted techniques, improved the ability to improve sinus function, physicians returned to sinus treatment as an aid to asthma management. Further aids to treatment have included newer antibiotics and emphasis on cilia function. Newer medications, such as the corticosteroids sprays, have given new directions for treatment. Indeed, many allergists now emphasize their role in treating sinusitis.

Pathophysiology: The physiology of mucus in individuals with asthma is similar to that of nasal mucus. Mucociliary clearance (MCC) involves cilia and the layers of mucus on the ciliated epithelium and refers to the movement of particles along a desired path for maximum health. In the upper respiratory tract, cilia propel the mucus and its trapped bacteria and particles to the nasopharynx, where it drops to the hypopharynx and is swallowed. The stomach acid then disposes of the unwanted invaders.

In the lower respiratory tract, the cilia that line the trachea and bronchial tree similarly move the mucus blanket up the trachea and into the hypopharynx for swallowing.

The science of rheology investigates the makeup of this liquid and studies its viscosity and elasticity. Two layers of mucus are present over the ciliated cell; an outer thick, viscoelastic, semisolid mucus layer, which the cilia do not strike directly, is found over a layer of watery serous fluid. Because of the lowered viscosity of the layer of watery serous fluid, the cilia are able to beat normally and to move the watery lower layer, thereby affecting movement of the upper thick layer. Changes of these properties affect movement of the mucus blanket and play a major role in pulmonary and sinus disease. If the movement of the blanket is slowed, bacteria are able to multiply as the mucus thickens and stagnates.

Frequency: In the United States, asthma and sinusitis are both increasing in frequency. Fifteen million individuals with asthma and 35 million persons with sinusitis live in the United States. No doubt, overlapping of the conditions occurs. Internationally, an increased incidence is reported in all countries. The incidence of sinusitis is higher in Japan, Indonesia, and Europe than in the United States.

An increasing incidence of both sinusitis and asthma occurring together is reported internationally as well as in the United States.

Certain areas have special conditions causing an increased sinusitis incidence (for example, the fires of Kuwait and Indonesia or the chromium content of the sands of Saudi Arabia). Asthma-free areas have been noted in certain sub-Saharan areas where hookworm is endemic.

Mortality/Morbidity: Despite the availability of effective antiasthmatic drugs, asthma is responsible for more than 100 million days of restricted activity and 470,000 hospitalizations annually. The most common disease of early childhood, asthma exacts a particularly high toll among persons who are economically disadvantaged.

Sinusitis, fortunately, has a low death rate. Death can occur in young children when the condition is unrecognized. In infants, the maxillary sinuses are well developed but are often unrecognized as a source of possible lethal infection. In adults, fatalities occur primarily as a result of complications of sinus infection to the brain, meninges, and the cavernous sinus.

Sex: Incidence of sinusitis appears to be equal between the sexes.

Age: Asthma and sinusitis can occur in very young children. Sinusitis in very young children is not appreciated because the presence of the maxillary and ethmoid sinuses is not always recognized. Once children start nursery school, the incidence of sinus and chest infections increases dramatically.

Clinical

History: Individuals with asthma often have a childhood history of allergy. Patients present with wheezing and coughing, and they report sleepless nights. These patients benefit from the use of an inhaler. Associated with these symptoms are symptoms of frequent sinus infections, heavy pus, or thick mucus drainage into the chest. Whenever individuals with asthma get a sinus infection, the asthma worsens. When accompanied by a sinus infection, the asthma does not clear with simple treatment. When the nose obstructs, these individuals breathe with the mouth open, which precipitates an asthma attack. Patients with asthma have a dry mouth all the time and are bothered by thick nasal phlegm dripping into the throat. The thick phlegm causes these patients to cough and try to clear the throat constantly. With a sinus infection, a much longer time period is required to clear the asthma.

Physical: In susceptible individuals, inflammation causes recurrent episodes of wheezing, breathlessness, chest tightness, and coughing, particularly at night or in the early morning. These episodes are usually associated with widespread, but variable, airflow obstruction that is often reversible either spontaneously or with treatment. The inflammation also causes an associated increase in the existing bronchial hyperresponsiveness to a variety of stimuli.

Causes

Asthma and sinusitis are increasing in frequency and morbidity, despite the advances made in understanding and treating these conditions. The following theories suggest what is causing these increases:

Overuse of Antibiotics

A current theory suggests that with overuse of antibiotics, the normal disease reaction is replaced by a hypersensitivity reaction. This theory notes a high incidence of disease in families with upper incomes; these individuals have full access to medical care, cleanliness, and dust proofing. The body's immune system is designed to fight parasites and infections, and if the antibiotic is administered at the first sign of illness, perhaps the normal immunity does not develop and alternate systems are produced (for example, asthma or poor resistance to infection).

Genetics

- When compared to sinusitis, asthma has more of a genetic etiology.
- Incidence of asthma increases when both parents have asthma.
- More individuals with asthma are having children.

Environmental Factors

These factors are becoming increasingly more important and include the following:

- The major environmental irritant, other than specific occupational substances, is tobacco smoke.
- Current theory attributes the increase of sinusitis and asthma to air pollution. When the air is polluted with smog, diesel, gasoline,

Sinusitis and Asthma

and other noxious products, the sun's heat and rays may combine them into dozens of products whose long-term effects are unknown at this time.

- Additionally, smog, diesel fumes, and sulfur dioxide all combine to interfere with good cilia function. Hypersensitivity reactions seem to occur when the individual has an overwhelming exposure and does not recover ciliary function. Unfortunately, new solvents are marketed daily and the effect on cilia function is not provided by the manufacturers. Even more unfortunate is the fact that despite the 50 million dollars spent by the Federal Drug Administration (FDA) on clinical evaluations, no drugs are evaluated as to their effect on mucociliary clearance.

- Known industrial toxins include chlorine, sulfur dioxide, cupric compounds, and chromium dusts.

- Fires are a known factor. When countrywide fires occur, such as in Kuwait or Indonesia, the incidence of sinusitis and asthma increases.

- Other environmental problems to be considered include pet allergens, house dust mite allergen, cockroach allergen (most significant in patients who live in the inner city), indoor fungi and molds, and outdoor allergens (for example, trees, grass, weed pollens, and seasonal mold spores).

Impaired Mucociliary Clearance

Sinusitis and asthma are inflammatory diseases and, as such, are caused or aggravated when mucociliary clearance is impaired. Factors that slow cilia include the following:

- cocaine
- antihistamines
- dehydration
- inhalation of air or steam hotter than 40 degrees Celsius
- heavy load of iced drinks
- chilling drafts
- sulfur dioxide, ozone, smog
- inhalation of chromium dusts
- cupric (copper) compounds

- nickel dusts
- chimney dusts
- formaldehyde
- late stages of allergy
- nasal polyps
- Skydrol (a solvent used in airplane maintenance)
- infections with *Pseudomonas* species, *Haemophilus influenzae*, and many viral pathogens
- hyperbaric oxygen
- reduction of airway diameter
- acquired immune deficiency syndrome (AIDS)

Gastroesophageal Reflux Disease (GERD)

In addition to the above factors, recognition of GERD as an irritant that brings on asthmatic symptoms, as well as throat and laryngeal symptoms, is increasing.

Bacteria

Little question exists that bacteria from the sinuses find their way to the lower respiratory system. Bacteria then act as an inflammatory agent.

Treatment

Medical Care: Whether sinusitis and asthma are caused by inflammation or allergies has been questioned. Today, sinusitis and asthma are attributed to inflammatory effect. An excellent example of this is the existence of nasal polyps. With administration of corticosteroids (both oral and topical), polyps may not shrink; however, if an antibiotic is added at the same time as the corticosteroids, clearing of the polyps from the nasal cavity with clearing of the blockage occurs in more than 90% of the author's patients. Patients prefer this form of treatment to surgery.

Treatment consists of using measures to increase mucociliary clearance. To help cilia movement in the chest and nose, a deep-throated "oooooommmmmm" vibration is useful to help break up thick mucus. Patients should drink enough fluids (for example, hot tea or hot chicken soup) to lighten the urine. Bacterial load should also be reduced. This

Sinusitis and Asthma

may be achieved by terbutaline, inhaled corticosteroids, various enzymes, pseudoephedrine, breathing and coughing exercises, flutter inhalation device, iodides, guaifenesin, irrigation, Locke-Ringer moisturizer spray, and exercise.

Many cases of sinusitis do not respond to treatment because (1) the wrong antibiotic is prescribed; (2) duration of the antibiotic is too short—treatment may require six weeks; (3) drainage, rest, and anti-inflammatories are not combined with treatment; (4) fungus is present; and (5) the mucociliary system fails. If infection does not clear in six weeks, referral to an ear, nose, and throat specialist is recommended.

Because bacteria and thick phlegm play a significant role, the physician can reduce the asthmatic symptoms from sinusitis by suctioning or irrigating in the office if pus is present in the nose or sinuses. Pulsatile irrigation may also be beneficial to the patient with allergies during the pollen season. Daily irrigation reduces the pollen load in the nose and the immunoglobulin E (IgE) levels in the nose and in the circulation.

If asthma and sinusitis are considered as being inflammatory diseases, treatment is clearly similar for both in regards to specific infection, inflammation, drainage, attention to thinning mucus, and restoring cilia and comfort to the patient. Treatment may include the following:

- Antibiotics

- Anti-inflammatory agents: Sinus pain is present when membranes are inflamed or swollen. Anti-inflammatory agents (for example, Naproxen) are useful.

- Steroids: One of the major advances in sinus and asthma treatment has been in the use of steroids. These are anti-inflammatory and serve well to reduce these factors.

- Mucolytic medications: Whenever stasis occurs, mucus thickens and bacteria multiply. Thinning the mucus is important in order to restore mucociliary clearance. Drinking hot tea with lemon and honey is one of the best treatments, as is ingesting chicken soup. Most cold drinks slow cilia.

- Decongestants: Pseudoephedrine (Sudafed) has long been a favorite to open a stuffy nose. It is contraindicated in hypertension and in persons who are kept awake by the drug. Strangely, this drug may make children younger than 12 years drowsy.

- Topical medications

- Irrigation/aspiration: Clearing sinus infection is indicated for the individual with asthma. Irrigation/aspiration at the first office visit is a useful step in order to reduce the bacterial load. When the sinus infection does not clear with antibiotics, a doctor may prescribe daily irrigation, mucolytics, and anti-inflammatory medications and follow with a CT scan of the sinuses.

Surgical Care: Sinusitis may require surgical care. Primarily, the disease is a matter of obstruction of sinus drainage. If sterile cotton is placed in the healthy nose, whichever sinus is blocked becomes purulent. This is because the blockage prevents drainage along the mucociliary pathways, macrophages do not have access to the area, and bacteria are free to multiply. Surgery is directed at making sinus drainage adequate and effective. The advances in functional endoscopic sinus surgery (FESS) surgery make it easier and safer to clear the source of sinus disease.

Consultations: When the patient has frequently not responded to antibiotic treatment and other measures, consultation with an otolaryngologist is indicated. When good treatment is unsuccessful, frequently, an anatomic defect with obstruction of drainage is found.

Diet: One of the common urban myths is that milk makes mucus. Of course, certain persons may be allergic to milk, but the popular belief that avoiding milk prevents sinusitis is a myth.

- **Hot tea:** For singers, actors, and speakers, emphasize that hot tea with lemon and honey helps thin mucus and move the cilia; this treatment is especially recommended before a performance. Adequate hydration not only helps the sinus and chest, it can also reduce nosebleeds that many performers get when traveling or in desert climates.

- **Iced drinks:** Iced drinks make the allergy worse and slow the cilia. Many allergy symptoms can be reduced by avoiding iced drinks and avoiding getting chilled.

- **Breakfast in bed:** The individual with allergies warms the body by the actions of sneezing, hacking, and coughing. These actions do work to warm the body, but they start the cascade of symptoms of allergy. Often, 50% of these symptoms can be avoided by drinking a hot drink (for example, tea) before getting out of

Sinusitis and Asthma

bed. Use a thermos or automatic percolator for the hot drink and eat a cookie or whatever else is desired. Afterwards, when the blankets are removed and the feet touch the cold floor, the body is already warmed and the coughing and sneezing are not necessary to warm the body. In addition, because of the tea stimulating the cilia, the dust that accumulated in the nose is removed and sneezing for dust removal is unnecessary.

Activity: For chest problems and postural drainage, breathing exercises are important. With shallow breathing, mucus can be trapped in distal tubules and generate bacterial infection. Stress deep breathing to remove distal air.

Follow-Up

- After 1–2 years, if sinusitis symptoms persist (for example, congestion, drainage, fever, pain), a repeat of the CT scan may be indicated.

- Following sinus surgery, the patient may report not getting enough air, burning in the nose, and dryness. These symptoms often reflect poor cilia function. The nasal membranes appear dry and irritable, and they look thin. Even though the airway is wide open, these symptoms persist with poor cilia function. Treatment is hydration, nasal moisturizer sprays, and ointments. Pulsatile irrigation provides relief and helps restore cilia activity.

- If the cilia of the nose remain normal, few sinus infections should occur; therefore, efforts should be directed to keeping the cilia of the nose normal. Use Locke-Ringer or saline (without Benzalkonium) solution to ensure moisture of the nose. Stress hydration, especially the intake of hot tea and/or chicken soup. Warm compresses to the sinus area are important.

- If sinus symptoms persist, review dust proofing of the bedroom with the patient.

- If cilia of the nose remain slow as shown by dry irritable membranes and thick phlegm, consider pulsatile irrigation with Locke-Ringer or saline solution in order to restore cilia. If cilia are permanently damaged (for example, by excess removal of mucosa, chlorine gas, other toxic substances), consider pulsatile irrigation daily to keep nose moist and remove thick phlegm and materials.

- Check for history of nasal polyps on an annual basis. Remind patients to avoid salicylates. Begin therapy if polyps are recurring.

- On waking up in the morning, the dust has accumulated in the nose and the body temperature is low. If an individual throws off the covers and touches the cold floor with the feet, a cascade of sneezing and hacking warms the body and removes the dust; however, this is an undesirable method to warm the body. Drinking hot tea before getting out of bed avoids this morning cascade of sneezing and hacking.

- Cold air and getting chilled can also trigger an asthma attack. Drinking hot tea before getting out of bed is an excellent preventative.

- The speed of the nasal cilia often reflects the action of the chest cilia. In difficult asthma with associated coughing, determine whether the nasal cilia are inactive. Seek the cause. After exposure to chlorine, chromium, or aldehydes, if the nasal cilia are affected, so are the chest cilia.

Preventing Recurrence

- Dust proofing is the best deterrence.

- Hot tea thins thick mucus. Thick mucus must be thinned by a moisturizer or pulsatile irrigation or proteolytic enzymes taken buccally.

- Elements of the workplace cause sinusitis and asthma. Certain chemicals are highly toxic to the cilia. These include chromium dust, sulfur dioxide, smog, ozone, and certain aldehydes.

- For allergic nasal or chest symptoms, antiallergy medication started six weeks before pollen season often is effective.

- Persons who experience burning or lack of benefit from prepared nasal moisturizers may be reacting to the preservatives (for example, benzalkonium). Switch to homemade products.

Chapter 23

Food Allergies and Asthma

While allergy to pollen or other environmental sources typically causes a lot of discomfort during spring, summer, and fall, food allergy is one condition that knows no season. According to the National Institutes of Health, true food allergy affects six to seven million Americans (approximately two percent of the U.S. population) and four to eight percent of young children, although surveys show that approximately one in three adults believe they have a food allergy.

People tend to diagnose themselves, believing they have allergic reactions to certain foods or food ingredients. Unfortunately, self-diagnosis of food allergy often leads to unnecessary food restrictions, nutrient deficiencies, and misdiagnosis of potential life threatening medical conditions other than food allergy. Therefore, experts urge people to see a board-certified allergist for proper diagnosis of food allergy.

Understanding Food Allergies

A food allergy is an adverse reaction to a food or food component that involves the body's immune system. There are also some adverse reactions to foods that involve the body's metabolism but not the immune system. These reactions are known as food intolerance. Examples of food intolerance are food poisoning or the inability to

---

"Background on Food Allergies and Asthma," © 2005 International Food Information Council. All rights reserved. Reprinted with permission.

properly digest certain food components, such as lactose or milk sugar. This latter condition is commonly known as lactose intolerance.

A true allergic reaction to a food involves three primary components:

1. contact with a food allergen (reaction-provoking substance, virtually always a protein);
2. immunoglobulin E (IgE-an antibody in the immune system that reacts with allergens); and
3. mast cells (tissue cells) and basophils (blood cells), which when connected to IgE antibodies release histamine or other substances causing allergic symptoms.

The body's immune system recognizes an allergen in a food as foreign and produces antibodies to halt the "invasion." As the battle rages, symptoms appear throughout the body. The most common reaction sites are the mouth (swelling of the lips), digestive tract (stomach cramps, vomiting, diarrhea), skin (hives, rashes or eczema), and the airways (wheezing or breathing problems).

Allergic reactions to food are rare and can be caused by any food. The most common food allergens, known as the "top 8" are fish, shellfish, milk, egg, soy, wheat, peanuts, and tree nuts (such as walnuts, cashews, etc.). Symptoms of a food allergy are highly individual and usually begin within minutes to a few hours after eating the offending food. People with true, confirmed food allergies must avoid the offending food altogether.

There are numerous misconceptions regarding allergy to food additives, preservatives, and ingredients. Although some additives and preservatives have been shown to trigger asthma or hives in certain people, these reactions are not the same as those reactions observed with food allergies. These reactions do not involve the immune system and, therefore, are examples of food intolerance or idiosyncrasy rather than food allergy. Most people consume a wide variety of food additives and ingredients daily, with only a very small number having been associated with adverse reactions.

Life-Threatening Reactions

Many allergic reactions to food are relatively mild. However, a small percentage of food-allergic individuals experience severe reactions, called anaphylaxis, that can be life-threatening. Anaphylaxis

Food Allergies and Asthma

is a rare but potentially fatal condition in which several different parts of the body experience food-allergic reactions simultaneously, causing hives, swelling of the throat, and difficulty breathing. It is the most severe allergic reaction.

Symptoms usually appear rapidly, sometimes within minutes of exposure to the allergen. Because they can be life-threatening, immediate medical attention is necessary when an anaphylactic reaction occurs. Standard emergency treatment often includes an injection of epinephrine (adrenaline) to open up the airway and blood vessels.

Diagnosing Food Allergy

Diagnosis usually begins with a thorough medical history, a complete physical examination, and selected tests to rule out underlying medical conditions not related to food allergy. Patients may also have to keep a food diary and record symptoms over a period of time.

Several tests are available to determine if a person is allergic to a certain food. In skin-prick testing, a diluted extract of the suspected food is placed on the skin, which is scratched or punctured. A blood test can provide information similar to skin testing. The gold standard for food allergy testing is the double-blind, placebo-controlled food challenge (DBPCFC). This test is performed by a board-certified allergist. The suspected allergen (for example, milk, fish, soy) is placed in a capsule or hidden in food, and fed to the patient under strict supervision. Neither the allergist nor the patient is aware of which capsule, or food, contains the suspected allergen—hence the name "double-blind." For the test to be effective, the patient must also be fed capsules or food which do not contain the allergen to make sure the observed reaction, if any, is to the allergen and not to some other factor—hence the term "placebo-controlled." These tests have enabled allergists to identify the most common allergens, and also to determine what foods and additives do not cause allergic reactions. These tests may also be used to determine if a child or individual has "outgrown" a certain allergy.

Managing Food Allergy

If a food allergy is diagnosed, the only proven therapy is avoidance of the offending food. Because there are no drugs or allergy shots on the market today to alter the long-term course of food allergy, elimination diets are prescribed. Each diet must consider the person's individual nutritional needs—ability to tolerate the offending food, caloric needs, and other factors. Strict adherence to an elimination diet and careful avoidance of the food allergen may, in some cases, hasten the disappearance of the food allergy.

Most life-threatening allergic reactions to foods occur when eating away from the home. It is important to explain your situation and needs clearly to your host or food server. If necessary, ask to speak with the chef or manager.

The Food and Drug Administration (FDA) requires that ingredients be listed on food labels. You can look at the ingredient listing on food labels to determine the presence of the eight major allergens (fish, shellfish, peanuts, tree nuts, soy, wheat, milk, and egg). Since food and beverage manufacturers are continually making changes, food-allergic people should read the food label for every product purchased each time it is purchased.

Do foods derived from food biotechnology have the potential to be allergenic?

Food biotechnology uses what is known about plant science and genetics to improve food and food production. Through recent advancements in gene transfer, scientists are able to produce tastier, more varied, and more wholesome foods. According to FDA guidelines, any company enhancing foods through biotechnology must evaluate the safety of the new food, including its potential to contain allergens. If unexpected allergens are found in the food, it must be properly labeled to alert individuals who may be sensitive to the specific allergen(s).

Asthma and Food

What is asthma?

Asthma, a chronic medical condition, results when triggers (or irritants) cause swelling of the tissues to the air passages of the lungs, making it difficult to breathe. Typical symptoms of asthma include wheezing, coughing, and shortness of breath.

What are the major triggers of asthma?

Asthma can be triggered by numerous factors, including allergens from dust, molds, pollen, animals, and, occasionally, food; air pollutants, such as cigarette smoke, auto exhaust, smog, or aerosol cleaners; colds and particularly respiratory infections; weather changes; exercise; or certain medications.

Food Allergies and Asthma

Can foods trigger asthma?

Only a few. For years it has been suspected that foods or food ingredients may cause or exacerbate symptoms in those with asthma. After many years of scientific and clinical investigation, there are very few confirmed food triggers of asthma. Sulfites and sulfiting agents in foods (found in dried fruits, prepared potatoes, wine, bottled lemon or lime juice, and shrimp), and diagnosed food allergens (such as milk, eggs, peanuts, tree nuts, soy, wheat, fish, and shellfish) have been found to trigger asthma. Many food ingredients such as food dyes and colors, food preservatives like BHA (butylated hydroxyanisole) and BHT (butylated hydroxytoluene), monosodium glutamate, aspartame, and nitrite, have not been conclusively linked to asthma.

How many Americans are affected by food-triggered asthma?

Food-triggered asthma is rare, occurring only among six to eight percent of children with asthma and less than two percent of adults with asthma.

What can individuals with asthma do to prevent a food-triggered asthma attack?

The best way to avoid food-induced asthma is to eliminate or avoid the offending food or food ingredient from the diet or from the environment. Reading ingredient information on food labels and knowing where food triggers of asthma are found are the best defenses against a food-induced asthma attack. The main objectives of an asthmatic's care and treatment are to stay healthy, to remain symptom free, to enjoy food, to exercise, to use medications properly, and to follow the care plan developed between the physician and patient.

Chapter 24

Gastroesophageal Reflux Disease (GERD) and Asthma

It is estimated that more than 75 percent of patients with asthma also experience gastroesophageal reflux disease (GERD). People with asthma are twice as likely to have GERD as those people who do not have asthma. Of those people with asthma, those who have a severe, chronic form that is resistant to treatment are most likely to also have GERD.

GERD is the backward flow of stomach acids into the esophagus. When this acid enters the lower part of the esophagus, it can produce a burning sensation, commonly referred to as heartburn. If left untreated, GERD can eventually lead to lung damage, esophageal ulcers, and in some instances Barrett's esophagus, a condition that can eventually lead to esophageal cancer.

Does GERD cause asthma?

Although studies have shown a relationship between asthma and GERD, the exact relationship is uncertain. GERD may worsen asthma symptoms, however asthma and some asthma medications may worsen GERD symptoms. On the other hand, treating GERD often helps to

---

"GERD and Asthma," © 2003 The Cleveland Clinic Foundation, 9500 Euclid Avenue, Cleveland, OH 44195, www.clevelandclinic.org. Additional information is available from the Cleveland Clinic Health Information Center, 216-444-3771, toll-free 800-223-2273 extension 43771, or at http://www.clevelandclinic.org/health.

also relieve asthma symptoms, further suggesting a relationship between the two conditions.

Doctors most often look at GERD as the cause of asthma when:

- asthma begins in adulthood;
- asthma symptoms get worse after a meal, after exercise, at night, or after lying down;
- asthma doesn't respond to the standard asthma treatments.

How can GERD affect my asthma?

As previously mentioned, the exact link between the two conditions is uncertain. However, there are a few possibilities as to why GERD and asthma may coincide. One possibility is that the acid flow causes injury to the lining of the throat, airways, and lungs, making inhalation difficult and often causing a persistent cough.

Another possibility for patients with GERD is that when acid enters the esophagus, a nerve reflex is triggered, causing the airways to narrow in order to prevent the acid from entering. This will cause a shortness of breath.

Aside from these possible relationships between asthma and GERD, one study showed there was an increase in the rate of GERD in patients with asthma who were treated with asthma medications known as beta-adrenergic bronchodilators. However, further studies must be done before the relationship between GERD and these drugs can be fully understood.

What should I do if I have asthma and GERD?

If you have both asthma and GERD, it is important that you consistently take any asthma medications your doctor has prescribed to you, as well as controlling your exposure to asthma triggers as much as possible.

Fortunately, many of the symptoms of GERD can be treated and/or prevented by taking steps to control or adjust personal behavior. Some of these steps include:

- Raise the head of your bed by six inches to allow gravity to help keep the stomach's contents in the stomach. (Do not use piles of pillows because this puts your body into a bent position that actually aggravates the condition by increasing pressure on the abdomen.)

Gastroesophageal Reflux Disease (GERD) and Asthma

- Eat meals at least three to four hours before lying down, and avoid bedtime snacks.
- Eat smaller meals with moderate portions of food.
- Maintain a healthy weight to eliminate unnecessary intra-abdominal pressure caused by extra pounds.
- Limit consumption of fatty foods, chocolate, peppermint, coffee, tea, colas, and alcohol—all of which relax the lower esophageal sphincter—and tomatoes and citrus fruits or juices, which contribute additional acid that can irritate the esophagus.
- Give up smoking, which also relaxes the lower esophageal sphincter.
- Wear loose belts and clothing.

Aside from these steps, over-the-counter antacids such as Tums, Rolaids, Maalox, Zantac, Tagamet, Pepcid, and Axid can often relieve GERD symptoms. However, if after two weeks these medications do not help with your symptoms, your doctor may need to prescribe medications that block or limit the amount of stomach acid your body produces. Under rare circumstances, GERD may only be treatable through surgery.

Chapter 25

Influenza Information for People with Asthma

Key Facts about Influenza

What is influenza?

Influenza, also called flu, is a contagious respiratory illness caused by influenza viruses. It can cause mild to severe illness, and at times can lead to death. The best way to prevent this illness is by getting a flu vaccination each fall.

Every year in the United States, on average:

- 5% to 20% of the population gets the flu;
- more than 200,000 people are hospitalized from flu complications, and;
- about 36,000 people die from flu.

Some people, such as older people, young children, and people with certain health conditions, are at high risk for serious flu complications.

Symptoms of flu include the following:

- fever (usually high)
- headache

This chapter includes excerpts from the following documents produced by the Centers for Disease Control and Prevention (CDC): "Key Facts about Influenza and the Influenza Vaccine," August 8, 2005; "Key Facts about Flu Vaccine," August 12, 2005; and "Asthma and Flu Shots," February 2005.

- extreme tiredness
- dry cough
- sore throat
- runny or stuffy nose
- muscle aches

Stomach symptoms, such as nausea, vomiting, and diarrhea, also can occur but are more common in children than adults.

Complications of flu can include bacterial pneumonia, dehydration, and worsening of chronic medical conditions, such as congestive heart failure, asthma, or diabetes. Children may get sinus problems and ear infections.

How does the flu spread?

Flu viruses spread in respiratory droplets caused by coughing and sneezing. They usually spread from person to person, though sometimes people become infected by touching something with flu viruses on it and then touching their mouth or nose. Most healthy adults may be able to infect others beginning one day before symptoms develop and up to five days after becoming sick. That means that you can pass on the flu to someone else before you know you are sick, as well as while you are sick. The single best way to prevent the flu is to get a flu vaccination each fall.

Key Facts about Flu Vaccine

There are two types of vaccines:

- The "flu shot": an inactivated vaccine (containing killed virus) that is given with a needle, usually in the arm. The flu shot is approved for use in people older than 6 months, including healthy people and people with chronic medical conditions.
- The nasal-spray flu vaccine: a vaccine made with live, weakened flu viruses that do not cause the flu (sometimes called LAIV for "Live Attenuated Influenza Vaccine"). LAIV is approved for use in healthy people 5 years to 49 years of age who are not pregnant.

Each vaccine contains three influenza viruses—one A (H3N2) virus, one A (H1N1) virus, and one B virus. The viruses in the vaccine change each year based on international surveillance and scientists'

Influenza Information for People with Asthma

predictions about which types and strains of viruses will circulate in a given year.

About 2 weeks after vaccination, antibodies that provide protection against influenza virus infection develop in the body.

When is the best time to get vaccinated?

October or November is the best time to get vaccinated, but you can still get vaccinated in December and later. Flu season can begin as early as October and last as late as May.

Who should get vaccinated?

In general, anyone who wants to reduce their chances of getting the flu can get vaccinated. However, certain people should get vaccinated each year. They are either people who are at high risk of having serious flu complications or people who live with or care for those at high risk for serious complications.

People at high risk for complications from the flu should get vaccinated each year:

- people 65 years and older
- people who live in nursing homes and other long-term care facilities that house those with long-term illnesses
- adults and children 6 months and older with chronic heart or lung conditions, including asthma
- adults and children 6 months and older who needed regular medical care or were in a hospital during the previous year because of a metabolic disease (like diabetes), chronic kidney disease, or weakened immune system (including immune system problems caused by medicines or by infection with human immunodeficiency virus [HIV/AIDS])
- children 6 months to 18 years of age who are on long-term aspirin therapy (Children given aspirin while they have influenza are at risk of Reye syndrome.)
- women who will be pregnant during the influenza season
- all children 6 to 23 months of age
- people with any condition that can compromise respiratory function or the handling of respiratory secretions (that is, a condition

that makes it hard to breathe or swallow, such as brain injury or disease, spinal cord injuries, seizure disorders, or other nerve or muscle disorders)

In addition, people 50 to 64 years of age should get vaccinated each year. Nearly one-third of people 50 to 64 years of age in the United States have one or more medical conditions that place them at increased risk for serious flu complications.

People who can transmit flu to others at high risk for complications should also get vaccinated each year. Any person in close contact with someone in a high-risk group should get vaccinated. This includes all health-care workers, caregivers of children 0 to 23 months of age, and close contacts of people 65 years and older.

Who should not be vaccinated?

There are some people who should not be vaccinated:

- people who have a severe allergy to chicken eggs
- people who have had a severe reaction to an influenza vaccination in the past
- people who developed Guillain-Barré syndrome (GBS) within 6 weeks of getting an influenza vaccine previously
- children less than 6 months of age
- people who are sick with a fever (These people can get vaccinated once their symptoms lessen.)

Is the flu vaccine effective?

The ability of flu vaccine to protect a person depends on the age and health status of the person getting the vaccine, and the similarity or "match" between the virus strains in the vaccine and those in circulation. Testing has shown that both the flu shot and the nasal-spray vaccine are effective at preventing the flu.

Does the flu vaccine have any side effects?

Different side effects can be associated with the flu shot and LAIV.

The flu shot: The viruses in the flu shot are killed (inactivated), so you cannot get the flu from a flu shot. Some minor side effects that could occur are:

Influenza Information for People with Asthma

- soreness, redness, or swelling where the shot was given;
- fever (low grade);
- aches.

If these problems occur, they begin soon after the shot and usually last one to two days. Almost all people who receive influenza vaccine have no serious problems from it. However, on rare occasions, flu vaccination can cause serious problems, such as severe allergic reactions. As of July 1, 2005, people who think that they have been injured by the flu shot can file a claim for compensation from the National Vaccine Injury Compensation Program (VICP). For more information go to http://www.hrsa.gov/osp/vicp.

LAIV: The viruses in the nasal-spray vaccine are weakened and will not cause severe symptoms often associated with influenza illness. (In clinical studies, transmission of vaccine viruses to close contacts has occurred only rarely.)

In children, side effects can include the following:

- runny nose
- headache
- vomiting
- muscle aches
- fever

In adults, these side effects can occur:

- runny nose
- headache
- sore throat
- cough

Asthma and Flu Shots

Adults with asthma are at high risk of developing complications after contracting the influenza virus, yet most adults with asthma do not receive an annual flu vaccination. Only one-third of all asthmatic adults and one-fifth of asthmatic adults younger than 50 years of age receive the flu vaccine annually, according to a study by the Centers for Disease Control and Prevention (CDC) that was published in the

September 2003 issue of *Chest* (the journal of the American College of Chest Physicians).

Respiratory infections like influenza are more serious in patients with asthma, and such infections can often lead to pneumonia and acute respiratory disease.

CDC researchers used data from the National Health Interview Survey, 1999 to 2001, to examine the prevalence of flu vaccinations among people who have asthma. The following percentage of survey respondents with asthma reported that they received the flu vaccine: 35.1% (1999), 36.7% (2000), and 33.3% (2001).

As study respondents with asthma aged, the number who were vaccinated increased, as indicated below:

- 18 to 49 years of age: 20.9% (1999), 22.7% (2000), and 21.1% (2001)

- 50 to 64 years of age: 46.2% (1999), 47.8% (2000), and 42.3% (2001)

- 65 years of age and older: 72.8% (1999), 71.2% (2000), and 64.8% (2001)

According to the survey, vaccination rates increased among those respondents with higher education. Sex and ethnicity also affected vaccination rates. Of those respondents interviewed in 2000, fewer men than women and fewer African Americans than whites reported having been vaccinated. In 2001, fewer Hispanics than whites reported having been vaccinated.

Annual flu vaccination rates among people with asthma need to be increased. The flu vaccine is safe and effective. All people who have asthma should be encouraged to get the flu vaccination as part of their routine care.

Chapter 26

Asthma and Bone Health

Asthma is a chronic lung disease. Typical asthma symptoms include coughing, wheezing, tightness in the chest, difficulty breathing, a rapid heart rate, and sweating. Children with asthma often complain of an itchy upper chest or develop a dry cough, which may be the only sign of an asthma.

Asthma itself, does not pose a threat to bone health. However, certain medications used to treat the disease, and some behaviors triggered by concern over the disease can have a negative impact on the skeleton. This chapter discusses approaches for optimizing bone health for people with asthma.

The Asthma-Osteoporosis Connection

People with asthma tend to be at increased risk for osteoporosis, especially in the spine, for several reasons. First, anti-inflammatory medications, known as corticosteroids, are commonly prescribed for asthma. Taken by mouth, these medications can decrease calcium absorbed from food, increase calcium loss from the kidneys, and decrease bone formation. Corticosteroids also interfere with the production of sex hormones in both women and men, which can contribute to bone loss, and they can cause muscle weakness, which can increase the risk of falling.

A fact sheet produced by the National Institutes of Health Osteoporosis and Related Bone Diseases~National Resource Center (www.osteo.org), September 2002.

Many asthma sufferers think that milk and dairy products trigger asthmatic attacks, although there is little evidence to support this belief unless the person has a dairy allergy. Unfortunately, this often results in an unnecessary avoidance of dairy products and is especially damaging for asthmatic children who need calcium to build bone.

Since exercise often can trigger an asthma attack, many people with asthma avoid weight-bearing physical activities that are known to strengthen bone. Those asthmatics who remain physically active often choose swimming as their first exercise of choice because it is the least likely activity to trigger an asthmatic attack. Unfortunately, swimming does not have the same beneficial impact on bone health as weight-bearing exercises that work the body against gravity, such as walking, jogging, racquet sports, basketball, volleyball, aerobics, dancing, or weight-training.

Medications for Asthma

Because of their effectiveness in controlling asthma with the fewest side effects, inhaled corticosteroid medication is preferred to oral forms for asthma. Oral corticosteroids, which can cause significant bone loss over time, may be necessary for some asthmatics. Asthma patients who are treated with 40 to 60 mg per day of oral corticosteroids for long periods of time are most likely to experience bone loss. Even those patients who take 10 mg per day are likely to experience some bone loss over time.

Strategies to Optimize Bone Health

The following tips can help individuals with asthma to maximize their bone health.

Use medications prudently: Bone loss tends to increase with increased glucocorticoid doses and prolonged use. No matter which form of medication is used, the lowest possible dose for the shortest period of time that controls asthma symptoms is recommended. There are other medications available that also may relieve symptoms without causing bone loss, although for some people steroids are necessary.

Reduce exposure to triggers: Reducing exposure to those stimuli that appear to trigger asthma attacks lessens the patient's reliance on medication.

Avoid infection: Avoid people with colds and other respiratory infections whenever possible.

Minimize exposure to irritants: Avoid cigarette smoke, strong odors, air pollution, aerosol sprays, paint fumes, red wine, beer, food coloring, food dyes, sulfite food preservatives, and extreme changes in temperature. Pay attention to air quality notices on your local weather stations.

Reduce contact with allergens: Since asthma symptoms can be triggered by allergies, avoid known allergens, and when possible remove allergens from the home, school, or work environment. Common household allergens include animal dander, dust mites, pollen, molds, and dust.

Monitor nutrition: A balanced diet with adequate amounts of calcium and vitamin D is critical for bone health. People with asthma who have a proven milk allergy should explore non-dairy sources of calcium and consider calcium supplementation in order to obtain enough calcium. The National Institutes for Health (NIH) recommends 400 to 600 mg of elemental calcium for infants, 800 to 1200 mg for children ages one to ten, and 1200 to 1500 mg for adolescents and young adults ages 11–24. For both children and adults on chronic corticosteroid therapy, some health care providers routinely recommend a daily elemental calcium intake of between 1000 and 1500 mg. Experts also recommend a daily vitamin D intake of between 400 and 800 IU per day.

Exercise: Weight-bearing activity, such as walking, running, weight-training, and team sports can all have a positive impact on bone health and participation should be encouraged. By improving muscle strength and coordination, exercise also can reduce the risk for falling and breaking bones. People who experience exercise-induced asthma should exercise in an environmentally controlled facility and participate in activities that fall within their limitations. They may also use medication when necessary to enable them to exercise.

Stress reduction: If asthma is triggered by emotional stress, patients should consider participating in stress reduction programs.

Making the Osteoporosis Diagnosis

Asthmatics who must rely on corticosteroids to manage their asthma are at significant risk for bone loss and may benefit from a bone density test, which is the only accurate way to measure current bone mass, diagnose osteoporosis, and predict future fracture risk. This information can help determine if medication is needed to prevent or treat bone loss. Since corticosteroids may increase bone resorption, blood or urine biochemical marker tests can be used to determine if bone is being broken down rapidly.

Medications to Prevent and Treat Bone Loss

Several medications are available for the prevention and/or treatment of osteoporosis. These medications can help prevent bone loss and reduce the risk of fracture. Asthmatics, particularly those taking corticosteroids, are encouraged to ask their health care providers whether they might be a candidate for an osteoporosis medication.

Part Three

Asthma Management: Working with Your Doctor

Chapter 27

Finding a Doctor for Asthma Care

Finding a Good Doctor

Most people start looking for a general practitioner in the directory their health insurance company distributes. Call your local hospital to see if they have a physician reference service, check with a hospital nurse, or scan the yellow pages. And since personal experience offers the strongest recommendation, ask your neighbors, co-workers, family, and friends who they use and like.

Decide what qualities are most important to you: experience, reputation, good bedside manner, office hours/location, or insurance coverage, for example. While the doctor with the highest grade point average may be the best choice for some, a physician's manner is more important to others.

Because no two asthma or allergy cases are the same, look for a physician who will help you sort through all possible allergens, irritants, or conditions—such as sinusitis (infection of the sinuses), gastroesophageal reflux (heartburn or regurgitation), or food allergies—that may be causing your symptoms. Your doctor should then develop a treatment plan you can understand and use.

What is the doctor's treatment philosophy? If he or she plans to treat your asthma just in the most severe instances, he or she is only

---

This chapter includes the following documents: "Finding a Good Doctor," "What Is a Specialist?" and "Your Doctor's Credentials," reprinted courtesy of Allergy & Asthma Network Mothers of Asthmatics (AANMA), 800-878-4403, www.breatherville.org, © 2001.

doing 50 percent of the doctor's job. Choose an assertive physician, one who takes a preventive approach. Expect a customized written asthma management plan that includes early intervention measures to prevent asthma episodes and attacks from occurring in the first place.

Look for a physician who will really listen to you. You may have already met the ones that breeze in and out of the exam room without giving you a chance to ask even one question. As a patient, you have the right to voice your comments, concerns, and questions. Only you know how you feel physically—and mentally. Describe your symptoms so your doctor can properly treat your asthma or allergies. Remember, the doctor is there to help you; the doctor should respect you enough to stop and listen.

A physician should be willing to share knowledge of asthma and allergies with you instead of leaving you to follow instructions blindly. The doctor should explain what happens physically during an asthma or allergy attack, why the prescribed medications and treatment plan were selected, and when to seek emergency help. By reviewing some of the basic facts with you, your physician empowers you to handle your daily healthcare needs outside the office. If the doctor throws around lengthy medical terms without explanation and fails to clearly outline your treatment options, that doctor is not the doctor for you.

Does the physician encourage you to learn more about your asthma and allergies? Does he or she offer reading lists, books, videos, or support group contact information? The doctor should.

What Is a Specialist?

Specialists are physicians who have been trained to treat a specific area of the body such as the lungs, heart, brain, or teeth. For people with asthma, doctors like allergists, immunologists, and pulmonologists focus on what's triggering the asthma symptoms. If allergies are the main trigger, for example, an allergist will identify what you're allergic to and help you combat the allergy. He or she may suggest avoiding the allergen, using medications, or starting allergy shots.

But which specialist is right for you? What do all of these doctors with fancy names really do?

Allergist: An allergist is a medical doctor with extensive training in allergy and immunology problems, including asthma. If your symptoms are not responding to current treatment, your triggers seem to have an allergy component, or your asthma is worsening, it's time to see an allergist.

Immunologist: An immunologist specializes in the diseases and disorders of the immune system. Since the two disciplines are closely interrelated, many doctors who specialize in allergy also specialize in immunology.

Pulmonologist: A pulmonologist focuses on diseases and congenital or structural disorders of the lungs and airways, including bronchopulmonary dysplasia (a chronic lung disease that develops in premature infants who have had extensive respiratory treatment), cystic fibrosis (a chronic lung infection), chronic obstructive pulmonary disease (a disease that causes a decrease in lung function), recurrent pneumonia, and asthma.

Otolaryngologist (OTO)/Head and Neck Surgeon: Once known as an ear, nose, and throat doctor (ENT), an OTO focuses on head and neck problems and surgery for the brain, eyes, nose, sinuses, teeth, neck, and spine. You may be referred to this doctor for evaluation, treatment, or surgery for problems associated with rhinitis (inflammation of the nasal passages), sinusitis, or hearing.

Gastroenterologist: A gastroenterologist specializes in diseases and disorders of the stomach and intestines. If your general practitioner suspects that gastroesophageal reflux or undiagnosed, persistent stomach pain is triggering your asthma, you should see a gastroenterologist.

Orthodontist: An orthodontist corrects abnormally aligned or positioned teeth. Visit an orthodontist if problems associated with allergies or nasal obstructions are affecting your facial development or jawbone structure.

Your Doctor's Credentials

Although most physicians are well trained, it never hurts to do some research before visiting a new doctor. Make sure the doctor trained at a reputable institution and has a current medical license.

After a doctor finishes medical school and his or her residency program, he or she must pass a state exam. A state board of medical examiners then licenses him or her to practice general medicine in that state. Without a medical license, a doctor is not legally allowed to treat patients.

Your state medical board can tell you if a doctor in your state has a valid medical license. Contact the Federation of State Medical Boards at 817-868-4000 or www.fsmb.org to locate the medical board in your state. On the Allergy and Asthma Network Mothers of Asthmatics website (www.aanma.org), you can also find out if a physician has had malpractice suits or complaints and whether he has ever practiced in another state. Most health insurance companies also offer this information if they have lists of participating physicians.

When you're selecting a specialist, look for one who is board certified. This certification is not a legal requirement for practicing medicine, but board-certified specialists are more committed to a specific area of medicine and are often more knowledgeable.

The American Board of Medical Specialties (ABMS) oversees 24 approved medical specialty boards in the United States that certify doctors. The American Board of Allergy and Immunology, for example, certifies doctors specializing in allergy and immunology, while the American Board of Otolaryngology certifies doctors specializing in otolaryngology/head and neck surgery.

Board-certified physicians must successfully complete an approved educational program and evaluation process and pass an exam that assesses knowledge, skills, and experience in their chosen area of expertise such as allergy, dermatology, or pediatrics. The certification is valid nationwide—not just in the state where the doctor practices.

Checking to see if your physician is board certified is easy. The ABMS offers a doctor verification service at www.abms.org or via its toll-free hotline at 866-ASK-ABMS. ABMS also annually publishes *The Official American Board of Medical Specialties Directory of Board Certified Medical Specialists*, which is available in most medical and public libraries. ABMS website offers contact information for each of the 24 medical specialty boards; they can provide written verification of a doctor's certification.

Chapter 28

You and Your Asthma Doctor: Roles, Rights, and Responsibilities

Asthma: You and Your Doctor

The Doctor's Role in Asthma Care

The doctor's role in asthma care begins with your diagnosis. Once a doctor decides that you have asthma, then you and the doctor can work together to control it.

During the diagnosis, a doctor will take your medical history, give you a physical checkup and do some lab tests. These tests may include a chest x-ray, blood and allergy tests, and lung function tests, such as spirometry. In spirometry, you blow into a device called a spirometer, which measures the air you breathe in and out of your lungs.

Once the doctor decides that you do, indeed, have asthma, then medical treatment can start. This means that the doctor chooses the best asthma medicines at the right doses for you.

The doctor, too, may recommend that you start using a peak flow meter at home. Ask your doctor about this.

In peak flow monitoring, you blow into a device, called a peak flow meter, which measures the greatest amount of air that you can exhale.

This chapter begins with "Asthma: You and Your Doctor," reprinted with permission © 2005 American Lung Association. For more information about the American Lung Association or to support the work it does, call 1-800-LUNG-USA (1-800-586-4872) or log on to www.lungusa.org. "Rights and Responsibilities of Patients with Asthma," by Miles Weinberger, M.D. is from *Managing Asthma for Patients and Families*, September 2004. This copyright protected material is used with permission of the author and the University of Iowa's Virtual Hospital, www.vh.org.

Peak flow meters are easy to use by yourself every day. These devices can help you to know if your breathing problems are starting even when you don't feel any asthma symptoms. That way, you know when to take your asthma medicine before your symptoms get worse.

After you start taking your asthma medicines, you need to see a doctor on a regular basis, not just when you're having problems. That way the doctor can make certain your medicines are working well.

The doctor needs to know if:

- you have breathing problems at night and you do not get a good night's sleep.
- your asthma makes it hard for you to do things during the day.
- you take more medicine than the doctor has prescribed. This is a danger sign. It means that something is not working right with your treatment.

There is no need for you to suffer. Once you talk with a doctor, you may find that a change in your asthma medicines is all that is needed to help you feel better.

So talk regularly to a doctor about your asthma. There are many things that can start asthma and asthma can change, sometimes getting better or worse.

You may find that your medicines need to be changed. Or, new medicines may be available that will work even better for you.

Your Role in Asthma Care

There are three things that you need to do to control your asthma:

- **First:** See a doctor or other primary care health provider regularly about your asthma. This is important because your symptoms can change over time. Your triggers can change, too. You may need different medicines to help keep you healthy. So regular contact with a doctor or other primary care health provider is an important part of controlling your asthma.
- **Second:** Take your asthma medicines as the doctor has prescribed, even when you feel well. That way, you keep breathing problems from happening.
- **Third:** Get educated about asthma. Find out what triggers it and what you must do to stay healthy. In fact, everyone in your family should know about asthma and know what to do when you need help.

You and Your Asthma Doctor: Roles, Rights, and Responsibilities

Start taking control of asthma:

- Learn your triggers and symptoms and what to do about them.
- Learn what to do for asthma attacks.
- Learn about your medicines so you know how quickly they should work.

Rights and Responsibilities of Patients with Asthma

The management of asthma is most successful when the patient and/or family assumes an active role. To begin to do this, the patient (and/or family) must be effectively assertive in both accessing the medical care system and assuming responsibility for the day-to-day management of the disease. There are reasonable expectations that patients and their families should have of their medical care providers, and they must also accept responsibilities for the actual administration of the care.

The Asthmatic's Bill of Rights

Asthma is the most frequent chronic disease in childhood and remains common throughout life. It is the leading cause of hospitalization in children, a frequent cause in adults, and an exceedingly frequent cause of emergency medical care at all ages. Asthma has been known to the medical profession for over 2,000 years. The number of medications effective for asthma has increased considerably since the 1970s, and the sales of those medications have been progressively increasing. There is a major disparity, however, in the effectiveness with which therapeutic measures have been applied. Well-intentioned but misguided practices, occasional indifference, and medical attention focused on the immediate problem, rather than a comprehensive approach, cause frustrations for patients and their families. State-of-the-art care usually results in a high degree of successful control of asthma with acceptably safe and reasonably convenient therapy. Patients should therefore not settle for less. They should insist on these things:

- the right to immediate care when needed for respiratory distress
- the right to intensive treatment until respiratory distress is relieved
- the right to measures that prevent the need for future emergency care
- the right to accurate scientific medical knowledge about asthma

- the right to a comprehensive evaluation to assure the diagnosis, characterize the pattern of symptoms, assess the severity, and identify the triggers of asthma
- the right to an organized rational therapeutic plan and instruction to implement that plan
- the right to medication that can safely, rapidly, and effectively relieve symptoms
- the right to measures that can prevent frequent return of troublesome symptoms without side effects of treatment
- the right to be able to take part in the same activities as non-asthmatics, including competitive athletics
- the right to a knowledgeable physician with interest and expertise in managing asthma

The Responsibilities of the Patient and/or Family

Asthma is a recurring or chronic problem. Treatment is best when applied by a patient or parent who understands the disease and its treatment. It is the physician's responsibility to determine the safest effective treatment and teach the patient how to apply that treatment. The patient has the following responsibilities:

- understand what asthma is and what it does
- know the names of the medications, both the generic name and brand name. (Please don't identify medications just by color. Colors for the same medication can vary with the manufacturer. All of the medications have names and should be clearly labeled. And besides, doctors often don't know what color they are.)
- know what each medication does for asthma
- know when each medication should be taken
- know possible side effects of each medication
- keep regularly scheduled appointments
- keep their asthma controlled
- know when to call the doctor for advice
- maintain a healthy active life-style if there are no other limiting medical problems
- discuss concerns regarding the asthma or its treatment with their physician

Chapter 29

Use of Asthma Diaries

An asthma diary can provide your physician with invaluable firsthand information regarding your asthma. As you well know, symptoms of asthma fluctuate and may not be present at all when you see your doctor. Your physician, however, must make decisions regarding the medical indications for adding, continuing, or withdrawing medication. The diary provides information that is more accurate than trying to remember what happened over weeks or months when you are seen for a scheduled medical appointment. This, in turn, results in better medical decisions.

A sample diary that can be copied, printed, and used is illustrated in Figure 29.1.

The question regarding asthmatic symptoms "last night" should be completed upon awakening in the morning. The second question line asks for a "morning peak flow" measurement. Not all patients are asked to keep track of peak flow measurements. The subsequent questions are completed at bedtime and ask about symptoms during the day. Keeping the diary and a pencil beside the bed and completing it at bedtime and on arising is probably the easiest way of not forgetting. Always bring the diary with you to appointments with your physician.

From "Managing Asthma for Patients and Families," by Miles Weinberger, MD, September 2004. This copyright protected material is used with permission of the author and the University of Iowa's Virtual Hospital, www.vh.org.

Asthma Diary for _____

Complete diary by checking the correct box or filling in the requested value

Month_____ Dates ___ – ___		Sn	M	Tu	W	Th	F	St
Last night	Good night							
	Slept well but some wheeze or cough							
	Awake briefly with wheeze or cough							
	Bad night, awake repeatedly							
Morning Peak Flow	(best of 3 efforts)							
Activity	Vigorous activity OK							
	Can run only briefly							
	OK for walking only							
	Must rest at home							
Wheeze	None							
	Briefly, not troublesome							
	Several times							
	Continuous							
Cough	None							
	Present but not troublesome							
	Interrupted activities once							
	Interrupted activities more than once							
Evening Peak Flow	(best of 3 efforts)							
Intervention	Inhaled bronchodilators (number of treatments)							
	Oral corticosteroid (dose)							

Figure 29.1. *A Sample Asthma Diary*

Interpreting the Allergy Evaluation

Asthma is not caused primarily by allergy. Neither are nasal symptoms necessarily caused by allergy. There first has to be a predisposition or sensitivity of the nose or lungs. However, inhaled allergens often aggravate the bronchospasm and airway inflammation of asthma and the stuffiness, congestion, and drainage from the nose. Allergens include such substances as pollens, mold spores, animal danders, substances in dusts (dust mite fomite), and sometimes specific types of exposures in the workplace. Allergens cause symptoms when they react with specific types of antibodies (of the IgE immunoglobulin class) that reside in the mucous membranes of the respiratory tract. This reaction results in the release of substances that cause constriction of muscle around the airway (bronchospasm) and inflammation of the mucous membrane of the airways which causes swelling of the tissues lining the airways and secretion of mucous into the airway. In the nose, this can result in sneezing, itchy nose, and runny nose. In the lungs, this results in tightness of the chest, coughing, wheezing, and labored breathing. It is important in managing asthma to identify the extent to which allergic factors contribute to the disease. And if allergic factors do contribute substantially to the disease, it is important to identify the specific allergic substances.

The evaluation for allergy involves a careful history of the environment and its relationship to your symptoms. Allergy testing identifies the type of antibody that causes allergic reactions in the airways. Both components of this evaluation are important in making clinical judgments regarding the importance of allergy in causing symptoms and in identifying what environmental factors, if any, may be causing problems with the nose or lungs.

There are two types of tests used to identify antibodies that cause allergic respiratory reaction. Allergy skin testing is most common. This involves exposing the tissues immediately below the outer surface of the skin to an extract of allergen (pollen, animal dander, dust mite, etc.) either by a superficial puncture, prick, or scratch or by injection of material just under the skin with a small needle. The size of local swelling and redness is then measured in 15 minutes. There are also blood tests for measuring the same type of antibody in a laboratory test. The blood tests are usually less sensitive, are no more accurate, and are usually more expensive than skin testing. They may be useful, however, when there is difficulty in interpreting skin tests.

The presence of positive skin tests or laboratory tests for the allergic antibodies do not, by themselves, indicate that usual natural exposure to those allergens will cause an allergic reaction. This depends on the degree of sensitivity of the airways, the degree of exposure, and perhaps other variables that we do not fully understand. The presence of the antibodies only indicates the potential for exposure to cause symptoms. The final decision as to whether exposure actually does cause symptoms is a clinical judgment based on evidence accumulated from the history and the allergy testing combined.

Not all environmental factors that aggravate respiratory problems are allergic. Cigarette smoking, whether by the patient or those around the patient, can cause respiratory symptoms through a direct irritant effect. Similar irritation may occur from open fires, such as those in fireplaces and wood stoves. Strong odors and chemical irritants may also trigger the sensitive airways of the asthmatic patient. Skin testing will not be useful in identifying the potential for these irritant substances to cause symptoms.

Chapter 30

Developing an Asthma Action Plan

During the mid-1980s, Sandra Fusco-Walker's life was filled with sleepless nights, ruined vacations, emergency room visits, and her children's frequent school absences. Two of her three children—all under age 6 at the time—had asthma.

"I was always worried about when the next bad thing would happen," says the Kinnelon, New Jersey, resident. "But that was before we had a plan."

The "plan" was an asthma action plan that guided her on how to track her children's symptoms, monitor their breathing, and give them medication. "A plan tells you what to do and when," she says. "Without it, asthma is out of control, and that's when the disease wreaks havoc on your life."

Asthma causes the airways to be inflamed or swollen, and the surrounding muscles are tight. When people with asthma react to various triggers—such as dust, pollen, or smoke—their airways become narrow, which causes labored breathing, wheezing, chest tightness, or coughing. About 15 million people in the United States have asthma and almost 5 million are children, according to the National Heart, Lung, and Blood Institute (NHLBI). Every year, asthma causes roughly 2

This chapter begins with excerpts from "Breathing Better: Action Plans Keep Asthma in Check," by Michelle Meadows, *FDA Consumer Magazine*, U.S. Food and Drug Administration (FDA), March–April 2003, updated in May 2004. "Make an Asthma Action Plan" is excerpted from "Help Your Child Gain Control Over Asthma," U.S. Environmental Protection Agency (EPA), November 2004.

million emergency room visits, up to 500,000 hospitalizations, and 4,500 deaths.

Fusco-Walker says she learned to control asthma after she followed her doctor's advice and called a nonprofit organization called Allergy and Asthma Network Mothers of Asthmatics (AANMA). The woman who answered the phone was Nancy Sander, who founded the organization in 1985 after facing challenges in dealing with her own daughter's asthma. Fusco-Walker says, "Nancy assured me that I wasn't going crazy."

With support and advice from AANMA, Fusco-Walker learned to look for patterns in her children's illness. For example, her kids got sick every time they visited her mother, and her mother smoked. Her oldest daughter had an asthma attack when she visited their horse barn. Fusco-Walker also learned to spot early warning signs of trouble. "I noticed that one of my daughters rubbed her nose when breathing became difficult," she says. "If I saw her rubbing her nose, I knew to get the peak flow meter." A peak flow meter is a small tool that measures how fast air moves out of the airways. Fusco-Walker attributes the success of her asthma action plan to the regular use of a peak flow meter.

By the time Fusco-Walker's youngest child was diagnosed with asthma at age 5, her family had a much better understanding of the disease. Shannon, who is now 16, Jared, 19, and Morgan, 21, grew up learning how to use their asthma medicine. "They know when to use their inhalers, they know when they need refills, and they know when they need to take medication before doing an activity," she says. They also grew up participating in just about any activity they wanted to, including football, swimming, soccer, and snowboarding.

Experts say most people with asthma can live a normal, active life. What it takes is avoiding the triggers that make your asthma worse, keeping track of your symptoms, and sticking to an effective treatment regimen. Many people with asthma need short-term medicine for when they experience symptoms, and also long-term daily medicine that reduces inflammation in the airways and helps prevent asthma attacks.

"I'll hear people say they skipped their medication because they haven't been coughing that much," says Richard L. Wasserman, M.D., Ph.D., clinical associate professor of pediatrics at the University of Texas Southwestern Medical School. "But I tell them they probably wouldn't have coughed at all if they kept to the regimen." He says it's important to understand that asthma is a chronic inflammatory lung disease. "Like high blood pressure, asthma is there all the time even when there are no symptoms."

Asthma Action Plan For ______________ Doctor's Name ______________ Date ________

Doctor's Phone Number ______________ Hospital/Emergency Room Phone Number ______________

GREEN ZONE: Doing Well
- No cough, wheeze, chest tightness, or shortness of breath during the day or night
- Can do usual activities

And, if a peak flow meter is used,
Peak flow: more than ______________
(80% or more of my best peak flow)

My best peak flow is ______________

Take These Long-Term-Control Medicines Each Day (include an anti-inflammatory)

Medicine	How much to take	When to take it

Before exercise ☐ ______________ ☐ 2 or ☐ 4 puffs 5 to 60 minutes before exercise

YELLOW ZONE: Asthma Is Getting Worse
- Cough, wheeze, chest tightness, or shortness of breath, or
- Waking at night due to asthma, or
- Can do some, but not all, usual activities

- Or -

Peak Flow: ________ to ________
(50% - 80% of my best peak flow)

FIRST **Add: Quick-Relief Medicine – and keep taking your GREEN ZONE medicine**

______________ ☐ 2 or ☐ 4 puffs, every 20 minutes for up to 1 hour
(short-acting beta$_2$-agonist) ☐ Nebulizer, once

SECOND **If your symptoms (and peak flow, if used) *return to GREEN ZONE* after 1 hour of above treatment:**
☐ Take the quick-relief medicine every 4 hours for 1 to 2 days.
☐ Double the dose of your inhaled steroid for ______________ (7-10) days.
- Or -
If your symptoms (and peak flow, if used) *do not return to GREEN ZONE* after 1 hour of above treatment:
☐ Take: ______________ ☐ 2 or ☐ 4 puffs or ☐ Nebulizer
(short-acting beta$_2$-agonist)
☐ Add: ______________ ________ mg. per day For ______ (3-10) days
(oral steroid)
☐ Call the doctor ☐ before/ ☐ within ________ hours after taking the oral steroid.

RED ZONE: Medical Alert!
- Very short of breath, or
- Quick-relief medicines have not helped, or
- Cannot do usual activities, or
- Symptoms are same or get worse after 24 hours in Yellow Zone

- Or -
Peak flow: less than ________
(50% of my best peak flow)

Take this medicine:
☐ ______________ ☐ 4 or ☐ 6 puffs or ☐ Nebulizer
(short-acting beta$_2$-agonist)
☐ ______________ ________ mg.
(oral steroid)

Then call your doctor *NOW*. Go to the hospital or call for an ambulance if:
- You are still in the red zone after 15 minutes AND
- You have not reached your doctor.

DANGER SIGNS
- Trouble walking and talking due to shortness of breath
- Lips or fingernails are blue

- **Take ☐ 4 or ☐ puffs of your quick-relief medicine *AND***
- **Go to the hospital or call for an ambulance (______________) NOW!**

Figure 30.1. *Sample Asthma Action Plan.*

National Asthma Education and Prevention Program; National Heart, Lung, and Blood Institute; NIH Publication No. 97-4053

Make an Asthma Action Plan

The action plan looks at what triggers or brings on your child's asthma. The plan also includes your child's daily medicine needs. And the plan lists rescue medicines for quick-relief during an attack or when asthma signs start. Work with your child's doctor and come up with a written action plan for managing your child's asthma.

- Share the asthma action plan with your child's school, teachers, babysitters, and family members.
- Talk it over with people in your child's life. In case of an asthma attack they will know what to do.

While asthma action plans may differ from doctor to doctor, most plans will address two areas: a daily program and a rescue program.

Follow the action plan. It can help lower the number of asthma attacks. Talk to your child's doctor if you need to make changes in the plan.

The action plan's daily program may list items such as the following:

- your child's asthma triggers
- daily medicines and how to use them
- peak flow meter chart

The action plan's rescue program may list items such as these:

- your child's warning signs
- your child's peak flow meter readings
- names of the rescue medicines used to treat asthma as an asthma attack gets worse
- steps to take if your child has an asthma attack and when to call the doctor
- emergency numbers and when to take your child to the emergency room

Make sure you know the right amount of medicine your child needs to take each day. Talk to your child's doctor if you have questions.

Does your child use an inhaler, a spacer or a peak flow meter? Ask the doctor to show you how to use these at home. Have your child practice a few times in front of the doctor.

Chapter 31

Using a Peak Flow Meter to Monitor Asthma

What is a peak flow meter?

A peak flow meter is a portable, inexpensive, hand-held device used to measure how air flows from your lungs in one "fast blast." In other words, the meter measures your ability to push air out of your lungs.

Peak flow meters may be provided in two ranges to measure the air pushed out of your lungs. A low range peak flow meter is for small children, and a standard range meter is for older children, teenagers, and adults. An adult has much larger airways than a child and needs the larger range.

There are several types of peak flow meters available. Talk to your doctor or pharmacist about which type to use.

Who can benefit from using a peak flow meter?

Many doctors believe that people who have asthma can benefit from the use of a peak flow meter. If you need to adjust your daily medication for asthma, a peak flow meter can be an important part of your asthma management plan.

Children as young as three years have been able to use a meter to help manage their asthma. In addition, some people with chronic bronchitis and emphysema may also benefit from the use of a peak flow meter.

"Peak Flow Meters," reprinted with permission © 2005 American Lung Association. For more information about the American Lung Association or to support the work it does, call 1-800-LUNG-USA (1-800-586-4872) or log on to www.lungusa.org.

Not all physicians use peak flow meters in their management of children and adults with asthma. Many doctors believe a peak flow meter may be of most help for people with moderate and severe asthma. If your asthma is mild or you do not use daily medication, a peak flow meter may not be useful for asthma management.

Who should I measure my peak flow rate?

Measurements with a peak flow meter can help you and your doctor monitor your asthma. These measurements can be important and help your doctor prescribe medicines to keep your asthma in control.

A peak flow meter can show you that you may need to change the way you are using your medicines. For example, peak flow readings may help be a signal for you to implement the medication plan you and your doctor have developed for worsening asthma.

On the other hand, if you are doing well, then measuring your peak flow may be helpful as you and your doctor try to lower the level of your medicines.

A peak flow meter can help you when your asthma is getting worse. Asthma sometimes changes gradually. Your peak flow may show changes before you feel them. It can allow your doctor to adjust your treatment to prevent urgent calls to the doctor, emergency room visits, or hospitalizations.

A peak flow meter may help you and your doctor identify causes of your asthma at work, home, or play. It may help parents to determine what might be triggering their child's asthma.

A peak flow meter can also be used during an asthma episode. It can help you determine the severity of the episode; decide when to use your rescue medication; and decide when to seek emergency care.

Knowing your "personal" peak flow rate allows you to elevate your readings. Being at your "best" can provide reassurance and make you feel more self-confident.

How do you use a peak flow meter?

Step 1: Before each use, make sure the sliding marker or arrow on the peak flow meter is at the bottom of the numbered scale (zero or the lowest number on the scale).

Step 2: Stand up straight. Remove gum or any food from your mouth. Take a deep breath (as deep as you can). Put the mouthpiece of the peak flow meter into your mouth. Close your lips tightly around

Using a Peak Flow Meter to Monitor Asthma

Name: _____ Week Beginning (Date) _____

Peak Flow Zones: Green Zone _____ Yellow Zone _____ Red Zone _____

Prescribed Medications (include dose and frequency) _____

Peak Flow Recording Times: _____ A.M. _____ P.M.

Day	Sunday		Monday		Tuesday		Wednesday		Thursday		Friday		Saturday	
Time	AM	PM	AM	PM	AM	PM	AM	PM	AM	PM	AM	PM	AM	PM
6:00														
5:50														
5:00														
4:50														
4:00														
3:50														
3:00														
2:50														
2:00														
1:50														
1:00														

Your Peak Flow Rates (liters/minute)

Changes in Medicine														
Notes														

Figure 31.1. Sample Chart

the mouthpiece. Be sure to keep your tongue away from the mouthpiece. In one breath blow out as hard and as quickly as possible. Blow a "fast hard blast" rather than "slowly blowing" until you have emptied out nearly all of the air from your lungs.

Step 3: The force of the air coming out of your lungs causes the marker to move along the numbered scale. Note the number on a piece of paper.

Step 4: Repeat the entire routine three times. (You know you have done the routine correctly when the numbers from all three tries are very close together.)

Step 5: Record the highest of the three ratings. Do not calculate an average. This is very important.
You can't breathe out too much when using your peak flow meter, but you can breathe out too little. Record your highest reading.

Step 6: Measure your peak flow rate close to the same time each day. You and your doctor can determine the best times. One suggestion is to measure your Peak Flow Rate twice daily between 7 and 9 A.M. and between 6 and 8 P.M.
You may want to measure your peak flow rate before or after using your medicine. Some people measure peak flow both before and after taking medication. Try to do it the same way each time.

Step 7: Keep a chart of your Peak Flow Rates. Discuss the readings with your doctor.

How do I chart my peak flow rates?

Chart the HIGHEST of the three readings. The chart could include the date at the top of the page with A.M. and P.M. listed. The left margin could list a scale, starting with zero (0) liters per minute (L/min) at the bottom of the page and ending with 600 L/min at the top.
You could leave room at the bottom of the page for notes to describe how you are feeling or to list any other thoughts you may have.

What is a "normal" peak flow rate?

A "normal" peak flow rate is based on a person's age, height, sex, and race. A standardized "normal" may be obtained from a chart comparing the patient with a population without breathing problems.

Using a Peak Flow Meter to Monitor Asthma

A personal best normal may be obtained from measuring the patient's own peak flow rate. Therefore, it is important for you and your doctor to discuss what is considered "normal" for you.

Once you have learned your usual and expected peak flow rate, you will be able to better recognize changes or trends.

How can I determine a "normal" peak flow rate for me?

Three zones of measurement are commonly used to interpret peak flow rates. It is easy to relate the three zones to the traffic light colors: green, yellow, and red. In general, a normal peak flow rate can vary as much as 20 percent.

Be aware of the following general guidelines. Keep in mind that recognizing changes from "normal" is important. Your doctor may suggest other zones to follow.

- **Green Zone:** 80 to 100 percent of your usual or "normal" peak flow rate signals all clear. A reading in this zone means that your asthma is under reasonably good control. It would be advisable to continue your prescribed program of management.

- **Yellow Zone:** 50 to 80 percent of your usual or "normal" peak flow rate signals caution. It is a time for decisions. Your airways are narrowing and may require extra treatment. Your symptoms can get better or worse depending on what you do, or how and when you use your prescribed medication. You and your doctor should have a plan for yellow zone readings.

- **Red Zone:** Less than 50 percent of your usual or "normal" peak flow rate signals a medical alert. Immediate decisions and actions need to be taken. Severe airway narrowing may be occurring. Take your rescue medications right away. Contact your doctor now and follow the plan he has given you for red zone readings.

Some doctors may suggest zones with a smaller range such as 90 to 100 percent. Always follow your doctor's suggestions about your peak flow rate.

Management Plan Based on Peak Flow Readings: It is important to know your peak flow reading, but it is even more important to know what you will do based upon that reading. Work with your doctor to develop an asthma management plan that follows your green-yellow-red zone guidelines.

Record the peak flow readings that your doctor recommends for your green zone, yellow zone, and red zone. Then work out with your doctor what you plan to do when your peak flow falls in each of those zones.

When should I use my peak flow meter?

Use of the peak flow meter depends on a number of things. Its use should be discussed with your doctor.

If your asthma is well controlled and you know the "normal" rate for you, you may decide to measure your peak flow rate only when you sense that your asthma is getting worse. More severe asthma may require several measurements daily—or twice a day.

Don't forget that your peak flow meter needs care and cleaning. Dirt collected in the meter may make your peak flow measurements inaccurate. If you have a cold or other respiratory infection, germs or mucus may also collect in the meter.

Proper cleaning with mild detergent in hot water will keep your peak flow meter working accurately and may keep you healthier.

Does using a peak flow meter have any side effects?

A peak flow meter is not a medicine. It has no major side effects. Sometimes pushing the air out of your lungs in a "fast blast" may cause you to cough or wheeze.

Check with your doctor before you start using a peak flow meter.

Using the meter is as simple as taking a deep breath and blowing out a candle. If used properly, it can only help.

You must realize that measuring peak flow is only one step in a program to manage asthma. Its importance must not be exaggerated or over-interpreted.

Using a peak flow meter is not a substitute for regular medical care. Ask your doctor to help you understand your peak flow measurements.

Ideas to Review

Now you are aware of some of the techniques for using and caring for peak flow meters. You also know how meters may help manage asthma and other breathing problems.

Discuss the use of a peak flow meter with your doctor. Make measuring your peak flow rate a part of your personal asthma management program.

Chapter 32

What Makes Asthma Worse?

Airways of people with asthma are often chronically inflamed (swollen). Therefore, the airways are sensitive to things that make asthma worse. These, either singly or together, cause symptoms in people with asthma. Identifying and controlling or treating things that make asthma worse is essential to good asthma management.

Common Things that Make Asthma Worse

Things that make asthma worse include: irritants, allergens, infections, weather, exercise, emotions, gastroesophageal reflux, and hormonal changes. These vary from person to person.

Irritants and Asthma: Common airway irritants include smoke (for example, tobacco smoke, smoke from wood-burning or kerosene stoves, and fireplaces), aerosol sprays, strong odors (for example, perfumes, cologne, gasoline fumes), dust, and air pollution. These substances found in the environment can irritate sensitive airways. Cigarette smoke is a very serious asthma trigger—do not allow smoking in your home or car and always look for non-smoking sections in public areas.

Allergens and Asthma: A variety of allergens can make asthma symptoms worse. It is important to note that not all people with asthma

---

© Copyright 2005 National Jewish Medical and Research Center. All rights reserved. For additional information, visit http://asthma.nationaljewish.org/ or call 1-800-222 LUNG.

have allergies. Reliable and valid allergy tests are available and a board-certified allergist can guide you through this process. Common allergens include animal dander, saliva and urine from feathered or furry animals, dust mites (a major component of house dust in humid climates), cockroaches, indoor and outdoor molds, pollens, foods, and chemicals. If you are allergic to any of those substances, making changes in your environment to control or avoid contact with the allergen is very important. Ask your healthcare provider about environmental control.

Infections and Asthma: Infections can also make asthma worse. Common cold viruses, respiratory infections, sinusitis, and influenza frequently cause an increase of asthma symptoms. Your healthcare provider may recommend an annual flu vaccination.

Exercise and Asthma: Exercise or physical activity can make asthma worse; for some it may be the only cause of asthma symptoms. However, exercise is important for everyone and should not be avoided. For many people, using a pre-treatment medication 10–15 minutes before exercise allows them to exercise without experiencing asthma symptoms. Discuss pre-treatment before exercise with your healthcare provider.

Weather and Asthma: There is not one best weather climate for people with asthma. However, there are certain types of weather that may cause problems for some people with asthma in any climate. Some weather situations that may make asthma symptoms worse include: extremely hot or cold temperatures, windy conditions, and changes in the humidity or barometric pressure.

Emotions and Asthma: Emotions do not cause asthma, but they can make asthma worse. Strong feelings can lead to changes in breathing patterns. Times of "good" stress and "bad" stress can cause problems for people with asthma. However, it is important to express your emotions, and good asthma management can minimize the effect of stress.

Changes in Breathing Patterns and Asthma: Sneezing, laughing, holding your breath, or sleep disorders may cause changes in breathing patterns which may make asthma worse. It is not always possible or desirable to avoid these situations; however, good asthma management may minimize these effects.

Hormonal Changes and Asthma: Some women with asthma have increased symptoms at a particular time during their menstrual cycle, such as pre-menstruation, or during pregnancy. This worsening results from a change in the balance of hormones that is occurring at that time. Your healthcare provider may adjust asthma medications during that time to reduce your symptoms.

Gastroesophageal Reflux and Asthma: Gastroesophageal reflux, or GER, occurs when the acidic contents of the stomach flow back up into the esophagus. This stimulates a reflex that may cause asthma to worsen. Symptoms of heartburn and breathing difficulty at night can indicate GER. Your healthcare provider can discuss preventive measures to reduce these symptoms.

Summary

As you can see, there are a number of factors that can make asthma worse. It is helpful to think about your last asthma episode; did you experience any of the situations described in this information? Please discuss this information with your healthcare provider who can help you identify what makes your asthma worse and teach you ways to control or avoid exposure to them.

Chapter 33

Exercise and Sports: Guidelines for People with Asthma

Questions and Answers about Exercising with Asthma

Is exercise recommended for patients with allergies and asthma?

In general, a patient with allergies or asthma is usually able to exercise as much as desired, as long as a few precautions are followed. Exercise should not be done if the patient is sick or not feeling well. A person should never push beyond his or her capabilities.

An exercise program should begin carefully, and it is a good idea to discuss such a program with your physician before starting. Once a patient is feeling well, has discussed an exercise program with his or her doctor, and is ready to start, the following suggestions and precautions should be used.

Why is breathing through the nose important?

The nose and sinus (upper airway) should be as clear as possible when exercising, so that nasal breathing can take place. This is important because the nasal passages contain a natural filtering and

---

This chapter begins with "Questions and Answers about Exercising With Allergies and Asthma," © 2005 American College of Allergy, Asthma and Immunology. All rights reserved. Reprinted with permission. The chapter continues with "Activity Guidelines for Youths and Adults with Asthma," Alberta Clinical Practice Guideline, September 1999. Reprinted with permission. Reviewed by David A. Cooke, M.D., January 2006.

humidifying system. This system will help keep the air at proper temperature and humidity. In addition, this nasal filtering system will help to keep out pollutants, irritants, and allergens.

If a person breathes through the mouth, this filtering and humidifying system is bypassed. Mouth breathing can introduce irritants to the bronchial tubes and lungs and the exercise program will be less effective.

It may be necessary or helpful for the allergic patient to use a medication that will keep the nasal airways open, such as an antihistamine, decongestant, nasal cromolyn sodium, or a nasal steroid spray. (Check with your doctor, as many of these are prescription medications.) The asthmatic patient may need to use medication for the bronchial tubes if exercise causes symptoms of chest tightness, cough, wheezing, or shortness of breath. This can commonly occur in patients with asthma, chronic bronchitis, or chronic obstructive pulmonary disease.

In addition to immediate bronchial constriction and wheezing, exercise has recently been shown to cause delayed reactions several hours after the initial exercise has been performed. Some common delayed symptoms include chest tightness, cough, and shortness of breath.

How can I control my symptoms during exercise?

Patients can often prevent these symptoms by taking medication prior to exercising. The type of medication used depends on the frequency and duration of physical activity, how often exercising is done throughout the day, and the practicality of taking medication before exercise.

An inhaler, such as albuterol or cromolyn, taken 5–10 minutes before exercise, is one type of medication that can be used. Sometimes theophylline or other bronchodilator tablets are recommended before exercise. A physician should be consulted on the best medication to use before exercise.

After the medication decision has been made, the choice of the exercise activity and the location are very important. If you have allergies, vigorous exercising should obviously not be done near a field full of grasses and weeds. It may be more appropriate to exercise indoors at certain times of the year.

If exercise is done outdoors, it should be in areas where there are not large concentrations of allergens (pollens, dust, mold, etc.). If allergens cannot be avoided, certain preventative methods, such as

Exercise and Sports: Guidelines for People with Asthma

medication taken before exercise or wearing of a mask, may be indicated.

Exercising should also be avoided in areas where there are large amounts of chemical irritants. For example, jogging and other vigorous sports should not be done near a heavy traffic area where there is a large amount of exhaust from vehicles or near factories that emit large amounts of pollutants in the atmosphere. Indoor areas where there are noxious or irritating odors should also be avoided.

What form of exercise is best?

The allergic or asthmatic individual should consider what form of exercise would best meet their needs. Exercise that has stop-and-go activity tends to cause less bronchial constriction than an exercise using continuous motion.

Continuous running most commonly causes bronchial constriction and spasm to those with respiratory problems, while swimming poses the least amount of respiratory irritation.

Weather conditions should also be considered when exercising. Cold and dry or very dry weather can be quite irritating to the bronchial tubes.

What special precautions are advisable?

Special precautions should be taken by those individuals who have severe allergies to stinging insects (such as bee, wasp, yellow jacket, etc.). If exercising is done outdoors, injectable epinephrine must be kept on hand. Another person should also be nearby to assist in an emergency.

Individuals with bee-sting allergy should avoid wearing bright-colored clothing or strong perfumes or lotions that may attract stinging insects and increase the risk of being stung.

Areas where stinging insects tend to inhabit should always be avoided. These include flower beds and flowering fields, bodies of water, and areas near garbage.

The most care should be taken by individuals who develop hives, swelling, or anaphylaxis when exercising. (Anaphylaxis is the most severe form of an allergic reaction and can be life threatening.) Patients must carry injectable epinephrine with them, should never exercise alone, and should not exercise or jog in remote areas where medical help is not nearby. These individuals may also find it necessary to take antihistamines or other medication before they exercise.

All the above factors should be taken into consideration before an exercise program is begun or before any type of physical activity is planned. These suggestions and precautions are not meant to discourage exercise, but to help in choosing suitable activities, taking into account different medical conditions and circumstances. Remember, patients with bronchial asthma have even participated (and won medals) in the Olympics. Exercise programs can be quite vigorous and helpful if undertaken with care and a physician's guidance.

Activity Guidelines for Youth and Adults with Asthma

Why should I exercise?

Exercise makes you strong, flexible, and healthy. It gives you more energy and makes you feel better about yourself.

Can I exercise if I have asthma?

Yes. Exercise may even help your asthma.

Can I ever become an athlete?

Yes. Just like anyone else. You can be involved in any number of activities if you learn to manage your asthma. People with asthma have won many Olympic medals and broken world records. One year, 15% of the U.S.A. Olympic athletes had exercised induced asthma and they captured 41 medals.

How can I tell how bad my asthma is?

By how you feel, your symptoms, and by how much you use your asthma medications. You may also monitor your asthma using a diary and/or a peak flow meter. This device measures how much air you can blow out. You can measure the difference when you feel good and when you feel short of breath. Your doctor, pharmacist, or respiratory therapist can help you choose one and teach you how to use it.

Which drugs are not allowed in sport competitions ("banned drugs")?

Drugs that are thought to give athletes an unfair advantage in competition or that may harm the user are considered 'banned'. All inhaler medicines for asthma are okay except Berotec (Fenoterol). However,

Exercise and Sports: Guidelines for People with Asthma

athletes need to declare the use of inhaler medications before competing. Many pills, liquid medicines, or injections are banned, including some non-prescription medicines. Check with your team doctor or pharmacist before taking any medicine if you are in serious competition and eligible for drug testing.

How can I control my asthma during exercise?

Keeping your asthma under control is an important first step. (Under control means you do not need to use your reliever medications very often, you are sleeping well, and your asthma symptoms are minimal.) By getting in shape you may be able to tolerate exercise better. An adequate warm up and cool down are important to prevent the asthma from getting worse during and after exercise. Keeping well hydrated by taking in fluids also helps. Finally, some people may need to take medication before exercise.

How can I use medicine to prevent asthma problems when I exercise?

First, you should try to have your asthma under good control before exercising or competing. For some individuals, treatment with Ventolin, Intal or Tilade about 20 minutes before exercising helps to stop problems with asthma. If Ventolin makes your heart beat faster, you must wait until it slows down before commencing.

How do I take my pulse?

You can count your pulse for 15 seconds on the side of your neck (carotid artery) or on your wrist (radial artery). To find the pulse on your neck, locate the midpoint of your jaw bone (half way between your chin and ear), move down about 4 cm, and use your fingers (not thumb) to count the beats.

To find the pulse on your wrist, place your palm upward and move your fingers about 4 cm down the outside of your wrist from your thumb. For a one minute count, multiply your 15 second count by 4.

What else can I do to prevent an asthma attack?

Warm up for 15–20 minutes before exercising. It helps to prevent attacks by creating a "refractory period" and prevents injury to muscles and ligaments. A refractory period is a time of a few hours when there is less chance of an attack.

What is a warm up?

A warm up is a light exercise that makes your body ready for strenuous exercise. You should gradually increase the heart rate and loosen muscles by game-like activity and stretching exercises for 15–20 minutes. It is the same activity you are going to do, but at lower intensity.

Here are some examples of warm up exercises that can be altered to suit your chosen activity and your own needs. If you cough or wheeze, slow down and consider using your reliever medication to help you.

- **Ice Hockey:** Skate easily for 8–10 minutes, working the puck. Stretch all the muscles. Then skate faster, mixing sprints with light skating.
- **Baseball:** Walk around the field, increasing to a slow jog for 7–10 minutes. Stretch then alternate slow and fast jogging and start throwing the ball. After each turn at bat, jog slowly to your position and warm up by throwing the ball.
- **Soccer:** Walk around the field, increasing to a slow jog for 7–10 minutes. Stretch. Then slow jog with the ball, passing, and doing other skills. Lastly, mix sprints with slow jogging with and without the ball.
- **Volleyball and Basketball:** Walk around the court. Then jog for 7–10 minutes. Stretch. Then do jumping and ball drills until the game.
- **Racquet Sports:** Start with easy strokes, hitting the ball to your partner. After 7–10 minutes, stretch. Then increase power and speed until you equal game conditions.
- **Running, Cycling and Swimming:** Go slow to start. After 7–10 minutes, stretch. Then return to your activity, gradually increasing the speed.
- **Gymnastics:** Walk around the mats and apparatus, increasing to a slow jog for 7–10 minutes. Stretch. Then do easy exercises on each apparatus increasing the intensity slowly.

How do I stretch properly?

Start to stretch after some warm up activity. A good stretching program involves all the major muscles in the body. During a warm

Exercise and Sports: Guidelines for People with Asthma

up, however, you may not have enough time to stretch all your muscles. If so, stretch the muscles you are going to use. Hold these stretches for about 10 to 15 seconds without bouncing. Concentrate on bringing your muscles to a gentle stretch where you feel mild pulling. Note that muscle tension varies from day to day. If you feel pain, check your body position and ease up a little. Remember all stretching should be pain-free. When you have more time, stretch all your muscles for longer periods of time. Hold the stretch for 15 seconds or longer, while breathing in and out easily.

How do I know if I'm doing too much?

By the way you feel. Unless you are in competition, you should feel comfortable. You should feel that you are working fairly hard to very hard, but not at maximum of very, very hard. Another way to tell—you should be able to talk to a companion without too much difficulty. You should feel "pleasantly tired" at the end of your workout. Increase the time you exercise by no more than 5–10 minutes/week for each session.

What do I do if I get a problem with asthma while I'm exercising?

Slow down or stop. Use your reliever medication, and if needed, wait for your pulse to slow down before starting again.

What sports or exercises are best for people with asthma?

Any sport you want to do is okay as long as you are prepared. Those sports that incorporate interval training and those involving breathing warm, moist air are best. Interval training is training that alternates strenuous and light exercise.

Try to avoid any sports that expose you to your allergens, such as grass and pollens.

Swimming is great, but some people have problems with chlorine. Other good sports include racquet sports, basketball, baseball, some track and field events, volleyball, soccer, or hockey. Long distance running or cycling with continuous hard effort may not be as easy and exercising in cold dry air may be difficult. But with suitable medication and training you can do those, too. Don't use asthma as an excuse for not participating. Be realistic as to how much you can do until you are conditioned.

How often should I work out?

Ideally, 3–6 times a week, or as much as you want. Start with 5–10 minutes and work up to half an hour or more per session. Remember to increase by no more than 5–10 minutes/week per session.

After exercise, then what?

Cool down. After vigorous activity don't stop suddenly, but slow down gradually over about fifteen minutes until you are breathing easily. Drink lots of cool fluids (not ice cold). This will help prevent more asthma symptoms later on. Before you get cold, you should also stretch again, as you did in the warm up.

Any other tips?

Yes, lots. However, common sense is your best guide. If you do something that makes you feel bad, stop it. Keep away from the things that set off an asthma attack.

- If you are allergic to trees or grasses, you may have to avoid woods or parks, use a mask, or exercise indoors.
- If your asthma is triggered by dust, smoke, or fumes, stay off main roads; try residential areas.
- If cold air makes you have an asthma attack, warm the air with a scarf or mask over your mouth and nose.
- If you can, choose the time of day and weather best suited to you; for example, ragweed is worst in the morning.
- Windy weather is usually cold or may create dust which may trigger an attack.
- If asthma symptoms develop during or after exercise, use your reliever medication to help relieve symptoms.
- Try to breath in through your nose and out your mouth whenever possible. The nose filters, warms, and moistens the air.

What should I tell my teacher or coach about my asthma?

- Tell them you have asthma and explain your symptoms.
- Tell them what medicines you are taking and how you use them.

Exercise and Sports: Guidelines for People with Asthma

- Let them know how you try to avoid symptoms and what to do if you experience them.

An action plan is what you do when you have asthma symptoms. It is best if your parents give a copy of the action plan to your teacher or coach. Also, agree on a signal with your coach to show you need to sit out. If you have a new teacher, make sure he or she is also told the same things.

Is it okay to take part in Physical Education class?

Yes, as much as you can as long as your asthma is well controlled. Remember to take your medication before you exercise, if needed, and warm up and cool down every time.

Should I always carry my medication with me?

Yes. Always keep your reliever medication with you because you never know when you may need it.

What else can I do?

Make sure you know what you can do to control your asthma. Work with your parent and doctor to keep it under control all the time. Learn how you can manage it so that you can enjoy doing anything you want. You should also include active living in your lifestyle: take the stairs instead of the elevator or escalator; ride a bike or walk instead of driving.

Chapter 34

Nutrition and Asthma

Eating Well and Maintaining a Healthy Weight

An important part of a healthy lifestyle is good nutrition. Good nutrition involves choosing healthy foods that can work to heal and repair your body and make it stronger against disease. We will explore eating healthy and give you practical suggestions for good nutrition.

In order to educate Americans about healthy eating, the U.S. Department of Agriculture (USDA) and the U.S. Department of Health and Human Services developed the *Dietary Guidelines for Americans* and a food guidance system. Following the *Dietary Guidelines* works for people of all ages, with and without chronic lung disease.

Pointers for a healthy diet are to include a variety of foods from each group in your diet. Each of the food groups provides nutrients that are important to you. Foods in one group can't replace those in another. Try to include each of the food groups in your daily diet. Choose a variety of foods within each food group and eat small amounts of fats, oils, and sweets. Talk with your doctor or dietitian about your specific nutritional needs. Eating a healthy diet can help you feel and breathe better.

© Copyright 2005 National Jewish Medical and Research Center. All rights reserved. For additional information, visit http://asthma.nationaljewish.org/ or call 1-800-222 LUNG.

Pull Up a Chair! It's Time to Eat

If you find yourself short of breath at mealtimes, this section is for you. Shortness of breath can make eating hard work. If you use all your energy preparing a healthy meal, you may find yourself unable to eat and/or enjoy what you have prepared. Here are a few practical suggestions on how to conserve energy and get the most from your meals.

- Eat six smaller meals instead of three big meals. Smaller, more frequent meals are recommended for people with chronic lung problems. Many people with chronic lung disease feel more short of breath when their stomach is full. This is because the diaphragm can not work as well when the stomach is full. You can satisfy your nutritional needs, keep your stomach comfortable,

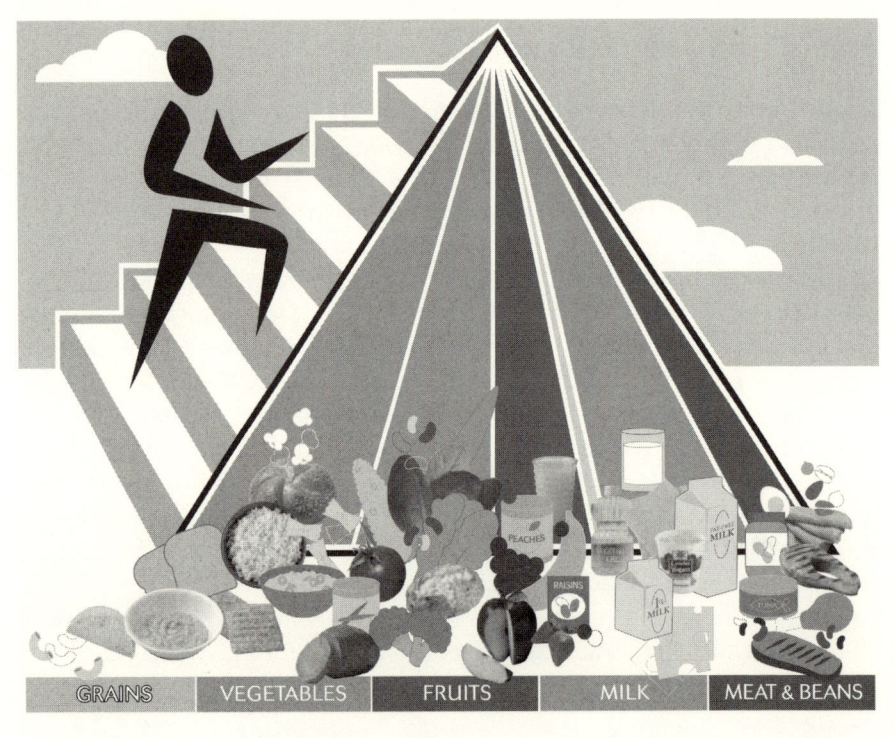

Figure 34.1. The MyPyramid Plan can help you choose the foods and amounts that are right for you. Visit http://www.mypyramid.gov for more information.

Nutrition and Asthma

and help your diaphragm to work better by eating smaller, more frequent meals. Small, frequent meals also reduce the chance of reflux.

- Plan to eat before you are too hungry or tired. Refuel before you hit empty.
- Breathe evenly while you are chewing and eating. Stop eating if you need to catch your breath. Relax at mealtime.
- When cooking or baking, double or triple your favorite recipes to keep your freezer full for times when you do not feel like cooking.
- Use prepared foods to save time and energy in the kitchen. Frozen meals, prepared foods, or take-out meals from a restaurant can make your life easier. Remember, the sugar, salt, or fat content of these foods may be higher than homemade. Be sure to ask if you are following a special diet.
- Do the tasks that require the most effort when you have the most energy. For example, many people would agree that grocery shopping is a tiring task. This chore can be done when you feel freshest, in the morning or after a rest. Better yet, have a friend or family member pick up your groceries for you.
- Don't stand in the kitchen when you can sit. Bring your chopping, cutting, and mixing projects over to the kitchen table and sit while you prepare the food or keep a barstool by the kitchen counter.
- Another way to avoid that "too full" feeling is to eat less of the foods that cause gas. The following foods are common offenders. Keep a food diary to find out if they are a problem for you.
    - asparagus
    - beans (pinto, kidney, navy, black)
    - broccoli
    - Brussels sprouts
    - cabbage
    - carbonated drinks
    - cauliflower
    - cucumbers
    - melons
    - garlic

- onions (raw)
- peas (split, blackeye)
- peppers
- radishes
- rutabagas
- sausage
- spicy foods
- turnips

Gastroesophageal Reflux Disease

Many people with chronic lung disease also suffer from gastroesophageal reflux (GER or GERD). In this condition, the valve between the stomach and esophagus (swallowing tube) is weak and acid leaks out of the stomach and into the esophagus, causing heartburn. Excess weight and overeating can contribute to reflux. Here are a few recommendations to decrease the risk of reflux and heartburn.

- Avoid overeating. Choose several small meals to balance your intake throughout the course of the day. A full stomach will put extra pressure on the valve causing it to open and allow acid into the esophagus.
- Eat low fat foods. Avoid fried foods, heavy sauces, and limit the use of butter or margarine. Choose low fat dairy products and lean meats.
- Avoid foods that you know cause your heartburn. These foods vary from person to person and may include spicy or acidic foods.
- Do not eat for two to three hours before lying down. Lying down increases the risk of heartburn.

Steroids and Nutrition

Some people with chronic lung disease, including asthma, take steroid pills on a regular basis. Steroid pills (such as prednisone or methylprednisolone) are strong medicines that decrease swollen airways. They also have some nutritional side effects to be aware of. Steroid therapy has the potential to interfere with the way the body uses specific nutrients, including calcium, potassium, sodium, protein, and vitamins D and C.

Nutrition and Asthma

If you take steroid pills for asthma, it is very important to eat a well balanced diet that meets the Food Pyramid Guidelines. A healthy diet that includes foods from each food group can make up for some of the nutritional effects of steroid therapy. Over a long period of time, steroid pills can increase the risk of osteoporosis (loss of calcium in the bones). Therefore, it is very important to eat foods high in calcium, such as dairy products. To prevent other side effects, limit the use of salt and foods that are high in sodium and decrease the amount of cholesterol and fats in your diet. In addition, certain supplements, such as calcium and a multivitamin may help. Talk with your doctor or a registered dietitian about specific concerns regarding steroids and your diet.

Asthmatic Children

Asthmatic children have the same nutritional requirements as other children. Aside from avoiding specific foods that you know trigger symptoms, no special kind of diet has been shown to be beneficial for asthma. Extra vitamins, over and above normal daily requirements, typically are not needed. Some children need extra calcium and vitamin D because of long-term steroid therapy, as mentioned above.

Chapter 35

The Weather and Asthma

Can the Weather Affect My Child's Asthma?

The effect of weather on asthma symptoms isn't fully understood, but there clearly is a link. Numerous studies have shown a variety of connections, such as increases in asthma-related emergency department visits when certain weather conditions are present. Some people find that their asthma symptoms get worse at specific times of year. For others, a severe storm or sudden weather change may trigger an attack.

Exposure to cold, dry air is a common asthma trigger and can quickly cause severe symptoms. People with exercise-induced asthma who participate in winter sports are especially susceptible. Hot, humid air can also trigger asthma symptoms in some people. In certain areas, heat and sunlight combine with pollutants to create ground-level ozone, which is also an asthma trigger.

Wet weather, which encourages the growth of mold spores, and dry, windy weather, which blows pollen and mold in the air, can cause problems as well. And a recent study showed that during thunderstorms,

---

This chapter begins with "Can the Weather Affect My Child's Asthma?" This information was provided by KidsHealth, one of the largest resources online for medically reviewed health information written for parents, kids, and teens. For more articles like this one, visit www.KidsHealth.org, or www.TeensHealth.org. © 2005 The Nemours Center for Children's Health Media, a division of The Nemours Foundation. "Researching a Possible Link between the Cold and Asthma" is from "What Do Racehorses, Asthmatics And Meatpackers Have In Common?" APS Press Release based on "Cold weather exercise and airway cytokine expression," *JAP* 98:2132-2136, 2005 by Davis et al. Used with permission of The American Physiological Society.

the daily number of emergency department visits for asthma increased by 15%. The study concluded that the problem was caused by the number of fungal spores in the air, which almost doubled. It wasn't rain, but the wind, that caused this increase. Changes in barometric pressure may also be an asthma trigger, although scientists aren't sure why.

If you suspect weather is playing a role in your child's asthma, keep a diary of asthma symptoms and possible triggers and talk to your child's doctor. Once you've determined what kind of weather affects your child, you can take steps to protect him or her:

- Watch the forecast for pollen and mold counts as well as other conditions (extreme cold or heat) that might affect your child's asthma.
- Limit your child's outdoor activities on peak trigger days.
- Make sure your child wears a scarf over his or her mouth and nose outside during very cold weather.
- Keep windows closed at night to keep pollens and molds out. If it's hot, use air conditioning, which cleans, cools, and dries the air.
- Keep your child indoors early in the morning (before 10 A.M.) when pollen is at its highest levels.
- Don't ask your child to mow the lawn and rake the leaves, and keep your child away from freshly cut grass and leaf piles.
- Dry clothes in the dryer (hanging clothes or sheets to dry can allow mold or pollen to collect on them).
- Make sure your child always has his or her rescue medication on hand.

Your child's written asthma action plan should list weather triggers and the steps you can take to handle them, including any seasonal increases in medication. If your child's asthma seems to be allergy-related, he or she may also need to see an allergist for medication or allergy shots.

Researching a Possible Link between the Cold and Asthma

When you exercise or work outside in winter, that dry feeling at the back of your throat indicates the cold air has irritated your throat.

The Weather and Asthma

Racehorses share a similar experience: exercising in below-freezing air causes mild airway injury.

Recent research suggests these kinds of experiences, also shared by winter athletes, sled dogs, meatpackers, and even fisherman, may be the beginning of a cascade of events leading to more serious conditions later.

Similarly, both athletes and horses seem open to infection after such strenuous bouts of activity as handicap races or marathons. Exercise physiologists and others have long thought that over-exertion might open a kind of "window of susceptibility" for sickness, but most of the evidence is anecdotal.

Physiologists at Oklahoma State University reporting on new research believe they may have found evidence that could link the problems suffered by horses, athletes, and cold-air workers that potentially could lead to progress in understanding the development and perhaps give hints toward cures for asthma and related diseases. Specifically, the Oklahoma State team reported that their research "data are the first to provide a specific mechanism for the exercise-induced open-window effect as a local pulmonary phenomenon."

The research involved horses exercising while breathing air at 23 degrees Fahrenheit and may "help explain why flu season occurs in the winter, how asthma develops in humans, and why race and other active horses get 'heaves,'" lead researcher Michael S. Davis said.

The study, entitled "Cold weather exercise and airway cytokine expression," appears in the June 2005 issue of the *Journal of Applied Physiology*, published by the American Physiological Society. The research was conducted by Michael S. Davis, Jerry R. Malayer, Lori VanDeventer, Christopher M. Royer, Erica C. McKenzie and Katherine K. Williamson of the Department of Physiological Sciences, Oklahoma State University, Stillwater.

Respiratory Responses to Cold Air Point to Asthma, 'Heaves' Links

The study showed "cold weather exercise can lead to asthma-like airway disease through the local induction of cytokines," small peptide protein hormones that direct and fine-tune the immune system, in a "profile associated with preferential production of antibodies and down-regulation of cell-mediated immunity...also characteristic of asthma."

They added that the "results support the novel contention that exercise while breathing cold air can actually contribute to the development of asthma." Specifically, they found that a group of cytokines of the TH2 phenotype were preferentially upregulated after cold air exercise by manifold amounts: Interleukin-4 (12-fold), IL-5 nine-fold, IL-10 10-fold, while other cytokines were upregulated less (IL-2 six-fold, IL-6 three-fold) or not at all.

Similarity of Human and "Equine" Athletes' Responses

The paper reported: "the potential effect of the cytokine expression shift described in this study and the resulting alteration in antigen responses are consistent with common pulmonary diseases of both equine and human athletes. Antibody-mediated pulmonary hypersensitivity (heaves) is common in horses and has been linked to increased expression of TH2 cytokine expression. The most prominent antigens identified in this syndrome are mold spores found in hay and straw bedding, thus closely linking the development of heaves to the horse's environment."

Furthermore, they note that like cold-induced human "ski asthma," the clinical signs of heaves (notably persistent coughing due to airway constriction) quickly diminish when the subject is removed from the offending environment. "In this regard, heaves is quite similar to human asthma, including the fact that the initial cause of the hypersensitivity has not been elucidated. The data of this study provide a compelling possibility: that strenuous exercise followed by exposure to environmental antigens promotes over-production of antibodies to those antigens," the report notes. Again it notes that this uncertain etiology is similar to that of "ski asthma," which Davis and others have also studied in sled dogs as an animal model for human asthma.

The current data "further raise the possibility of local suppression of cell-mediated immunity through the increased expression of IL-10" supporting the concept of the open window "of transient immune suppression after strenuous exercise (as well as) increased susceptibility to respiratory viruses in animals after strenuous exercise."

Conclusion and Next Steps

The authors conclude, stating: "We believe our data are the first to provide a specific mechanism for the exercise-induced open-window effect as a local pulmonary phenomenon. The potential deleterious effect of increased IL-10 expression is increased susceptibility to pathogens, particularly those that are normally cleared by cell-mediated immunity. On the other hand, it is possible that the increase in IL-10 is an appropriate response that moderates the net effect of the increased proinflammatory cytokine expression.

"These issues warrant further investigation, for which the equine model is ideally suited," the study notes. Some other "next steps" include:

- Looking at viral immunity in these cold-air scenarios, including "challenging" horses to see if blocking short-term inflammation perhaps could block pathogenesis, particularly in heaves.
- Challenging horses with influenza virus after a cold-air challenge.
- Further studying equine airway response to cold air to determine the cell populations active in these responses; that is, to determine the mast cell activation process and role of resident airway lymphocytes.
- Determining if heaves is more prevalent in colder climates, and among athletic horses (or formerly athletic ones) than in sedentary ones.
- Determining the range of air temperatures where airway damage occurs.

Davis notes that horses are particularly good models of human exercise and especially pulmonary functions. "As athletic animals, horses' ventilation requirements actually increase more than humans under comparable conditions, but we're able to get valid data from horses without running them at their maximum exertion points. Another advantage with horses is that most of our monitoring is noninvasive, and because they're hardy and well-cared for, they actually can serve as their own controls in most experiments."

An additional benefit of using animal models, he said, is obvious from the fact that while it looks like "we could make progress from our research in human chronic and acute conditions, probably the first direct beneficial application will be in the area of heaves, which affects many horses, especially as they age."

Chapter 36

Asthma and Outdoor Air Pollution

About Outdoor Air Pollution

Small particles and ozone come from things like exhaust from cars and factories, smoke, and road dust. When inhaled, outdoor pollutants can aggravate the lungs, and can lead to chest pain, coughing, shortness of breath, and throat irritation. Outdoor air pollution may also worsen chronic respiratory diseases, such as asthma. On days when ozone air pollution is highest, ozone has been associated with 10–20% of all respiratory hospital visits and admissions.

Watch for the Air Quality Index, or AQI, during your local weather report. The AQI is a tool that offers you clear information every day on whether air quality in your area could be a health risk. The AQI uses colors to show how much pollution is in the air. Green and yellow mean air pollution levels are low. Orange, red or purple mean pollution is at levels that may make asthma worse.

Actions You Can Take

State agencies will use television and radio to notify citizens of ozone alerts. On days when your state or local air pollution control agency calls an Ozone Action Day, people with asthma should limit prolonged physical activity outdoors. Consider adjusting outdoor activities to early in the morning or later in the evening.

This chapter includes text from "Outdoor Air Pollution," 2005, and "Asthma and Outdoor Air Pollution," 2004, produced by the U.S. Environmental Protection Agency (www.epa.gov).

Also, on Ozone Action Days, you can do the following ten things to help keep ozone formation to a minimum:

- Instead of driving, share a ride, walk, or bike.
- Take public transportation.
- If you must drive, avoid excessive idling and jackrabbit starts.
- Don't refuel your car or only do so after 7 P.M.
- Avoid using outboard motors, off-road vehicles, or other gasoline powered recreational vehicles.
- Defer mowing your lawn until late evening or the next day. Also avoid using gasoline-powered garden equipment.
- Postpone chores that use oil-based paints, solvents, or varnishes that produce fumes.
- If you are barbecuing, use an electric starter instead of charcoal lighter fluid.
- Limit or postpone your household chores that will involve the use of consumer products.
- Conserve energy in your home to reduce energy needs.

Facts about Outdoor Air Pollution and Asthma

Air pollution can make asthma symptoms worse and trigger attacks.

If you or your child has asthma, have you ever noticed symptoms get worse when the air is polluted? Air pollution can make it harder to breathe. It can also cause other symptoms, like coughing, wheezing, chest discomfort, and a burning feeling in the lungs.

Two key air pollutants can affect asthma. One is ozone (found in smog). The other is particle pollution (found in haze, smoke, and dust). When ozone and particle pollution are in the air, adults and children with asthma are more likely to have symptoms.

You can take steps to help protect your health from air pollution.

Get to know how sensitive you are to air pollution: Notice your asthma symptoms when you are physically active. Do they happen more often when the air is more polluted? If so, you may be sensitive to air pollution. Also notice any asthma symptoms that begin

Asthma and Outdoor Air Pollution

up to a day after you have been outdoors in polluted air. Air pollution can make you more sensitive to asthma triggers, like mold and dust mites. If you are more sensitive than usual to indoor asthma triggers, it could be due to air pollution outdoors.

Know when and where air pollution may be bad: Ozone is often worst on hot summer days, especially in the afternoons and early evenings. Particle pollution can be bad any time of year, even in winter. It can be especially bad when the weather is calm, allowing air pollution to build up. Particle levels can also be high near busy roads, during rush hour, and around factories, and when there is smoke in the air from wood stoves, fireplaces, or burning vegetation.

Plan activities when and where pollution levels are lower: Regular exercise is important for staying healthy, especially for people with asthma. By adjusting when and where you exercise, you can lead a healthy lifestyle and help reduce your asthma symptoms when the air is polluted. In summer, plan your most vigorous activities for the morning. Try to exercise away from busy roads or industrial areas. On hot, smoggy days when ozone levels are high, think about exercising indoors.

Change your activity level: When the air is polluted, try to take it easier if you are active outdoors. This will reduce how much pollution you breathe. Even if you can't change your schedule, you might be able to change your activity so it is less intense. For example, go for a walk instead of a jog. Or, spend less time on the activity. For example, jog for 20 minutes instead of 30.

Listen to your body: If you get asthma symptoms when the air is polluted, stop your activity. Find another, less intense activity.

Keep your quick-relief medicine on hand when you're active outdoors: That way, if you do have symptoms, you'll be prepared. This is especially important if you're starting a new activity that is more intense than you are used to.

Consult your health care provider: If you have asthma symptoms when the air is polluted, talk with your health care provider.

- If you will be exercising more than usual, discuss this with your health care provider. Ask whether you should use medicine before you start outdoor activities.

- If you have symptoms during a certain type of activity, ask your health care provider if you should follow an asthma action plan.

Get up-to-date information about your local air quality.

Sometimes you can tell that the air is polluted—for example, on a smoggy or hazy day. But often you can't. In many areas, you can find air quality forecasts and reports on local TV or radio. These reports use the Air Quality Index, or AQI, a simple color scale, to tell you how clean or polluted the air is. You can also find these reports on the internet at: www.epa.gov/airnow. You can use the AQI to plan your activities each day to help reduce your asthma symptoms.

Chapter 37

Indoor Environmental Asthma Triggers

Americans spend up to 90% of their time indoors. Therefore, indoor allergens and irritants can play a significant role in triggering asthma attacks. It is important to recognize potential asthma triggers in the indoor environment and reduce your exposure to those triggers. You may not be affected by all of the triggers listed in this chapter. Your doctor can help you to determine which triggers affect your asthma and develop a customized asthma management plan.

When you and your doctor make the plan, be sure to include the following:

- your child's asthma triggers
- instructions for asthma medicines
- what to do if your child has an asthma attack
- when to call your doctor
- emergency telephone numbers

Some of the most common indoor asthma triggers include secondhand smoke, dust mites, mold, cockroaches and other pests, household pets, and combustion byproducts.

This chapter contains text from "Indoor Environmental Asthma Triggers," "Secondhand Smoke," "Dust Mites," "Molds," "Cockroaches and Pests," "Pets," and "Nitrogen Dioxide (NO_2)," U.S. Environmental Protection Agency (www.epa.gov), May 2005.

Secondhand Smoke

What is secondhand smoke?

Secondhand smoke, also known as environmental tobacco smoke (ETS), consists of exhaled smoke from smokers and side stream smoke from the burning end of a cigarette, cigar or pipe. Secondhand smoke contains more than 4,000 substances, including over 40 compounds that are known carcinogens.

How does secondhand smoke affect asthma?

Secondhand smoke can trigger asthma episodes and increase the severity of attacks. Secondhand smoke is also a risk factor for new cases of asthma in preschool aged children who have not already exhibited asthma symptoms. Scientists believe that secondhand smoke irritates the chronically inflamed bronchial passages of people with asthma. Secondhand smoke is linked to other health problems, including lung cancer, ear infections and other chronic respiratory illnesses, such as bronchitis and pneumonia.

Many of the health effects of secondhand smoke, including asthma, are most clearly seen in children because children are most vulnerable to its effects. Most likely, children's developing bodies make them more susceptible to secondhand smoke's effects and, due to their small size, they breathe more rapidly than adults thereby taking in more secondhand smoke. Children receiving high doses of secondhand smoke, such as those with smoking mothers, run the greatest relative risk of experiencing damaging health effects.

What can you do?

- Choose not to smoke in your home or car and don't allow others to do so.
- Choose not to smoke in the presence of people with asthma.
- Choose not to smoke in the presence of children, who are particularly susceptible to the harmful effects of secondhand smoke.
- Do not allow baby-sitters, caregivers or others who work in your home to smoke in your house or near your children.
- Talk to your children's teachers and day care providers about keeping the places your children spend time smoke-free.

Indoor Environmental Asthma Triggers

Dust Mites

What are dust mites?

Dust mites are tiny insects that are invisible to the naked eye. Every home has dust mites. They feed on human skin flakes and are found in mattresses, pillows, carpets, upholstered furniture, bedcovers, clothes, stuffed toys and fabric and fabric-covered items. Body parts and feces from dust mites can trigger asthma in individuals with allergic reactions to dust mites, and exposure to dust mites can cause asthma in children who have not previously exhibited asthma symptoms.

What can you do?

- Cover mattresses and pillows with dust proof ("allergen-impermeable") zippered covers.
- Wash bedding (sheets, blankets and bedcovers) once per week in hot water.
- Choose washable stuffed toys, wash them often in hot water and dry them thoroughly.
- Keep stuffed toys off beds.
- Maintain low indoor humidity, ideally between 30–50% relative humidity. Humidity levels can be measured by hygrometers which are available at local hardware stores.

Common house dust may contain asthma triggers. When you are treating your house for dust mites, try these simple steps as well.

- Remove dust often with a damp cloth.
- Vacuum carpet and fabric-covered furniture to reduce dust build-up.
- Using vacuums with high efficiency filters or central vacuums may be helpful.
- People with asthma or allergies should leave the area being vacuumed.

Molds

What are molds?

Molds are microscopic fungi that live on plant and animal matter. Molds can be found almost anywhere; they grow on virtually any substance when moisture is present.

Molds produce tiny spores to reproduce, just as plants produce seeds. Mold spores waft through the indoor and outdoor air continually. When mold spores land on a damp spot indoors, they may begin growing and digesting whatever they are growing on in order to survive. Some molds can grow on wood, paper, carpet, foods and even dynamite.

There is no practical way to eliminate all molds indoors; the way to control indoor mold growth is to control moisture. If you think you have a mold problem and can see mold growth, you do not need environmental testing to determine what kind of mold you have. Instead, simply clean the mold from the surface it's growing on and dry the surface thoroughly.

How does mold affect asthma?

For people sensitive to molds, inhaling mold spores can cause an asthma attack.

What can you do?

If mold is a problem in your home, you need to clean up the mold and eliminate sources of moisture.

- Wash mold off hard surfaces and dry completely. Absorbent materials, such as ceiling tiles and carpet, may have to be replaced if they are contaminated with mold.
- Fix leaky plumbing or other sources of water.
- Keep drip pans in your air conditioner, refrigerator and dehumidifier clean and dry.
- Use exhaust fans or open windows in kitchens and bathrooms when showering, cooking or using the dishwasher.
- Vent clothes dryers to the outside.

Maintain low indoor humidity, ideally between 30–50% relative humidity. Humidity levels can be measured by hygrometers, which are available at local hardware stores.

Cockroaches and Pests

How do cockroaches and other pests affect asthma?

Droppings or body parts of cockroaches and other pests can trigger asthma. Certain proteins, called allergens, are found in cockroach

Indoor Environmental Asthma Triggers

feces and saliva and can cause allergic reactions, or trigger asthma symptoms, in some individuals. Cockroaches are commonly found in crowded cities and the southern regions of the United States. Cockroach allergens likely play a significant role in asthma in many inner-city areas.

What can you do?

An important key to pest management is to remove places in your home for pests to hide and to keep exposed areas free of food and water. But remember, pesticides you may spray to prevent pests are not only toxic to pests, they can harm people too. Try to use pest management methods that pose less of a risk. Here are some tips to prevent pests:

- Do not leave food or garbage out.
- Store food in airtight containers.
- Clean all food crumbs or spilled liquids right away.
- Wash dishes as soon as you are done using them.
- Keep counters, sinks, tables and floors clean and clear of clutter.
- Fix plumbing leaks and other moisture problems.
- Seal cracks or openings around or inside cabinets.
- Remove piles of boxes, newspapers and other hiding places for pests from your home.
- Make sure trash is stored in containers with lids that close securely, and remove trash daily.
- Try using poison baits, boric acid or traps first before using pesticide sprays.
- If sprays are used:
  - limit the spray to the infested area.
  - do not spray where you prepare or store food, or where young children play, crawl or sleep.
  - carefully follow instructions on the label.
  - make sure there is plenty of fresh air when you spray and keep people with asthma out of the room while spraying.
  - after spraying, the room should be thoroughly aired out.

Pets

How do pets affect asthma?

Your pet's dead skin flakes, urine, feces, saliva and hair can trigger asthma. Dogs, cats, rodents (including hamsters and guinea pigs) and other mammals can trigger asthma in individuals with an allergic reaction to animal dander. Proteins in the dander, urine or saliva of warm-blooded animals (for example, cats, dogs, mice, rats, gerbils, birds, etc.) have been reported to sensitize individuals and cause allergic reactions or trigger asthma episodes in individuals sensitive to animal allergens.

The most effective method to control animal allergens in the home is to not allow animals in the home. If you remove an animal from the home, it is important to clean the home (including floors and walls, but especially carpets and upholstered furniture) thoroughly.

Pet allergen levels are reported to stay in the home for several months after the pet is removed even with cleaning. Isolation methods to reduce animal allergen in the home have also been suggested by reputable health authorities (for example, keeping the animal in only one area of the home, keeping the animal outside or ensuring that people with allergies or asthma stay away from the animal) but the effectiveness of these methods has not been determined. Several reports in the literature indicate that animal allergen is carried in the air and by residents of the home on their clothing to all parts of the home, even when the animal is isolated. In fact, animal allergen is often detected in locations where no animals were housed.

Often, people sensitive to animal allergens are advised to wash their pets regularly. Recent research indicates that washing pets may only provide temporary reductions in allergen levels. There is no evidence that this short term reduction is effective in reducing symptoms and it has been suggested that during the washing of the animal the sensitive individual may be initially exposed to higher levels of allergens.

Thus, the most effective method to control exposure to animal allergens is to keep your home pet free. However, some individuals may find isolation measures to be sufficiently effective. Isolation measures that have been suggested include keeping pets out of the sleeping areas, keeping pets away from upholstered furniture, carpets, and stuffed toys, keeping the pet outdoors as much as possible and isolating sensitive individuals from the pet as much as possible.

Indoor Environmental Asthma Triggers

What can you do?

- If pets are one of your asthma triggers, strongly consider finding a new home for your pets.
- Keep pets out of the bedroom and other sleeping areas at all times and keep the door closed.
- Keep pets away from fabric-covered furniture, carpets and stuffed toys.
- Vacuum carpets, rugs and furniture two or more times per week.

Nitrogen Dioxide (NO_2)

What is nitrogen dioxide?

Nitrogen dioxide (NO_2) can be a byproduct of fuel-burning appliances, such as gas stoves, gas or oil furnaces, fireplaces, wood stoves and un-vented kerosene or gas space heaters. NO_2 is an odorless gas that can irritate your eyes, nose, and throat and cause shortness of breath. In people with asthma, exposure to low levels of NO_2 may cause increased bronchial reactivity and make young children more susceptible to respiratory infections. Long-term exposure to high levels of NO_2 can lead to chronic bronchitis.

What can you do?

- Properly ventilate a room where a fuel-burning appliance is used and use appliances that vent to the outside whenever possible.
- Do not idle the car inside your garage.
- Have the entire heating system—including furnace, flues and chimneys—professionally inspected and cleaned annually.
- Always open the flu on your fireplace before building a fire to ensure that smoke escapes through the chimney.
- Make sure the doors are tight fitting on your wood-burning stove and follow the manufacturer's directions for starting, stoking and putting out the fire.
- Follow the manufacturer's directions for proper fuel use on un-vented kerosene or gas space heaters and keep the heater properly

adjusted. Open a window slightly or use an exhaust fan in the room while using the heater.

- Install and use an exhaust fan over a gas stove and vent it outdoors.

Chapter 38

Air Filters: What People with Asthma Should Know

What do I need to know about air filters?

When we think of air pollution, we usually associate it with outdoor air. With the growing epidemic of asthma and allergies in the United States in the last 20 years, however, especially among infants and children who spend most of their time inside, much attention has been given to indoor air. In fact, the United States Environmental Protection Agency (EPA) ranks indoor air pollution as "a high priority public health risk."

Indoor air "pollution" can include airborne allergens, such as pet or rodent dander, mold spores, pollen, and cockroach or dust mite droppings. It can also include airborne irritants, such as tobacco smoke, chemicals, nitrogen oxides (NOx), volatile organic compounds (VOCs), other gases, outdoor pollution that comes inside through windows and doors, and more.

The EPA recommends three strategies for improving indoor air quality:

- controlling the sources that cause airborne allergens and irritants
- ventilating rooms and the entire house adequately
- cleaning/filtering indoor air

"Air Filters," reprinted with permission from the Asthma and Allergy Foundation of America, © 2005. All rights reserved. For additional information about asthma and related topics visit the AAFA website at http://www.aafa.org.

Before you make any changes to your indoor home environment or purchase any air filtration products, make sure to speak with a doctor who knows your personal medical history and current condition.

Will air filters really help my asthma or allergies?

Although the EPA recommends air filtration, controlling the sources that cause airborne allergens and irritants inside is more important than air filtration alone. Air filters are worth considering, but not as a solution to your asthma or allergy problems by themselves. Rather, air filters should only be considered as one small part of a total allergen avoidance and prevention plan. Talk to your doctor about developing a personal plan for your home.

While many allergens and irritants remain suspended in household air as the air naturally circulates, there are far more resting on surfaces like rugs, furniture, and countertops. Keeping such areas clean is an important step in preventing these substances from getting into the air in the first place. The most effective action, however, is to eliminate the sources that cause these allergens and irritants before they ever get into your home.

Good to know: Before you decide to buy an air filter, talk to your doctor about whether or not air filtration is right for you and about the best type of filter for your home.

Are there national standards for air filter performance?

No. The U.S. Food and Drug Administration (FDA) has asked groups of experts to recommend national standards, but no federal standards have yet been adopted. So far they have concluded there isn't enough research data on the relationship between air filtration and actual health improvement to recommend national standards.

When you shop for air filters, you will find several rating systems that compare filters. These are not health-related rating systems. They are standards used by manufacturers or manufacturers' organizations, and they provide little guidance for the health-conscious shopper.

Although the FDA has no health-related standards, it does consider some portable air filtration systems to be Class II medical devices. In the United States, nothing can claim this status without FDA approval. To get approval, a manufacturer must show two things: (1) that the device is safe, usually indicated by the Underwriters Laboratory

Air Filters: What People with Asthma Should Know

(UL) seal, and (2) that it has a medical benefit. If you are seeking a medical-quality air filtration device, look for both the UL seal and a statement of the FDA's Class II approval. If no FDA statement is available with the device, check the FDA's medical device listing before buying and always ask your doctor for guidance.

Keep in mind: Some air cleaners are Class II medical devices so ask your health plan if they will help to pay for the cost if your doctor recommends air filtration.

Are there different kinds of air filters?

Yes. Many homes have whole-house air filtration systems, but there are also several types of single-room air filters on the market. Five basis types of room air filters are described below:

Mechanical filters: These force air through a special mesh that traps particles, including allergens like pollen, pet dander, and dust mites. They also capture irritant particles like tobacco smoke. The fans in these types of devices produce ozone byproduct and are usually within the acceptable level. Make sure to ask for proof from the manufacturer that the product is within the acceptable level of ozone byproduct. (The standards for acceptable levels of ozone byproduct are found in section 21:801.415 of the Code of Federal Regulations (CFR) and Underwriters Laboratory (UL) standard 867.)

Electronic filters: These use electrical charges to attract and deposit allergens and irritants. If the device contains collecting plates, the particles are captured within the system. The ion-chargers in these types of filters produce more ozone byproduct than fans in mechanical filters, but they may still be within the acceptable level. Make sure to ask for proof from the manufacturer that the product is within the acceptable level of ozone byproduct.

Hybrid filters: These contain the elements of both mechanical and electronic filters.

Gas phase filters: These remove odors and non-particulate pollution, such as cooking gas, gasses given off by paint or building materials, and perfume. They cannot remove allergenic particles.

Ozone generators [not recommended]: Although pure ozone molecules (made up of three oxygen atoms) technically can "clear" the air of some particles, most experts, including the American Allergy Foundation of America (AAFA), do not recommend these. These devices exceed the acceptable level for ozone.

Remember: No air filter can fully protect you from the dangers of secondhand smoke. The most effective way get rid of "secondhand" smoke is to get rid of the source: get smokers in your family to quit.

What is a HEPA filter?

A HEPA filter is a kind of mechanical filter—a "high-efficiency particulate air" filter. HEPA was invented during World War II to prevent the escape of radioactive particles from laboratories. To qualify as a true HEPA filter, it must be able to trap at least 99.97% percent of all particles 0.3 microns in diameter or larger.

What are 'ozone' and 'ozone byproduct'?

Ozone is a molecule made up of three atoms of oxygen (O_3). The oxygen we breathe—the oxygen that is so important for life—consists of molecules that contain two atoms of oxygen (O_2). Ozone is different because of the presence of the third oxygen atom. In the outdoor environment, O_3 is found everywhere. It often mixes with gases, air pollution, and particulate matter (PM) to create smog that is unhealthy to breathe, especially on hot summer days. The U.S. Environmental Protection Agency (EPA) sets standards for outdoor ozone levels to help measure and determine air quality on a daily basis. EPA's standard level for outdoor ozone is 80 parts per billion (ppb) (also written as .08 parts per million [ppm].)

Inside, high ozone levels like those found outside are rare, but "ozone byproduct" (small, trace amounts of ozone indoors) is common. People are advised keep indoor ozone byproduct levels to a minimum. Many electronic devices in your home make ozone byproduct—kitchen mixers, ceiling fans, hair dryers, computers, TVs, copiers, and more. The EPA has adopted standards for indoor ozone byproduct levels for certain household devices which is written in the Code of Federal Regulations (CFR) as a maximum acceptable level of 50 parts per billion (ppb) (also written as .05 parts per million [ppm]), or lower.

Keep in mind: Beware of machines called "ozone generators" which directly produce ozone molecules—not as a byproduct, but as a direct product—and blow them into the room to "clean" the air. These

Air Filters: What People with Asthma Should Know

"ozone generator" machines can produce ozone up to 10-times more than the acceptable standard. AAFA and other groups, therefore, recommend that you do not use "ozone generator" machines in your home.

Can air filters protect me from secondhand smoke?

The only effective way to eliminate environmental tobacco smoke (ETS)—also called "secondhand" smoke—is to eliminate the source of smoke: Get smokers in your family to quit smoking. Some air cleaners may help to reduce secondhand smoke to a limited degree, but no air filtration or air purification system can completely eliminate all the harmful constituents of secondhand smoke. The U.S. Surgeon General has determined that secondhand smoke causes heart disease, lung cancer, and respiratory illness. Also, a simple reduction of secondhand smoke does not protect against the disease and death caused by exposure to secondhand smoke.

What else should I consider before buying an air filtration system?

If your home is heated or air conditioned through ducts, it may be possible to build filters into your air handling system. This has the advantage of the great force with which air will pass through the filter. It also eliminates a space-consuming appliance and an additional sound in your home. On the other hand, the filters may be more expensive and more difficult to handle, and they may need to be changed more often. Consult your doctor and your heating service on this alternative to a portable system.

What type of air filter works best for people with asthma or allergies?

The most effective filter is a kind of mechanical filter called the high-efficiency particulate air (HEPA) filter. A HEPA filter is a type of filter—not a product name. Many different air filtering devices or products can contain a HEPA filter. When buying a HEPA filter, insist on a system that meets "true HEPA" filtration standards (that is, be able to trap at least 99.97% percent of all particles 0.3 microns in diameter or larger).

Be aware: Air filtration will not eliminate your asthma or allergies. Air filters should only be considered as one small part of a total asthma and allergy prevention plan, and not total solution.

Does health insurance cover the cost of air filters purchased to help with controlling asthma or allergies?

Probably not, but a limited number of filters are classified as Class II medical devices and a portion of the cost may be deductible or reimbursable by your health plan carrier. Check with your health plan for details first, and don't rely on information from air filter sales people who don't know your health plan. Also, to help with the cost, consider using funds from a health savings account to purchase an air filter device needed for medical reasons. (You'll need to take a look at the terms of the account for rules on spending.) You may also want to talk with your accountant about the possibility of deducting the cost of an air filter under medical expenses.

Do you want to know more about asthma or allergies?

The Asthma and Allergy Foundation (AAFA) is a not-for-profit organization providing practical information and community based services and support through education, materials, and a national network of chapters and educational support groups. AAFA also sponsors research to find cures and better treatments for asthma and allergic diseases.

AAFA offers more than 50 fact sheets about aspects of asthma and allergies. Visit the AAFA website at http://www.aafa.org, write by e-mail to info@aafa.org, or call the Information Helpline at 800-7-ASTHMA (800-727-8462).

Chapter 39

How to Create a Dust-Free Bedroom

If you are dust-sensitive, especially if you have allergies and/or asthma, you can reduce some of your misery by creating a "dust-free" bedroom. Dust may contain molds, fibers, and dander from dogs, cats, and other animals, as well as tiny dust mites. These mites, which live in bedding, upholstered furniture, and carpets, thrive in the summer and die in the winter. They will, however, continue to thrive in the winter if the house is warm and humid. The particles seen floating in a shaft of sunlight include dead mites and their waste products. The waste products actually provoke the allergic reaction.

The routine cleaning necessary to maintain a dust-free bedroom also can help reduce exposure to cockroaches, another important cause of asthma in some allergic people.

You probably cannot control dust conditions under which you work or spend your daylight hours. To a large extent, however, you can eliminate dust from your bedroom. To create a dust-free bedroom, you must reduce the number of surfaces on which dust can collect.

In addition to getting medical care for your dust allergy and/or asthma, the National Institute of Allergy and Infectious Diseases suggests the following guidelines.

Preparation

- Completely empty the room, just as if you were moving.

National Institute of Allergy and Infections Diseases (http://niaid.nih.gov), August 2004.

- Empty and clean all closets and, if possible, store contents elsewhere and seal closets.
- Keep clothing in zippered plastic bags and shoes in boxes off the floor, if you cannot store them elsewhere.
- Remove carpeting, if possible.
- Clean and scrub the woodwork and floors thoroughly to remove all traces of dust.
- Wipe wood, tile, or linoleum floors with water, wax, or oil.
- Cement any linoleum to the floor.
- Close the doors and windows until the dust-sensitive person is ready to use the room.

Maintenance

- Wear a filter mask when cleaning.
- Clean the room thoroughly and completely once a week.
- Clean floors, furniture, tops of doors, window frames and sills, etc., with a damp cloth or oil mop.
- Carefully vacuum carpet and upholstery regularly.
- Use a special filter in the vacuum.
- Wash curtains often at 130 degrees Fahrenheit.
- Air the room thoroughly.

Carpeting and Flooring

Carpeting makes dust control impossible. Although shag carpets are the worst type to have if you are dust sensitive, all carpets trap dust. Therefore, health care experts recommend hardwood, tile, or linoleum floors. Treating carpets with tannic acid eliminates some dust mite allergen. Tannic acid, however, is not as effective as removing the carpet, is irritating to some people, and must be applied repeatedly.

Beds and Bedding

Keep only one bed in the bedroom. Most importantly, encase box springs and mattress in a zippered dust-proof or allergen-proof cover. Scrub bed springs outside the room. If you must have a second bed in the room, prepare it in the same manner.

How to Create a Dust-Free Bedroom

Use only washable materials on the bed. Sheets, blankets, and other bedclothes should be washed frequently in water that is at least 130 degrees Fahrenheit.

- Lower temperatures will not kill dust mites.
- If you set your hot water temperature lower (commonly done to prevent children from scalding themselves), wash items at a Laundromat which uses high wash temperatures.

Use a synthetic, such as Dacron, mattress pad and pillow. Avoid fuzzy wool blankets or feather- or wool-stuffed comforters and mattress pads.

Furniture and Furnishings

Keep furniture and furnishings to a minimum.

- Avoid upholstered furniture and blinds.
- Use only a wooden or metal chair that you can scrub.
- Use only plain, lightweight curtains on the windows.

Air Control

Air filters—either added to a furnace or a room unit—can reduce the levels of allergens. Electrostatic and HEPA (high-efficiency particulate absorption) filters can effectively remove many allergens from the air. If they don't function right, however, electrostatic filters may give off ozone, which can be harmful to your lungs if you have asthma.

A dehumidifier may help because house mites need high humidity to live and grow. You should take special care to clean the unit frequently with a weak bleach solution (1 cup bleach in 1 gallon water) or a commercial product to prevent mold growth. Although low humidity may reduce dust mite levels, it might irritate your nose and lungs.

Children

In addition to the above guidelines, if you are caring for a child who is dust-sensitive here are some guidelines to protect the child:

- Keep toys that will accumulate dust out of the child's bedroom.
- Avoid stuffed toys.

- Use only washable toys of wood, rubber, metal, or plastic.
- Store toys in a closed toy box or chest.

Pets

Keep all animals with fur or feathers out of the bedroom. If you are allergic to dust mites, you could also be allergic or develop an allergy to cats, dogs, or other animals.

Although these steps may seem difficult at first, experience plus habit will make them easier. The results—better breathing, fewer medicines, and greater freedom from allergy and asthma attacks—will be well worth your effort.

Chapter 40

Asthma and Smoking

People with asthma have sensitive airways inside their lungs. Certain 'triggers' can make these airways narrow. If you have asthma, smoking can lead to more asthma symptoms and more frequent asthma attacks. Smoking also damages your airways.

Damage to the Airways

Your lungs are lined by tiny hairs called cilia. These move in a wave-like motion to sweep dust, pollens, and other irritants out of your lungs when you cough. Cigarette smoke damages these tiny hairs. This means your lungs will be less able to clean themselves. A person with asthma who smokes is prone to chest infections, which can worsen their asthma or bring on asthma attacks.

Passive Smoking

Breathing in other people's cigarette smoke can also be harmful to a person with asthma, especially children. Secondhand cigarette smoke can:

- trigger an asthma attack;

© 2004 Better Health Channel, Victoria, Australia. This information was provided by the Better Health Channel. Material on the Better Health Channel regularly updated. For the latest version of this information please visit: www.betterhealth.vic.gov.au.

- increase the frequency of asthma attacks;
- increase your need for asthma medication;
- make your airways more sensitive to other triggers like pollen;
- reduce your lung function.

Pregnant Women Who Smoke

If a woman smokes when she is pregnant, the chemicals in the cigarette smoke are passed to the developing baby via the umbilical cord. The baby's lungs can be affected, which increases the baby's risk of developing wheezing symptoms early in life. Smoking during pregnancy is also linked to many other problems, such as low birth weight, premature labour, and increased risk of fetal death and stillbirth.

Smoking around Children

Children exposed to passive smoking are more likely to develop asthma in childhood. Children of smokers are more likely to develop chest infections and other respiratory illnesses. Repeated chest infections in infancy may be an indicator of an increased likelihood of developing asthma.

Reducing the Risk

You can reduce the risk of worsening your asthma by avoiding cigarette smoke. Some suggestions include:

- quit smoking;
- make your home smoke free—ask guests not to smoke in your house;
- avoid smoky places, like pubs and bars;
- when going out choose smoke free venues, such as restaurants, cafes, cinemas, and smoke free dance parties and gigs.

When Smoky Places Are Unavoidable

If you can't always keep away from smoky places, it is important to manage your asthma on a daily basis. If you need to take your reliever medication more than three or four times a week (excluding 'before exercise' medication) then you should visit your doctor. Your

Asthma and Smoking

asthma management plan might need to be adjusted. Remember to take your reliever medication with you when you visit a smoky place.

Things to Remember

- Cigarette smoke is a trigger for people with asthma.
- Asthma is more common in people who smoke.
- Women who smoke during pregnancy are harming the development of their baby's lungs.
- If you have asthma, avoid smoky places whenever possible.

Chapter 41

Traveling with Asthma

Whether you're taking a holiday or a work trip, you can still maintain good management of your asthma with some forward planning.

Travel Insurance

Read the fine print to make sure your travel insurance covers you for any health care costs related to pre-existing asthma.

Special Considerations

When you plan your trip, remember:

- Weather can bring on asthma symptoms, especially when the air is cold and dry.
- Temperature changes can bring on asthma symptoms.
- All beds and pillows harbor dust mites—unless they are treated with a microbial compound (for example, UltraFresh) which inhibits their growth. Be wary of hotels that look unclean.
- Scuba diving is dangerous for a person with asthma and should be avoided completely—go snorkeling instead.

"Asthma and Travel," © 2005 Better Health Channel, Victoria, Australia. This information was provided by the Better Health Channel. Material on the Better Health Channel is regularly updated. For the latest version of this information please visit: www.betterhealth.vic.gov.au.

Visit Your Doctor before You Go

Prior to taking your trip, visit your doctor for a check-up. It's important that your day-to-day asthma is under control before you leave home. Make sure your management and action plans are up to date. If you don't already know, ask your doctor about strategies to handle your asthma if it deteriorates while on your trip.

Get a Written Record

Ask your doctor to write up a report on your asthma. This report should include your medical history, the severity of your condition, and what treatment you need in case of medical attention. Carry this document with you at all times in case of an emergency. You might need to present your doctor's report to international customs officials if they question your medication.

Your Medications

It is a good idea to:

- take a little more medication than you think you'll need, just in case.
- always keep a supply of your medication with you in your carry bag.
- consider taking a prescription in case you lose all or some of your supplies.
- take copies of your prescriptions with you to prove the medicine is for your own personal use.

Equipment

A spacer device is cheap and portable, which makes it a better choice for traveling than a nebulizer. If you need a nebulizer pump, allow for different voltages and power points when traveling overseas. You will need to make prior arrangements with the airline if you need to use your nebulizer on board the aircraft. Alternatively, you can use a foot-powered nebulizer or one that is operated by sealed dry cell battery. Make sure you thoroughly understand how to use any unfamiliar equipment before you leave.

Physical Activity

If your asthma is normally well controlled, you should be able to go sightseeing, trekking, swimming, and generally enjoy any other leisure activity you wish. If your asthma is manageable at sea level, then you should have no problems in areas of higher altitude. Remember, scuba diving is dangerous for a person with asthma and should be avoided.

Things to Remember

- Make sure your day-to-day management of asthma is under control before you travel.
- Visit your doctor for a check-up and to fine tune your management and action plans.
- Take more medication than you think you'll need and always carry some with you.

Part Four

Treating Asthma: Medications and Delivery Devices

Chapter 42

How Is Asthma Treated?

You and your doctor together can decide about your treatment goals and what you need to do to control your asthma. Asthma treatment includes the following:

- Avoiding things that bring on your asthma symptoms or make symptoms worse. Doing so can reduce the amount of medicine you need to control your asthma. Allergy medicine and allergy shots in some cases may help your asthma.
- Using asthma medicines.

With proper treatment, you should ideally have the following results:

- Your asthma should be controlled.
- You should be free of asthma symptoms.
- You should have fewer attacks.
- You should need to use short-acting bronchodilators less often.
- You should be able to do normal activities without having symptoms.

This chapter includes "How Is Asthma Treated" and "Can Asthma Be Prevented" from the Diseases and Conditions Index, National Heart Lung, and Blood Institute, 2004.

Your doctor will fill out an action plan for your asthma. Your action plan will tell you what medications you should take and other things you should do to keep your asthma under control.

Medications for Asthma

There are two main types of medicines for asthma.

1. Quick relief medicines give rapid, short-term treatment and are taken when you have worsening asthma symptoms that can lead to asthma episodes or attacks. You will feel the effects of these medicines within minutes.

2. Long-term control medicines are taken every day, usually over long periods of time, to control chronic symptoms and to prevent asthma episodes or attacks. You will feel the full effects of these medicines after taking them for a few weeks. People with persistent asthma need long-term control medicines.

Quick relief medicines are used only when needed. A type of quick relief medicine is a short-acting inhaled bronchodilator. Bronchodilators work by relaxing tightened muscles around the airways. They help open up airways quickly and ease breathing. They are sometimes called "rescue" or "relief" medicines because they can stop an asthma attack. These medicines act quickly but their effects only last for a short period of time. You should take quick relief medicines when you first begin to feel asthma symptoms like coughing, wheezing, chest tightness, or shortness of breath. Anyone who has asthma should always have one of these inhalers in case of an attack. For severe attacks, your doctor may use steroids to treat the inflammation.

Long-term control medicines: The most effective, long-term control medication for asthma is an inhaled corticosteroid because this medicine reduces the swelling of airways that makes asthma attacks more likely.

- Inhaled corticosteroids (or steroids for short) are the preferred treatment for controlling mild, moderate, and severe persistent asthma. They are safe when taken as directed by your doctor. Inhaled medicines go directly into your lungs where they are needed. There are many kinds of inhalers that require different techniques, and it is important to know how to use your inhaler correctly. In some cases, steroid tablets or liquid are used for

How Is Asthma Treated?

short times to bring asthma under control. The tablet or liquid form may also be used to control severe asthma.

- Long-acting beta-agonists are another kind of long-term control medication. They are bronchodilators, not anti-inflammatory drugs. These medicines are used to help control moderate and severe asthma and to prevent nighttime symptoms. Long-acting beta-agonists are taken together with inhaled corticosteroid medicine.

- Leukotriene modifiers (montelukast, zafirlukast, and zileuton) are long-term control medicines used either alone to treat mild persistent asthma or together with inhaled corticosteroids to treat moderate persistent asthma or severe persistent asthma.

- Cromolyn and nedocromil are also long-term control medicines used to treat mild persistent asthma.

- Theophylline is a long-term control medication used either alone to treat mild persistent asthma or together with inhaled corticosteroids to treat moderate persistent asthma. People who take theophylline should have their blood levels checked to be sure the dose is appropriate.

If you stop taking long-term control medicines, your asthma will likely worsen again.

Many people with asthma need both a short-acting bronchodilator to use when symptoms worsen and long-term daily asthma control medication to treat the ongoing inflammation. Over time, your doctor may need to make changes in your asthma medication. You may need to increase your dose, lower your dose, or try a combination of medications. Be sure to work with your doctor to find the best treatment for your asthma. The goal is to use the least amount of medicine necessary to control your asthma.

Use a Peak Flow Meter

As part of your asthma action plan, you may use a hand-held device called a peak flow meter at home to measure lung function. To use it, you take a deep breath and blow hard into a tube to find out how fast you can blow out. This gives you a peak flow number. You will need to find out your "personal best" peak flow number by recording the peak flow number daily for a few weeks until your asthma is under control. The highest number you get during that time is your personal best peak flow. Then you can compare future peak flow measurements to your personal best peak flow, and that will show if your asthma is staying under control or not.

Your doctor will tell you how and when to use your peak flow meter and how to use your medication based on the results. You may be asked to use your peak flow meter each morning to keep track of how well you are breathing. The peak flow meter can help warn of a possible asthma attack even before you notice symptoms. If your peak flow meter shows that your breathing is getting worse, you should follow your action plan. Take your quick relief or other medication as your doctor directed. Then you can use the peak flow meter to see how your airways are responding to the medication.

Managing your asthma: Ask your doctor about how you can help take care of your own asthma. You should know the following:

- how to take your long-term daily medication correctly
- what things tend to make your asthma worse and ways to avoid them
- early signs to watch for that mean your asthma is starting to get worse (like a drop in your peak flow number or an increase in symptoms)
- how and when to use your peak flow meter
- what medication and how much to take to stop an asthma attack and how to use it correctly
- when to call or see your doctor
- when you should get emergency treatment

Treating Asthma in Special Circumstances

Treating asthma in children: Children with asthma, like adults with asthma, should see a doctor for treatment. Treatment may include allergy testing, finding ways to limit contact with things that cause asthma attacks, and taking medication.

Young children will need help from their parents and other caregivers to keep their asthma under control. Older children can learn to care for themselves and follow their asthma action plan with less supervision.

Medications for asthma in children are like those adults use, but doses are smaller. Children with asthma may need both a quick-relief

How Is Asthma Treated?

(or "rescue") inhaler for attacks and daily medication to control their asthma. Children with moderate or severe asthma should learn to use a peak flow meter to help keep their asthma under control. Using a peak flow meter can be very helpful because children often have a hard time describing their symptoms.

Parents should be alert for possible signs of asthma in children, such as coughing at night, frequent colds, wheezing, or other signs of breathing problems. If you suspect asthma or that your child's asthma is not in good control, take your child to a doctor for an exam and testing.

Your doctor will choose medication for your child based on the child's symptoms and test results. If your child has asthma, you will need to go to the doctor for regular follow-up visits and make sure that your child uses the medication properly.

Treating asthma in older adults: Older adults may need to have adjustments in their asthma treatment because of other diseases or conditions they have. Some medicines (like beta blockers used for treating high blood pressure and glaucoma, aspirin, and nonsteroidal anti-inflammatory drugs) can interfere with asthma medications or even cause asthma attacks. Be sure to tell your doctor about all medications that you take, including over-the-counter ones. Using steroids may affect bone density in adults, so ask your doctor about taking calcium and vitamin D supplements and other ways to help keep your bones strong.

Treating asthma in pregnancy: If you are pregnant, it is very important to both you and your baby to control your asthma. Uncontrolled asthma can lower the oxygen level in your blood, which means that your baby gets less oxygen too. Most asthma medications are safe to take during pregnancy. If you are pregnant or thinking about becoming pregnant, talk to your doctor about your asthma and how to have a healthy pregnancy.

Treating exercise-induced asthma: Regular physical exercise is important for good health. If exercise brings on asthma symptoms, work with your doctor to find the best way to avoid having symptoms when you exercise. Some people with asthma use inhaled quick relief medication before exercising to keep symptoms under control. If you use your asthma medication as directed and learn how to pace yourself, you should be able to take part in any physical activity or sport you choose. Many Olympic athletes have asthma.

Preventing Asthma

We don't yet know how to prevent asthma, but there are some things that can lower the chances of an asthma attack.

To prevent asthma symptoms do the following:

- Learn about your asthma and how to control it.
- Use medications as directed by your doctor to prevent or stop attacks.
- Avoid things that make your asthma worse, as much as possible.
- Get regular checkups from your doctor.
- Follow your asthma action plan.

Scientists do not yet know how to prevent the inflammation of the airways that leads to asthma. Scientists are exploring some theories that include the following:

- Babies exposed to tobacco smoke are more likely to get asthma. If a mother smokes during pregnancy, her baby may also be more likely to get asthma.
- Personal smoking may also cause asthma.
- Obesity may be linked to asthma as well as other health problems.

Chapter 43

What Medications Are Used to Treat Asthma?

Quick-Relief Medications

These medications quickly control acute asthma attacks.

Short-Acting Beta2-Agonists

Beta2-agonists do not reduce inflammation or airway responsiveness but serve as bronchodilators, relaxing and opening constricted airways during an acute asthma attack. They are used alone only for patients with mild and intermittent asthma. Patients with more severe cases should use them in combination with other agents.

Asthma is a disease in which inflammation of the airways causes airflow into and out of the lungs to be restricted. When an asthma attack occurs, mucus production is increased, muscles of the bronchial tree become tight, and the lining of the air passages swells, reducing airflow and producing the characteristic wheezing sound.

Specific short-acting beta2-agonists include the following:

- Albuterol (Proventil, Ventolin), called salbutamol outside the U.S., is the standard short-acting beta2-agonist in America. Other similar beta2-agonists are isoproterenol (Isuprel, Norisodrine, Medihaler-Iso), metaproterenol (Alupent, Metaprel), pirbuterol (Maxair), terbutaline (Brethine, Brethaire, Bricanyl), and

Excerpted from "Asthma in Adults," © 2005 A.D.A.M., Inc. Reprinted with permission.

bitolterol (Tornalate). Isoetharine (Bronkometer, Bronkosol is available in nebulizers.

- Newer beta2-agonists, including levalbuterol (Xopenex), have more specific actions than the standard agents. Studies have indicated that levalbuterol is as effective as albuterol with fewer side effects.

Short-acting bronchodilators are generally administered through inhalation and are effective for three to six hours. They relieve the symptoms of acute attacks, but they do not control the underlying inflammation. If asthma continues to worsen with the use of these agents, then patients should discuss corticosteroids or other drugs to treat underlying inflammation.

Side Effects of Beta2-Agonists: Side effects of all beta2-agonists include the following:

- Anxiety
- Tremor
- Restlessness
- Headache
- Patients may experience fast and irregular heartbeats. A physician should be notified immediately if such side effects occur, particularly in people with existing heart conditions. Such patients face an increased risk for sudden death from cardiac related causes. This risk is higher with oral or nebulized agents, but there have also been reports of heart attacks and angina in some patients using inhaled beta2-agonists.

Beta2-agonists have serious interactions with certain other drugs, such as beta-blockers, and patients should tell the physician about any other medications they are taking. Individuals with diabetes, existing heart disease, high blood pressure, hyperthyroidism, an enlarged prostate, or a history of seizures should take these drugs with caution.

Loss of Effectiveness and Overdose: There has been some concern that short-acting beta2-agonists become less effective when taken regularly over time, increasing the risk for overuse. Over time some patients may become tolerant to many effects of short-acting beta2-agonists. The degree to which this affects the airways is uncertain.

What Medications Are Used to Treat Asthma?

Table 43.1. Medications for Treatment and Prevention of Asthma

Medication Purpose: Quick-Relief Medications (control acute attacks)

Drug Class	Generic Name	Brand Names	Administration
Short-Acting Beta-2 Agonists	Albuterol	Proventil, Ventolin, AccuNeb	Inhaler, nebulizer
	Levalbuterol	Xopenex	Nebulizer
	Metaproterenol	Alupent	Inhaler
	Pirbuterol	Maxair	Inhaler
	Ipratropium/ Albuterol	Combivent	Inhaler
Anticholinergics	Ipratropium	Atrovent	Inhaler
	Tiotropium	Spiriva	Inhaler
Systemic Corticosteroids	Cortisone	Cortone	Pill
	Dexamethasone	Decadron	Pill
	Hydrocortisone	Cortef	Pill
	Methylprednisolone	Medrol	Pill
	Prednisolone	Orapred, Prelone	Syrup
	Prednisone	Various	Pill
	Triamcinolone	Aristocort	Pill

Medication Purpose: Long-Term Relief Medications (prevent attacks and control chronic symptoms)

Drug Class	Generic Name	Brand Names	Administration
Inhaled Corticosteroids	Beclomethasone	QVAR	Inhaler
	Budesonide	Pulmicort	Inhaler, nebulizer
	Flunisolide	AeroBid	Inhaler
	Fluticasone	Flovent	Inhaler
	Fluticasone/ Salmeterol	Advair	Inhaler
	Mometasone	Asmanex	Inhaler
	Triamcinolone	Azmacort	Inhaler
Long-Acting Beta2-Agonists	Formoterol	Foradil	Inhaler
	Salmeterol	Serevent	Inhaler
Anti-inflammatories	Cromolyn	Intal	Nebulizer
	Nedocromil	Tilade	Inhaler
IgE-inhibitor	Omalizumab	Xolair	Injectable
Leukotriene Modifiers	Montelukast	Singulair	Pill
	Zafirlukast	Accolate	Pill
	Zileuton	Zyflo	Pill
Methylxanthine	Theophylline	Uniphyl, Quibron, Theo-24	Pill, syrup

In some studies, the duration of action has declined but the peak effect appears to be preserved, making these drugs still useful for acute attacks. Regular use of long-acting beta 2-agonists may reduce the effect of short-acting forms.

A 2005 landmark study suggested that patients' differing clinical response to albuterol may be based on their genotype. Albuterol targets the beta-adrenergic receptor. In the Beta-Adrenergic Response by Genotype (BARGE) trial, researchers studied the effects of albuterol on patients with two different forms of this receptor. The results suggested that patients with the arginine form of the receptor did not respond to albuterol. These patients' asthma symptoms actually improved when albuterol was not used. By contrast, patients with the glycine form of the receptor had improved asthma control with albuterol.

Patients who perceive beta2-agonists as being less effective may overuse them. Overdose can be serious and in rare cases even life-threatening, particularly in patients with heart disease.

Anticholinergic Agents

Inhaled ipratropium bromide (Atrovent) acts as a bronchodilator over time. Ipratropium bromide alone is only modestly beneficial for acute asthma attacks. In fact, the drug is not approved specifically for asthma. It may, however, have benefits in certain cases:

- It may be useful for certain older asthma patients who also have emphysema or chronic bronchitis.

- A combination with a beta2-agonist might be helpful for patients who do not initially respond to treatment with a beta2-agonist alone.

Systemic Corticosteroids

Common oral corticosteroids include prednisone, prednisolone, methylprednisolone, and hydrocortisone. They very effectively reduce inflammation but are generally used only after hospitalization for an acute attack. In some severe cases, they may be used as maintenance.

Adverse effects of prolonged use of oral steroids include cataracts, glaucoma, osteoporosis, diabetes, fluid retention, susceptibility to infections, weight gain, hypertension, capillary fragility, acne, excess hair growth, wasting of the muscles, menstrual irregularities, irritability, insomnia, and psychosis. Osteoporosis is a common and particularly severe long-term side effect of prolonged steroid use. Medications that can prevent osteoporosis include calcium supplements, parathyroid hormone, bisphosphonates, or hormone replacement therapy in postmenopausal women. Vitamin C and E may help reduce the risk of cataracts.

Osteoporosis is a condition characterized by progressive loss of bone density, thinning of bone tissue and increased vulnerability to fractures. Osteoporosis may result from disease, dietary or hormonal deficiency or advanced age. Regular exercise and vitamin and mineral supplements can reduce and even reverse loss of bone density.

Long-term use of oral steroid medications suppresses secretion of natural steroid hormones by the adrenal glands. After withdrawal from these drugs, this so-called adrenal suppression persists and it can take the body a while (sometimes up to a year) to regain its ability to produce natural steroids again. It should be noted that there have been a few cases of severe adrenal insufficiency that occurred when switching from oral to inhaled steroids, which, in rare cases, has resulted in death.

No one should stop taking any steroids without consulting a physician first, and if steroids are withdrawn, regular follow-up monitoring is necessary. Patients should discuss with their physician measures for preventing adrenal insufficiency during withdrawal, particularly during stressful times, when the risk increases.

Long-Term Relief Medications

These medications are taken on a regular basis to prevent asthma attacks and control chronic symptoms.

Inhaled Corticosteroids

Corticosteroids, also called glucocorticoids or steroids, are powerful anti-inflammatory drugs. Steroids are not bronchodilators (that is, they do not relax the airways) and have little effect on symptoms. Instead, they work over time to reduce inflammation and prevent permanent injury in the lungs. Many studies have now shown that the use of inhaled corticosteroids in patients with moderate to severe asthma significantly reduce the rate of re-hospitalizations and deaths from asthma. Nevertheless, they are still significantly under-prescribed in the patients who need them most.

Inhalation of corticosteroids makes it possible to provide effective local anti-inflammatory activity in the lungs with minimal systemic effects. (Oral steroids have considerable side effects.) They are currently recommended as the primary therapy under the following circumstances:

- For any asthmatic condition more serious than occasional episodes of mild asthma: Low-doses of inhaled steroids may even be safe and effective for some people with mild asthma, particularly those who find themselves using beta2-agonists daily.

- When treatment with bronchodilators is not effective

Examples of inhaled corticosteroids include the following:

- The most recent generation of inhaled steroids include (in order of potency) fluticasone (Flovent), budesonide (Pulmicort), triamcinolone (Azmacort and others), and flunisolide (AeroBid). In general, the newer agents are more powerful than the older generation of inhaled agents. Experts have some concern, then, that these potent agents, particularly fluticasone, may produce major side effects similar to oral agents. Studies are now suggesting, however, that the same benefits can be achieved with low doses of fluticasone as with high doses, thus reducing risks for serious side effects. (Of note, budesonide has been given a pregnancy approval rating.)

- A new inhaled corticosteroid, mometasone furoate (Asmanex) was approved by the FDA in 2005.

- The older corticosteroid inhalants are beclomethasone (Beclovent, Vanceril) and dexamethasone (Decadron Phosphate Respihaler and others). They are less powerful than the newer steroids when delivered with standard inhalers. New inhaler systems, such as QVAR, which uses extra fine formulations of beclomethasone to allow deep delivery into the lungs, may prove to be as effective as the newer, more potent steroids. Beclomethasone is believed to be safe during pregnancy.

- Inhalers that combine both long-acting beta2-agonists and corticosteroids are now available.

Traditionally, patients have been advised to take corticosteroids on a daily basis. However, a 2005 study suggested that intermittent corticosteroid therapy may be appropriate for some patients with mild persistent asthma. In the Improving Asthma Control Trial (IMPACT), researchers found that patients with mild persistent asthma who used an inhaled corticosteroid (budesonide) on an as-needed basis to control acute symptoms had similar lung function and quality of life outcomes as patients who used the drug daily. The researchers emphasize that patients with severe asthma should adhere to a daily dosage schedule, and that all asthmatic patients should consult with their physician to discuss any changes in medication regimen.

Optimal timing of the dose is important and may vary depending on the medication. Most of the newer inhaled steroids and even some older ones are now available as a single daily dose.

Inhaled steroids are generally considered safe and effective and only rarely cause any of the more serious side effects reported with prolonged use of oral steroids. Side effects of inhaled steroids are the following:

- The most common side effects are throat irritation, hoarseness, and dry mouth. These effects can be minimized or prevented by using a spacer device and rinsing the mouth after each treatment.

- Rashes, wheezing, facial swelling (edema), fungal infections (thrush) in the mouth and throat, and bruising are also possible but are not common with inhalators.

- A 2001 study, however, reported a higher risk for cataracts in patients over age 40. (No higher risk was observed in younger people.)

- Some studies are reporting a higher risk for bone loss in patients who take inhaled steroids regularly, which is known to occur with oral steroids. (A number of bone-preserving medications are now available that might safely offset this effect.) Medications are available to help prevent bone loss.

- There is some concern that the more potent agents, particularly fluticasone, suppress the adrenal system (which secretes natural steroids) to a greater degree than other steroid inhalants. (This is a serious side effect of oral steroids.)

Long-Acting Beta2-Agonists

Long-acting beta2-agonists, including salmeterol (Serevent) or formoterol (Foradil), plus inhaled corticosteroids are now the preferred preventive treatment for adults and children with moderate to severe asthma. Long-acting beta2-agonists are used for preventing an asthma attack (not for treating symptoms). The effects of one dose of a long-acting beta2 agonist last for about 12 hours, so they are particularly effective during the night. These agents also may be used for prevention of exercise-induced asthma in people and to protect against aspirin-induced asthma.

In comparison studies, salmeterol and formoterol appear to be equally beneficial. Formoterol has a much faster action, however, and may achieve better control of nighttime asthma. Formoterol, in fact, works almost as fast as the short-acting albuterol and is sometimes used to treat asthma symptoms. Salmeterol should never be used for treatment of acute episodes. For this purpose, short-acting bronchodilators should be used. (Formoterol has a faster action and may, in some cases, be used for treating symptoms, but patients should check with their physician.)

Long-acting forms are not used alone on any regular on basis, since they may reduce the effectiveness of the short-acting beta2-agonists (the mainstays for treating acute attacks). In patients with moderate to severe asthma, the long-acting beta2 agonists are best used in combination with anti-inflammatory drugs. In fact, unlike short-acting forms, these beta2-agonists may even have anti-inflammatory properties.

Single devices that contain both agents are now available in the U.S. (Advair) and parts of Europe (Seretide, Symbicort). These inhalers appear to be safe and possibly more effective than either agent used alone for patients who do not respond well to other agents.

Side Effects: Side effects of long-acting beta2-agonists are similar to the short-acting agents.

Specific Warning on Salmeterol: In 2003 a "black box" warning was added to product packaging for drugs that contain salmeterol, including Serevent Inhalation Aerosol, Serevent Diskus, and Advair Diskus. The warning urges caution based on a 2003 study that demonstrated a higher incidence of serious and even fatal asthma episodes in patients who used the drug than in patients who used a placebo. Salmeterol requires up to 20 minutes to achieve effectiveness, and there is a danger of overdose if a patient is not aware of this delay and takes additional doses to achieve faster relief. (Overdose has been fatal only in rare cases.) The risk for serious asthma episodes with salmeterol appears to be highest in African-American and elderly patients with severe asthma.

What Medications Are Used to Treat Asthma?

Salmeterol should never be used for stopping an attack. Patients should NOT stop taking salmeterol as long-acting treatment without first talking to their physician.

Cromolyn and Similar Drugs

Cromolyn sodium (Intal) serves as both an anti-inflammatory drug and has antihistamine properties that block asthma triggers such as allergens, cold, or exercise. Nedocromil (Tilade) is similar to cromolyn. A cromolyn nasal spray called Nasalcrom has been approved for over-the-counter purchase, but only to relieve nasal congestion caused by allergies. Asthmatic patients should not use it for self-medication without the advice of a physician.

Candidates: Cromolyn is often used in children with allergic asthma, but it has also been an important treatment for exercise-induced asthma (EIA) in all age groups, for pregnant women, and possibly for preventing allergic asthma in adults as well as children. Both cromolyn and nedocromil appear to be useful for patients with aspirin-induced asthma. These agents do not effectively treat asthma once an attack is underway. They also have very little long-term benefits on lung function compared to inhaled corticosteroids.

Side Effects: Side effects of cromolyn include nasal congestion, coughing, sneezing, wheezing, nausea, nosebleeds, and dry throat. Nedocromil has an unpleasant taste and some people have complained of nausea, headache, and spasms in the airways, but no serious side effects have been reported.

Leukotriene-Antagonists

Leukotriene-antagonists (also called anti-leukotrienes or leukotriene modifiers) are oral medications that block leukotrienes. Leukotrienes are powerful immune system factors that, in excess, produce a battery of damaging chemicals that can cause inflammation and spasms in the airways of people with asthma. As with other anti-inflammatory agents, leukotrienes are used for prevention and not for treating acute asthma attacks.

The leukotriene-antagonists include zafirlukast (Accolate), montelukast (Singulair), zileuton (Zyflo), and pranlukast (Ultair, Onon). These agents are proving to be effective for long-term prevention of asthma, including exercise-induced asthma and aspirin (or NSAID)-induced asthma. Unfortunately, most studies to date are still reporting better success with inhaled corticosteroids than with the leukotriene-antagonists. Their anti-inflammatory actions are different from those of steroids, however, and combinations of the two agents are being tried. A 2002 analysis of 13 studies, however, reported only modest benefits when anti-leukotrienes were added to corticosteroids. The combination did improve asthma control in some of the studies, but they did not reduce corticosteroid use. (In all but one of these studies the subjects were adults.)

Side Effects and Complications: Gastrointestinal distress is the most common side effect of leukotriene-antagonists. Very few other side effects have been reported. In general, these agents appear to be safe and well tolerated.

Of some concern are reports of Churg-Strauss syndrome in a few people taking zafirlukast or montelukast. Churg-Strauss syndrome is very rare, but it causes blood vessel inflammation in the lungs and can be life threatening. Oral steroids quickly resolve the problem. In fact, usually the syndrome has occurred in patients who were tapering off steroids and changing over to the leukotrienes-antagonists. Some experts believe that, in such cases, the steroids may simply have masked the presence of the disorder, which then developed when the steroid drugs were withdrawn. Symptoms include severe sinusitis, flu-like symptoms, rash, and numbness in the hands and feet.

Other concerns are indications of liver injury in patients taking zileuton and zafirlukast when taken at higher than standard doses. No adverse effects on the liver have been reported to date with montelukast.

Theophylline

Theophylline: Theophylline (Theo-Dur, Theolair, Slo-Phyllin, Slo-bid, Constant-T, and Respbid) relaxes the muscles around the bronchioles and also stimulates breathing. One study reported that it may also have anti-inflammatory qualities even in low doses. Available in tablet, liquid, and injectable forms, some theophylline sustained-release tablets and capsules have a long duration of action and can, therefore, be taken once or twice a day with good results.

If theophylline is not taken exactly as prescribed, an overdose can easily occur. Toxicity can cause nausea, vomiting, headache, insomnia, and, in rare cases, disturbances in heart rhythm and convulsions. A physician should be contacted immediately if any of these side effects occur.

What Medications Are Used to Treat Asthma?

The risks for these adverse effects are small if the drug is taken exactly as prescribed but the following precautions should be noted:

- Chronic smokers metabolize theophylline much more quickly and require higher doses of the drug than nonsmokers; prolonged-release versions are helpful for such people.

- Too much caffeine can increase the concentration of this drug and the amount of time it stays in the body.

- Theophylline also interacts with many other drugs that are taken for other common medical conditions, including asthma. Caution should be exercised if beta2-agonists and theophylline are used together.

- Theophylline should not be taken by anyone who has a peptic ulcer and should be taken with caution by the elderly and by individuals with heart disease, liver disease, hypertension, seizure disorders, or congestive heart failure. Of special note, people with heart conditions who take theophylline orally face an increased risk for sudden death from heart-related causes.

Omalizumab

Omalizumab (Xolair) is now FDA approved for patients age 12 and older who have moderate to severe persistent allergic asthma. The first agent of this type to be approved for asthma, omalizumab is a monoclonal antibody (MAb), or a genetically developed agent designed to attack very specific targets.

Omalizumab prevents the antibody immunoglobulin E (IgE) from triggering the inflammatory events that lead to asthmatic attacks. Studies have shown excellent benefits of the drug, including a reduced need for corticosteroids, fewer hospitalizations, and significant symptomatic improvements. Because IgE may play an important role in causing childhood asthma, omalizumab may prove to be even more helpful for children than adults; further study is underway.

Omalizumab is administered by injection every two to four weeks. Because of its high cost, it is presently being reserved for patients with severe asthma and whose symptoms are difficult to control even with corticosteroids. Experts predict that the applications of this therapy will likely expand in time, however, because it is a powerful modifier of severe seasonal and food allergies (in patients with or without asthma). A 2005 meta-analysis of omalizumab clinical trials found that omalizumab reduced the rate of asthma worsening by 38% and reduced the rate of total emergency visits by 47%.

Other Treatments

Some agents are being investigated that have anti-inflammatory effects, which might help reduce dependence on corticosteroids. Certain antibiotics, such as clarithromycin (Biaxin), may improve lung function in asthmatic patients who show evidence of infection with the atypical organisms *Mycoplasma* or *Chlamydia pneumoniae*. Dapsone, an agent known as a sulfone is also under investigation. According to data presented at recent annual meetings of the American Academy of Allergy, Asthma & Immunology, the humanized monoclonal antibody Daclizumab significantly improved asthma control in patients with treatment-resistant asthma, as well as patients with moderate to severe chronic persistent asthma.

Alternative Treatments

Alternative therapies are being widely used by children, adolescents, and adults with asthma. In one study, nearly half of asthma or allergy sufferers resorted to alternative treatments. To date, however, evidence does not support any value from most alternative therapies, including high-dose vitamins, urine injections, homeopathic remedies, and most herbal remedies.

Relaxation and Stress-Reduction Techniques: Patients report benefits from many stress reduction techniques, such as acupuncture, hypnosis, breathing relaxation techniques, massage therapy, and meditation practices.

Acupuncture, hypnosis and biofeedback are all alternative ways to control pain. Acupuncture involves the insertion of tiny sterile needles, slightly thicker than a human hair, at specific points on the body.

The Buteyko Breathing Method: The Buteyko breathing method is an experimental approach designed to increase levels of carbon dioxide in the body. To do this, patients are trained to reduce their volume of breath and to avoid hyperventilation (over-breathing). Some studies are reporting that patients use this method reduce their use of medications and improve their quality of life. The system originated in Australia and is not yet widely available in the U.S.

What Medications Are Used to Treat Asthma?

Probiotics: Probiotics are beneficial bacteria that may help protect against allergies and asthma. Antibiotic over-use and modern hygiene may specifically be reducing these helpful organisms. Probiotics can be obtained in active yogurt cultures and in supplements, which are being studied for protection.

Herbal Remedies: Herbal remedies have been used with apparent success in Eastern nations, but few have been studied rigorously in the United States. Butterbur (also known as *Petasites hybridus*, butter dock, blatterdock, bog rhubarb, and exwort), a traditional herbal remedy, is used for seasonal allergies and asthma. In a 2002 study, it was as effective and less sedating than a commonly prescribed antihistamine for treating seasonal allergies over a two week period. More research is needed. Even when natural remedies appear to be effective in trials, there are no standards or regulations in the U.S. to guarantee their quality, effectiveness, or safety. Of great concern are their growing use and the possibilities of serious drug interactions. Patients who try alternative treatments must be sure to inform their physician.

Warnings on Alternative and So-Called Natural Remedies

Alternative or natural remedies are not regulated and their quality is not publicly controlled. In addition, any substance that can affect the body's chemistry can, like any drug, produce side effects that may be harmful. Even if studies report positive benefits from herbal remedies, the compounds used in such studies are, in most cases, not what are being marketed to the public. There have been a number of reported cases of serious and even lethal side effects from herbal products. In addition, some so-called natural remedies were found to contain standard prescription medication.

The following are special concerns for people with asthma and allergic rhinitis:

- Grapeseed extract is sometimes touted as a natural antihistamine. A 2002 study, however, reported no benefits from it.

- A 2002 study found no benefits with homeopathy immunotherapy for asthmatic patients allergic to dust mites.

- Some allergic patients have reported worse symptoms after drinking herbal teas, which may contain leaves or pollens that the patient is sensitive to. In fact herbal remedies themselves can trigger an allergic reaction. For example, echinacea is of special concern. This herbal remedy actually boosts the immune system. People with nasal congestion may mistakenly take it because it is often used to treat colds. In the case of allergies, however, echinacea may worsen symptoms or even trigger them in people who haven't experienced them. People with autoimmune diseases or who have plant allergies should particularly avoid it.

- Aller Relief Chinese herbal cold and allergy contains trace amounts of aristolochic acid, a chemical that is toxic to the kidneys and a carcinogen. Products containing aristolochic acid have been associated with several reports of kidney failure in Europe. Of specific concern are studies suggesting that up to 30% of herbal patent remedies imported from China having been laced with potent pharmaceuticals such as phenacetin and steroids. Most reported problems occurred in herbal remedies imported from Asia, with one study reporting a significant percentage of such remedies containing toxic metals.

- Aromatherapy is now often used for relaxation. Some exotic plant extracts in these formulas have been associated with a wide range of skin allergies.

Chapter 44

Why People Don't Take Their Asthma Medication

Asthma rates are increasing nationwide, and asthma is a particularly alarming problem in inner-city African-American communities. In fact, African Americans are at least twice as likely to be hospitalized and to die from asthma as white Americans.

Although there are good medications that can prevent and treat airway constriction, a hallmark of the disease, studies have found that many people do not take their asthma mediation regularly, but their reasons are not always clear. In a small study published in the May 2003 *Journal of Allergy and Clinical Immunology*, Dr. Andrea Apter, associate professor of medicine at the University of Pennsylvania, and Maureen George, MSN, RN, AE-C, coordinator of the Comprehensive Asthma Care Program at the University of Pennsylvania, asked low-income, urban African Americans with asthma why they did not regularly use their mediation.

The study authors found that there are many barriers to adherence, some of which can be addressed through improved doctor-patient communication. Below, Dr. Apter and George share their study findings as well as strategies for maintaining a drug schedule.

What were you hoping to learn from this study?

Dr. Andrea Apter: Understanding why patients don't take their medicines is a very complicated issue. As providers, we only see one

---

"Sticking to the Schedule: Why People Don't Take Their Asthma Medication," by Christine Haran, © 2004 Healthology, Inc. All rights reserved. Additional information is available at www.healthology.com.

aspect of the patient: when the patient comes to clinic. We don't know about all the things in their life that impact whether they take their medicines.

Maureen George: We have these great medications that people don't seem to have accepted. Before we design interventional studies to try and improve compliance, we wanted to conduct these focus groups to get a better understanding of the attitudinal beliefs that may influence patients' decision making.

What were some of the reasons people weren't taking their medicine consistently?

George: Many of the patients skipped their medicines when they came home late because they believed it was safer to omit a dose than to take a dose late. And yet, if you were to ask any asthma provider, we would say it would be much wiser to take that dose than to skip a dose.

There were also some specific fears of the side effects of the medications that weren't true, such as the belief that the medication could cause organ damage, cancer, and infertility or sterility.

One of the barriers that was specific to this population was the belief that the patient's assessment of their disease control was superior to that of their provider.

Apter: Insurance coverage was another barrier. Some patients get 28 days worth of medicine through their insurance because that's considered a months' worth. They can't get those extra two days refilled until the new month, so they run out. That causes patients to not take their medication one day so that they have it when they really need it.

What are the consequences of not maintaining an asthma regimen?

George: The risk of under-treating asthma is, at best, suboptimal control and, at worst, death. Suboptimal control could include more acute asthma attacks and the risk of developing permanent damage to the lungs. It could also include more acute care needs—such unplanned doctor visits or intensive care admissions—absenteeism from work or school, poor exercise tolerance, poor quality of life, and nocturnal awakenings.

What strategies did patients find helpful?

George: Asthma educators and clinicians have been told by the experts that patients should just leave their medication at home and take it when they get up in the morning and go to bed at night. The patients in this study told us that they felt that the provider should encourage them to carry their medicines with them because they have chaotic lifestyles. Another theme was to offer fewer medicines that can be taken less frequently.

Apter: Different people had different solutions. For example, one woman thought of taking her medicine when her children took theirs. A man who went to work early in the morning put his medicine in the car and would take it on the way to work.

What did patients say about their relationship with their doctors?

Apter: Our patients liked their physicians, who came from one practice. But many of them described experiences in the past where they didn't feel that a physician listened to them. They felt the physician or the provider wasn't empathetic or didn't provide them the time and the individualized attention that they needed.

How can caregivers or family members help a patient stay on schedule?

Apter: If the patient's family has the time, coming with the patient to appointments is always helpful because they can support the patient. If that is not possible, a phone conversation with doctor, while the patient listens, could be helpful.

George: Some patients said, "My family members don't trust these medicines and don't trust the doctors." But many of the patients also felt that the family members were actually tougher on them. They didn't want their family members to know that they hadn't been taking their medicine. If family members came to the doctor with the patient, they'd have a better understanding of the burden of the disease and the complexity of the regimen. Family members might then learn to be more understanding of lapses in therapy and still provide some motivation for the patient to stay on the straight and narrow.

Chapter 45

What's the Difference between Rescue and Controller Medications?

Asthma medicine comes in two main types: controller medicine and rescue medicine. Rescue medications, also called quick-relief or fast-acting medications, work immediately to relieve asthma symptoms when they occur. These types of medicines are often inhaled directly into the lungs, where they open up the airways and relieve symptoms such as wheezing, coughing, and shortness of breath, often within minutes. But as effective as they are, rescue medications don't have a long-term effect.

Controller medications, also called preventive or maintenance medications, work over a period of time to reduce airway inflammation and help prevent asthma symptoms from occurring. They may be inhaled or swallowed as a pill or liquid.

Rescue Medications

Quick-acting bronchodilators, usually given through an inhaler or a nebulizer, loosen the tightened muscles around inflamed airways and are the most often-prescribed rescue medications. The most common of these are called beta2-agonists. These medications are related

---

This information was provided by KidsHealth, one of the largest resources online for medically reviewed health information written for parents, kids, and teens. For more articles like this one, visit www.KidsHealth.org, or www.Teens Health.org. © 2004 The Nemours Center for Children's Health Media, a division of The Nemours Foundation.

to adrenaline and usually work within minutes to provide temporary relief of symptoms.

If the bronchodilator alone doesn't resolve a severe flare-up, other medications may be given by mouth or injection to help treat it.

If your child has been prescribed rescue medication, it's important to keep these medicines on hand. That means at home, at the mall, at sport practice, and even on vacation.

Rescue medications, although an important part of asthma treatment, can be overused. Talk with your child's doctor about how often your child uses the rescue medication. If it's too much, the doctor also may prescribe a controller medicine, designed to prevent asthma flare-ups from happening.

Controller Medications

Because your child's airways may be inflamed even in between flare-ups, controller medications may be needed to prevent unexpected asthma flare-ups. Slower-acting controller medicines can take weeks to start working, but when they do, they prevent airway inflammation and keep the lungs from making too much mucus.

There are a variety of controller medications, but inhaled corticosteroids are most common. They're usually given through an inhaler or nebulizer. Despite their name, corticosteroids are not the same as performance-enhancing steroids used by athletes. They are a safe and proven form of treatment for asthma.

In fact, inhaled corticosteroids are the preferred long-term treatment for children with frequent asthma symptoms. Research shows that they improve asthma control and their risk of causing long-term negative effects is minimal. (But corticosteroids that are swallowed in liquid or pill form may cause side effects if used daily over a long period of time.)

Long-acting bronchodilators can also be used as controller medications. These relax the muscles of the airways for up to 12 hours, but can't be used for quick relief of symptoms because they don't start to work immediately.

Even if your child takes controller medicine regularly, rescue medication will still be needed to handle flare-ups when they occur.

Working with the Doctor

Your child's doctor will determine which type of medicine your child needs, depending on how frequent and how severe the asthma symptoms are. Both the type and dosage of medication that your child needs

The Difference between Rescue and Controller Medications?

are likely to change, with the goal being to have your child on the lowest amount of medication necessary for effective asthma management.

Because you spend more time with your child than the doctor will, you're an important player in your child's asthma treatment. For example, you can track how well the medicine is working by using a peak flow meter. You also can record information in an asthma diary and ask your doctor to create an asthma action plan, if you don't already have one. By reporting any concerns or changes in your child's symptoms, you can provide information that will help the doctor select the best course of treatment.

Chapter 46

What You Should Know about Corticosteroids

In 1935, the Mayo Clinic reported a research breakthrough that would affect millions of lives. Doctors had isolated the hormone cortisone from the adrenal glands, the walnut sized glands sitting on top of the kidneys. Cortisone produced by the adrenal glands reduces inflammation in the body.

The Mayo Clinic physicians first used cortisone to treat people with severe rheumatoid arthritis. Improvements were so dramatic in soothing swollen joints that patients crippled from the disease were actually able to walk again.

Pharmaceutical companies have since produced corticosteroid medications that mimic the hormone cortisone. For people with asthma, corticosteroids literally can be lifesavers by preventing or reversing inflammation in the airways, making them less sensitive to triggers. The drugs, sometimes referred to as "preventive" or "long-term control" medicines, work effectively to keep asthma episodes in check. They are not the same as anabolic steroids, which some athletes take illegally to build muscle mass.

Corticosteroid Safety

Oral, or systemic, corticosteroids quickly help out-of-control asthma, but more than two weeks of daily use may sometimes lead to serious

---

"Corticosteroids," reprinted with permission from the Asthma and Allergy Foundation of America, © 2005. All rights reserved. For additional information about asthma and related topics visit the AAFA website at http://www.aafa.org.

side effects. Inhaled corticosteroids are considered much safer for lengthier treatment. Unlike the oral forms that must travel throughout your body to reach your lungs, inhaled corticosteroids are delivered directly to the airways in small doses with less chance of reaching other parts of the body. The National Institutes of Health (NIH) calls inhaled corticosteroids "the most effective long-term therapy available for patients with persistent asthma. In general [they] are well tolerated and safe at the recommended dosages."

You have probably read or heard varying reports about the risks of corticosteroid use. The bottom line is that the relatively few side effects are usually balanced by the good they do for your asthma. Steroids are safe when used in the lower dosage range. Problems generally arise with high doses over long periods of time. As consumers and patients, it's important to know what specific side effects may occur and how we can work with our physicians to control them and our asthma.

Localized Risks

Oral candidiasis (thrush): Only 10 percent to 30 percent of inhaled steroid doses actually reach the lungs. The remainder is left in the mouth or throat or is swallowed, sometimes resulting in thrush, a fungal infection that produces milky white lesions in the mouth. Clinical thrush is far less common in lower dosages and affects more adults than children.

Physicians recommend using a spacer or holding chamber with your inhaler and rinsing your mouth with water after each treatment to reduce the amount of the inhaled steroid deposited in the mouth and throat. If you develop thrush, your doctor may also prescribe a less frequent dose and/or topical or oral antifungal medication.

Dysphonia (hoarseness): This condition is associated with increasing dosages of inhaled corticosteroids and vocal stress. Treatment may include using a spacer/holding chamber, less frequent dosing, and/or temporarily decreasing medication.

Systemic Risks

Slowed growth in children: Some studies have shown that medium-dose inhaled corticosteroids may affect a child's growth. It is not certain that this results in shorter stature in adulthood, but in general, the higher the dose, the greater the risk.

What You Should Know about Corticosteroids

In a 1995 study of 7 to 9-year-olds treated daily with 400 micrograms of beclomethasone for seven months, growth was significantly decreased in both boys and girls. There was no evidence of catchup growth after a five month period without medication. Yet a 1994 study of inhaled beclomethasone found no significant adverse effects on achieving adult height.

The National Institutes of Health (NIH) advises physicians to carefully monitor a young patient's height and to "step down" therapy when possible. NIH notes that even high doses of inhaled corticosteroids with children experiencing severe, persistent asthma create less risk of delayed growth than treatment with oral systemic corticosteroids (pills or capsules).

Osteoporosis (bone disease): In some people, high corticosteroid usage can reduce bone-mineral density, leading to osteoporosis. Links have been found between steroid use and inhibiting bone formation, calcium absorption, and the production of sex hormones that

Table 46.1. What are Considered Low, Medium and High Corticosteroid Dosages?

A = adult; C = child

All dosages are daily, in micrograms (mcg)

Drug	A/C	Low	Medium	High
Beclomethasone	A	168–504	504–840	840+
dipropionate	C	84–336	336–672	672+
Budesonide	A	200–400	400–600	600+
Turbuhaler	C	100–200	200–400	400+
Flunisolide	A	500–1000	1000–2000	2000+
	C	500–750	1000–1250	1250
Fluticasone	A	88–264	264–660	660+
	C	88–176	176–440	440+
Triamcinolone	A	400–1000	1000–2000	2000
acetonide	C	400–800	800–1200	1200

Source: NIH *Guidelines of the Diagnosis and Management of Asthma*, April 1997.

help keep bones vital. Brief courses of systemic corticosteroids or low-dose inhaled steroids are not dangerous, but inhaling 1500 micrograms of beclomethasone per day can lead to bone loss. The doses of other inhaled steroids, which may constitute a risk for osteoporosis, have not been studied.

Even if you need to take steroids for your asthma, you can take measures to protect yourself against osteoporosis. Here are some recommendations:

- Take the lowest dose possible and use inhaled steroids rather than oral preparations.

- Get about 1,500 milligrams (mg) of calcium daily through nutrition or supplements. Because vitamin D helps the body absorb calcium, it may help to take 800 international units (IU) daily of vitamin D.

Disseminated varicella (chickenpox): The U.S. Food and Drug Administration (FDA) reported that long-term or high-dose oral corticosteroid treatment might place people exposed to chickenpox or measles at increased risk of unusually severe infections or even death. That's because some doses suppress the immune system. "Children who are on immunosuppressant drugs are more susceptible to infections than healthy children," said the FDA. Yet, the NIH Guidelines said there is no evidence that recommended doses of inhaled corticosteroids suppress the immune system.

NIH advises that children who have not had chickenpox and periodically take oral corticosteroids should receive the varicella vaccine after they've been steroid-free for at least one month. Kids who have finished a short course of prednisone may receive the vaccine immediately. For un-immunized adults and children who are exposed to chickenpox while being treated with immunosuppressive levels of steroids, there are immunoglobulin and acyclovir.

Cataracts: The risk of cataracts in patients taking systemic corticosteroids has been well identified, but reports among those taking inhaled steroids are rare. In a notable exception, the *New England Journal of Medicine* published findings of a recent Australian study of inhaled corticosteroid users between the ages of 49 and 97. The authors concluded that the use of inhaled steroids is associated with an increased risk for development of cataracts. Patients taking moderate to high doses of inhaled corticosteroids especially should have regular eye exams.

What You Should Know about Corticosteroids

Other Risks

The NIH *Guidelines* also list a few other rare but potential risks of high dose corticosteroid use. In some cases, oral steroid use has been linked with adrenal suppression, effects on glucose metabolism, and hypertension. Serious medical complications have also been recorded in people on high doses of oral steroids with tuberculosis.

None of the above risks have been reported with inhaled corticosteroids. However, their use in moderate to high doses has been found to contribute to thinning and bruising of the skin, especially among women.

Oral (Systemic) Corticosteroids

- Generally for short-term use
- Quickly controls persistent asthma
- Forms: pills, tablets or liquid (for children)
- Medications: Methylprednisolone, Prednisolone, Prednisone

Inhaled Corticosteroids

- For long-term asthma prevention; suppress, control and reverse inflammation
- Forms: dry powder or aerosol
- Medications: Beclomethasone dipropionate, Budesonide, Flunisolide, Fluticasone propionate, Triamcinolone acetonide

Chapter 47

Asthma and Bronchodilators

Wheezing and difficult breathing in asthma are caused by narrowing of the air passageways—called bronchial tubes—of the lungs. One of the important causes of narrowing of the bronchial tubes is contraction of the muscles that are present in a ring around these tubes. In asthma, contraction of these muscles causes the bronchial tubes to become more narrow than normal.

Medications to Open Bronchial Tubes Wider

Bronchodilators are medications that cause the bronchial muscles to relax and, as a result, the bronchial tubes to open wider or dilate. When these muscles relax, the bronchial tubes can usually open fully again and breathing can become normal. We say "usually" because sometimes the bronchial tubes themselves are swollen and filled with mucus. If this swelling and plugging of the bronchial tubes is present, then a bronchodilating medication will only bring partial relief of asthma symptoms. In this case, even when the bronchial muscles are made to relax, the bronchial tubes remain partially narrowed and blocked.

In this chapter we discuss the various types of bronchodilating medications and their effects in asthma. First, to understand better

---

This information is reprinted with permission from the Partners Asthma Center, http://www.asthma.partners.org, © 2005. All rights reserved.

how bronchodilators work, it is necessary to explore a little more about the bronchial muscles.

Bronchial Muscles Are "Involuntary" Muscles

Muscles in our body over which we have conscious control are called "voluntary" muscles. If we want to, we can make our arms and legs move by causing contraction of the voluntary muscles in our arms and legs. On the other hand, many muscles in our body are controlled unconsciously. For instance, we have no conscious control over the beating of our heart muscle or the contractions of our stomach muscles. Like these muscles, the muscles around our bronchial tubes are "involuntary" muscles; they are under the control of our nervous system but are not controlled by the thinking parts of our brain.

Contraction of the Bronchial Muscles

Although the bronchial muscles do not work quite as fast as the voluntary muscles, they can squeeze or contract over approximately a minute or two. Anyone with asthma who has experienced the rapid onset of chest tightness and labored breathing and wheezing—for instance, after running on a cold day or being exposed to smoke or strong fumes—knows the effect of bronchial muscle contraction and the rapidity with which it can develop. The good news here is that relaxation of these bronchial muscles can occur equally rapidly, over a period of just a few minutes, allowing the bronchial tubes to widen again and breathing to occur freely.

Bronchodilators and Exercise

If asthma symptoms develop after running on a cold day, the bronchial muscles, left unstimulated, will usually gradually relax on their own over approximately an hour or less and the symptoms of asthma will go away. Bronchodilators are useful medications because they speed this process of relaxation of the bronchial muscles and can sometimes be used to prevent or block the contraction of the bronchial muscles in the first place. You may have made these observations yourself. If you use your bronchodilator medication before exercising, you can avoid developing wheezing, cough, and shortness of breath. If you use your bronchodilator after exercising has caused symptoms, the medication generally relieves the symptoms within 5 minutes or less. And if you simply stop exercising and wait, you gradually get better again over the next 30–60 minutes or so.

Asthma and Bronchodilators

Choices among Bronchodilators

Bronchodilators can be taken in different forms. They can be breathed in as a spray or mist, swallowed as a tablet or capsule, and sometimes given as an injection or intravenous medication (through a needle in a blood vessel). The advantage of inhaling bronchodilators is that the medication goes rapidly and directly to the bronchial muscles; it does not have to pass through the stomach and blood vessels to get there. As a result, inhaled bronchodilators are usually stronger and have fewer unpleasant side effects than swallowed bronchodilators.

Beta-agonist Bronchodilators: Like most medicines, bronchodilators can be grouped into general "families" or groups of medicines based on their chemical properties. The most widely used family of bronchodilators at the present time is called the beta-adrenergic agonists or beta agonists for short. Beta, the Greek letter "B," simply distinguishes this family of medications from a different group labeled with an "A." Agonists describe medications that stimulate something, and in this case refer to stimulation of the bronchial muscles to relax. Adrenergic refers to the adrenaline-like properties of these medicines. Examples of beta-agonist bronchodilators that can be inhaled are familiar to you: they include the generic names albuterol, metaproterenol, pirbuterol, terbutaline, formoterol, and salmeterol and the brand names Ventolin®, Proventil®, Alupent®, Metaprel®, Maxair®, Brethaire®, Foradil® and Serevent®.

Some of the beta-agonist bronchodilators are also available in tablet form. Although it often is more convenient to swallow a tablet than to use an inhaler, these same medications when taken by mouth generally are not as strong and tend to have more unpleasant side effects than when breathed in. The most common side effects of the beta agonists are raciness, jitteriness, heart pounding, tremulousness, and a nervous feeling. The beta agonists do not cause high blood pressure.

Theophylline Family of Bronchodilators: Another family of bronchodilator medications is only available to swallow or inject intravenously: the theophylline family. The special advantage of this group of bronchodilators is that with some of them the bronchodilator stays in the blood for 12–24 hours after taking the tablet or capsule, making possible use once or twice a day with continuous benefit throughout the day. There are several disadvantages to theophylline bronchodilators, however. They are not as strong as the beta agonists; they often have unpleasant side effects, especially stomach discomfort, loose bowels, sleeplessness, and jitteriness; and occasionally they can have dangerous effects (abnormal heart rhythms and seizures) when excessive amounts of theophylline get into the blood (an overdose). The amount of theophylline bronchodilator in the blood can be measured with a blood test, referred to as the "theophylline level." Many brand name examples of theophylline exist, including Theo-Dur®, Uni-Dur®, Uniphyl®, Slo-Phyllin®, Slo-bid®, and others. Theophylline is the generic name for all of these medicines.

Anticholinergic Bronchodilators (Used to Treat Emphysema and Chronic Bronchitis): One other family of bronchodilators is used in patients with emphysema and chronic bronchitis but is not usually recommended in asthma. The inhaled bronchodilator ipratropium (brand name, Atrovent®) is not as effective in asthma as are the beta agonist bronchodilators; it is weaker and takes longer to begin to work. Only in certain special circumstances would we recommend this type of bronchodilator for persons with asthma.

What Bronchodilators Do Not Do

It is important to remember that not all of asthma is corrected by causing the bronchial muscles to relax. Swelling of the bronchial tubes and their blockage with mucus—the aspects of asthma that we refer to as "inflammation," do not go away when bronchial muscles relax. If you use your bronchodilator medication and don't obtain relief of your asthma symptoms, the problem may not be with the bronchodilator. Bronchodilators cannot fix inflamed bronchial tubes. Other medications are available to treat this other aspect of asthma, the anti-inflammatory medications. Remember: if you are having difficulty with your asthma that is not fixed with use of your bronchodilator, other types of treatments are available and are likely to be needed. Your doctor can prescribe them for you and help guide you in how to use them.

Chapter 48

What You Should Know about Medication Delivery Devices

Puffs, Sprays, Powders, and Mists

Because aerosol asthma medications target the airways, they are the cornerstones of asthma therapy. Yet the technology that makes them work remains a deep mystery to most people who use them.

Television commercials made it look easy: press the inhaler and breathe. How complicated could it be? That's what I thought 20 years ago when my internist prescribed my first inhaler. With only a prescription in hand and no instruction, I was on my own.

Many asthma attacks later, I learned my timing was off; I was supposed to start a slow deep breath a split second before pressing the top of the inhaler. How could something so simple make such a difference?

This chapter begins with "Puffs, Sprays, Powders, and Mists, oh my!" by Nancy Sander, 2003. Reprinted courtesy of Allergy & Asthma Network Mothers of Asthmatics (AANMA), 800-878-4403, www.breatherville.org, © 2003. It continues with "How To Use Medication Devices." This section includes text from "Using Your Puffer Tip Sheet," "Pressured Metered Dose Inhaler," "Spacer," "Turbuhaler," "Diskhaler," and "Diskus," reprinted with permission from the Asthma Society of Canada, © 2003, all rights reserved. For additional information about asthma, visit http://www.asthma.ca/adults/ or http://asthma-kids.ca (illustrations redrawn with permission by Alison DeKleine). The chapter concludes with "Nebulizer Treatment and Cleaning." This information is reprinted with permission from the Cincinnati Children's Hospital Medical Center website, http://www.cincinnatichildrens.org. © 2005 Cincinnati Children's Hospital Medical Center. All rights reserved.

Inhaled medications can't work unless they reach the airways. And they won't reach the airways unless you know how to use the technology inside these powerful devices.

It's What's Inside

Just remember this—a mist is not just a mist. Inhalation technology is a science that couples white, crystalline asthma medication (the formulation) with an inhalation delivery system, the mechanical packaging. For example, metered dose inhaler (MDI) formulations employ a propellant-driven system consisting of a pressurized canister (a metering chamber or reservoir, valves, rings, and other components) that fits inside a plastic actuator, sometimes called a boot or sleeve because of its shape.

Dry powder inhaler (DPI) formulations are housed in breath-activated, plastic-encased auto- or manual-loading devices.

Nebulizers use several different types of technologies to break liquid formulations into a fine mist that is inhaled over 5 to 20 minutes. Jet nebulizers use compressed air, ultrasonic models use sound waves, and yet another type uses vibration technology.

There is no "one-size-fits-all" perfect aerosol delivery system. Some people use all three delivery systems while others use just one type. Furthermore, not all asthma medications are formulated for use in all types of delivery devices.

Reading the Fine Print

Even when inhalation delivery devices look similar or contain comparable formulations, there are distinct differences among them detailed in the patient instruction sheet packaged with each prescription. I'm sure you've seen it—it's the tissue-thin folded paper with all the tiny print. Open the paper and look for the heading "Patient Instructions."

For example, both Proventil® HFA and Ventolin® HFA contain the identical active ingredient, racemic albuterol, and a hydrofluoroalkane (HFA) propellant. After that, they're quite different. Ethanol (alcohol) and oleic acid (made from palm oil) are added to Proventil HFA to keep medication and propellants from clumping together. Ventolin HFA does not require anti-clumping agents and other additives.

Beyond ingredients used, other notable differences among formulations and inhalation devices include the number of doses contained, cleaning advisories, number of priming doses required, inhalation techniques, and storage recommendations.

What You Should Know about Medication Delivery Devices

Whole Lotta Shakin' Goin' On

Common to all MDIs is the instruction to "SHAKE THE INHALER WELL immediately before each use." It's an important step, one that's simple enough to do but so easy to forget.

Why is a shake-up so important? Most people do not know that the medication contained in each MDI starts out as a crystalline powder. Shaking the MDI vigorously a few times before use mixes the contents so that each dose contains the right blend of medication, propellant, and other ingredients. This blend is called a suspension.

DPIs, on the other hand, need no mixing and should never be shaken. In fact, if you shake it after a dose is loaded into the inhalation chamber, you may lose the dose entirely.

Most nebulizer solutions do not need shaking. However, Pulmicort Respules™ (budesonide) package instructions show patients how to swirl the single-dose vial in an upright circular motion to blend contents thoroughly before using.

Ready for Prime Time

Both Proventil HFA and Ventolin HFA MDI instructions advise the user to "prime the inhaler before using the first time and in cases where the inhaler has not been used for more than two weeks." (Note: Priming instructions and frequency vary among MDI formulations.)

Priming the inhaler loads a single dose into a metering chamber or reservoir. To prime a Proventil HFA or Ventolin HFA inhaler, the instructions tell you to shake and spray "four [yes, it says four] doses of medication into the air away from your face." Actuating the inhaler releases a single dose of medication from the metering chamber in the form of a mist. After each spray, the metering chamber is automatically primed for the next dose.

But why must you prime Proventil HFA and Ventolin HFA if you haven't used it for two weeks? I asked the question of several experts and got great but heavily technical answers, so bear with me here.

When the MDI has not been used for a while, the formulation separates and active medication settles to the bottom of the canister and the metering chamber. Shaking the MDI may not produce turbulence sufficient to re-blend the ingredients in the smaller chambers. Discarding the first few doses ensures the next one you inhale contains the labeled amount of medication.

As Is

The patient instruction sheet pictures a patient using the MDI exactly as approved by the U.S. Food and Drug Administration (FDA), with the MDI placed directly into the mouth. The patient closes his lips tightly around the mouthpiece. "While breathing in deeply and slowly through the mouth, fully depress the top of the metal canister with your index finger," say the instructions.

While the closed-mouth technique works, others may work better for you. If you notice that the medication winds up on your tongue and tonsils, tastes bad, or the propellant sprays out too quickly, your medical care provider can show you other inhalation techniques using the same device.

One method is to place the MDI about two inches in front of your open mouth and begin a slow, deep inhalation a split-second before pressing the top of the inhaler with your index finger. Continue the inhalation until your lungs are fully expanded, hold your breath a few seconds, and then slowly release it. If your physician has prescribed taking a second dose, wait one minute, shake the inhaler, and repeat the steps above.

However, if split-second timing isn't your thing, many medical professionals suggest using the MDI with a valved holding chamber, a hollow device fitted with a one-way flap that traps and suspends medication long enough to inhale over a 3-to-5 second period.

There are many different types of holding chambers, and as you might expect, results vary among device brands and formulations. While valved holding chambers are FDA-regulated medical devices, few studies document their effectiveness across all MDI brands and formulations available today. Your medical care provider can help you select the best inhalation device and/or valved holding chamber for you or your child.

Never attempt to use a holding chamber with a DPI. When using a DPI, simply load the dose (usually with a twist of the hand or flick of a finger), place the device in your mouth, and inhale as directed in the patient instruction sheet. Your inhalation draws tiny medicated grains into your airways so gently you may not even notice any sensation of taking a medication.

Boot Swap

Like hand-in-glove, each brand of MDI canister (the metal cylinder containing medication) is designed and FDA-approved for use only

What You Should Know about Medication Delivery Devices

with the actuator (the plastic boot-shaped sleeve in which the canister fits) supplied by the manufacturer.

The only time you should remove the canister from the boot is when cleaning the actuator. Never insert the canister into a different actuator.

Good Clean Fun

Got an MDI handy? Choose one you use daily or have used more than a dozen times. Remove the mouthpiece cap and look inside. Do you see that tiny little hole where the medication comes out?

See the white, crusty stuff forming around the hole? You are looking at crystalline medication. When dried crystals accumulate around the hole, less medication gets through to the airways.

Always clean the MDI exactly as directed in the package insert. Most MDIs should be cleaned weekly, but a few designs should be cleaned daily. Never place the MDI canister in water. To clean, carefully remove the canister from the boot and run warm water through the top and bottom of the plastic boot for 30 seconds. Never place the boot in boiling water or in the dishwasher. Excessive heat is not necessary and may cause the boot to distort.

It's best to clean MDIs after taking an evening dose. Allow the MDI boot to dry on the countertop before replacing the canister the next morning.

DPIs should never come in contact with water. Nebulizer cups should be cleaned after every use. Tubing should be replaced as often as instructed in the package insert. Some air compressor units have small felt-like filter disks that need to be replaced at specific intervals posted in the patient use materials. Order these and other replacement parts long before they are needed. Instructions vary among nebulizer brands; check and follow manufacturers recommendations.

Dry Dock Your Inhaled Medications

Dry powder inhalers are low-maintenance medications. Keep them moisture-free (in a resealable plastic bag if stored in the bathroom medicine cabinet) and watch the dose indicator countdown until time for a refill.

Some nebulized medications must be stored in a refrigerator or used within a specific period of time before discarding.

Never leave back-up medications, whether MDIs, DPIs or nebulizer vials, in the glove compartment of your car. Temperature extremes affect all inhaled medications; MDIs can explode in extreme heat conditions or fail to fire properly in cold climates.

Running on Empty and in the Dark

Contrary to popular belief, MDI formulations are not good to the last drop. Once you've used the number of doses posted in the package insert (also printed on the canister label), the quality and content of any additional doses released cannot be ensured to contain the labeled amount of medication. At this point, the package insert says to throw the canister away even when it is not empty.

However, unless you keep track of every dose taken and each priming dose released, it's impossible to know when you've reached or exceeded this magic number. It's a little like driving the family car without a gas gauge and odometer—stressful and dangerous.

Short of carving notches into the side of your MDI, how do you keep track of every actuation? Try this simple formula to calculate MDI refill dates for medications used on a daily basis (such as inhaled corticosteroids and Serevent®). You won't need a pocket abacus (or Palm Pilot), just paper and pencil:

- Write down the total number of labeled doses, then subtract the number of priming doses recommended. Divide this by the number of doses you plan to use each day. The result will give you the number of days you can use your MDI.

For example, an MDI corticosteroid canister containing 200 doses will last 49 days if used twice each morning and evening: 200 total doses minus four priming doses equals 196 total doses. Divide this by four doses a day to get 49 days. After that, even though the canister doesn't feel empty, it's time to throw it away.

Computing refill dates for bronchodilators, however, is downright tricky. You don't use them every day (and if you do, it's time to see your doctor—now). You use them now and then; when symptoms first creep up on you or when you're hit by a blast of secondhand cigarette smoke. Or when a cold settles into your chest. Or when your 10-year-old can't stop coughing at 2:00 A.M. Or before your morning jog.

Both Proventil HFA and Ventolin HFA (as well as generic albuterol MDIs) are factory-filled to deliver 200 quality-assured doses of medication. (Maxair™ Autohaler™ holds 400.) Will these MDIs last you a year or a month or somewhere in between? How many days-worth of priming doses will be discarded?

What You Should Know about Medication Delivery Devices

You simply won't know when this symptom-halting, lifesaving MDI is running on empty unless you keep a daily symptom diary, or make tic marks on the side of the MDI with each actuation including priming doses.

There is another alternative: a digital, battery-powered counter called The Doser™. It attaches to the top of most inhalers. It extends the height of the inhaler making it clumsy to use for small hands, and you need one device for each type of inhaler you are using, but for those so inclined to spend $25.00 or more per MDI, it is a good retrofit. For information, call 800-863-9633, or visit www.doser.com.

Solve Your Mysteries

There's more to aerosol technology than meets the eye. So go ahead, open that patient instruction sheet and bravely tackle the fine print. Like Sherlock Holmes, you might have to use a magnifying glass, but you'll learn how to get the most from your inhaled medications.

How To Use Medication Devices

Using Your Inhaler

Your inhaler is the tool you use to take the medication that takes care of your asthma, so its pretty important to use it properly. Here are some tips to keep in mind every time you use your inhaler.

- **Stand Up Straight:** You can use your inhaler either sitting down or standing up, but either way, make sure you have a super straight back.
- **Empty The Tank:** You want to make some room in your airways for your medicine, and the more air you let out of your lungs, the more mist you can take in. So breathe out fully before you breathe your mist in.
- **Breathe In Deeply:** Take a deep breath as you take your medication. You want to make sure the medication reaches all your airways, so don't stop breathing in until your lungs are full.
- **Hang on:** When you've breathed in as much as you can, hold your breath for about 10 seconds before you breathe out again. Ten seconds is about as long as it takes for you to count to ten slowly.

- **Let It Go, But Slow:** When you're done, breathe out slowly. If you need to take a second dose, wait 30 seconds before starting over.

- **Check It:** When you've taken your dose, check your inhaler to see how much is left.

- **Stash It:** Put your inhaler in a safe place where you'll remember it for next time.

Pressured Metered Dose Inhaler Or Metered Dose Inhaler

A pressured metered dose inhaler or metered dose inhaler can be called "pMDI" or "MDI" for short. Here are some special tips for using your MDI:

- Give your inhaler a good shake before you use it. Three or four shakes should do the trick.
- Take off the cap.
- Breathe out, away from your inhaler.

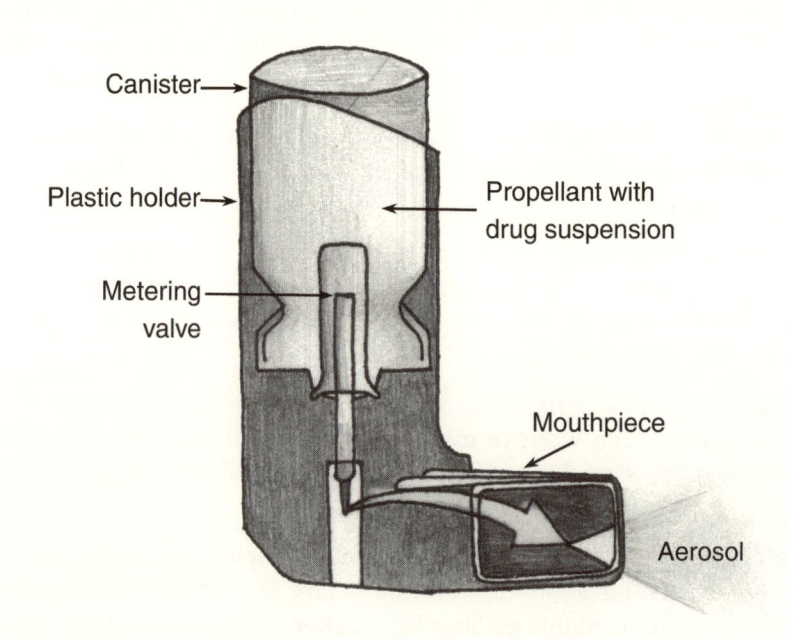

Figure 48.1. A metered dose inhaler looks like this.

What You Should Know about Medication Delivery Devices

- Bring the inhaler to your mouth. You can either put the mouthpiece gently between your teeth and close your lips around it, or you can hold it two finger-widths in front of your open mouth.
- Start to breathe in slowly.
- Press the top of your inhaler once and keep breathing in slowly until you've taken a full breath.
- Hold your breath for about 10 seconds, then breathe out slowly.

If you need a second puff, shake your inhaler again, and repeat after 30 seconds.

Always write down the number of puffs you've taken. This is the best way to tell how much medicine you have left.

Spacer

If you use a pressurized metered dose inhaler (pMDI) then your doctor may want you to use a spacer device so you can get more medicine into your airways. Here are some special tips for using your pMDI with a spacer:

- Give the inhaler a good shake before you use it. Three or four shakes should do the trick.
- Take the cap off your inhaler, and off your spacer too, if it has one.
- Put the inhaler into the spacer.
- Breathe out, away from the spacer.
- Bring the spacer to your mouth and put the mouthpiece gently between your teeth and close your lips around it. Be careful not to cover the air holes with your hands or mouth.
- Press the top of your inhaler once.
- Breathe in slowly until you've taken a full breath. If you hear a whistle sound, this means you are breathing in too fast. Slowly breathe in.
- Hold your breath for about 10 seconds, then breathe out slowly.

If you need a second puff, shake your inhaler again, and repeat after 30 seconds.

Always write down the number of puffs you've taken. This is the best way to tell how much medicine you have left.

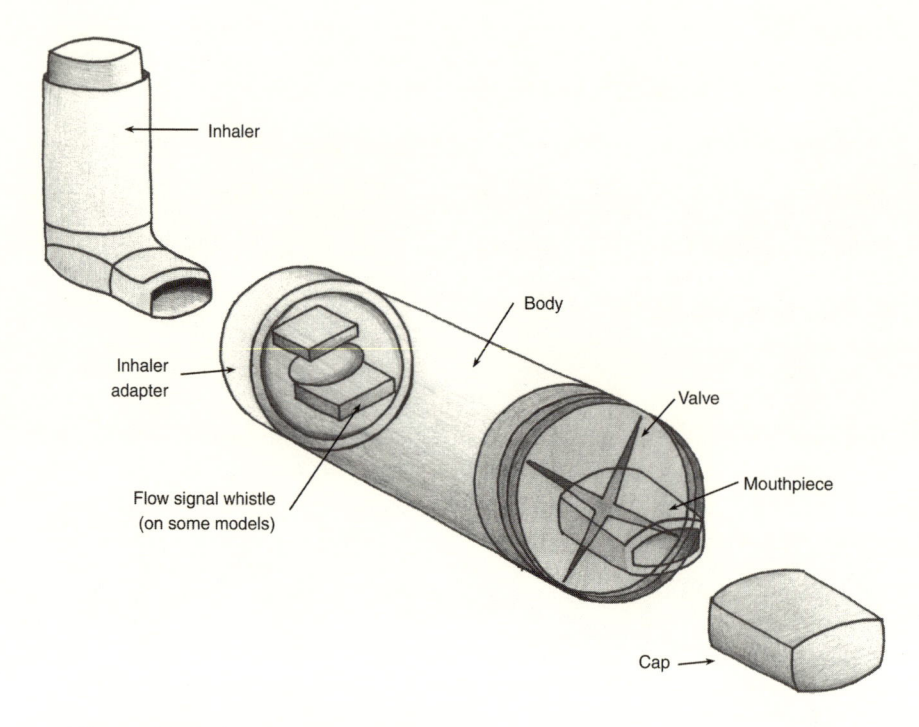

Figure 48.2. A spacer looks like this.

Turbuhaler

Here are some special tips for using your Turbuhaler:

- Unscrew the cap and take it off.
- Twist the bottom of your Turbuhaler as far as you can, then twist it all the way back. You'll know you've done it right when you hear a click.
- Put the mouthpiece between your teeth, close your lips around it.
- Breathe in very fast until you've taken a full breath.
- Hold your breath for about 10 seconds, then breathe out slowly.

What You Should Know about Medication Delivery Devices

Always check to see how much medicine is left by looking in the window under the mouthpiece. When you start to see a red color, your medicine is running out.

Diskhaler

Here are some special tips for using your Diskhaler:

- Take the cover off your mouthpiece.

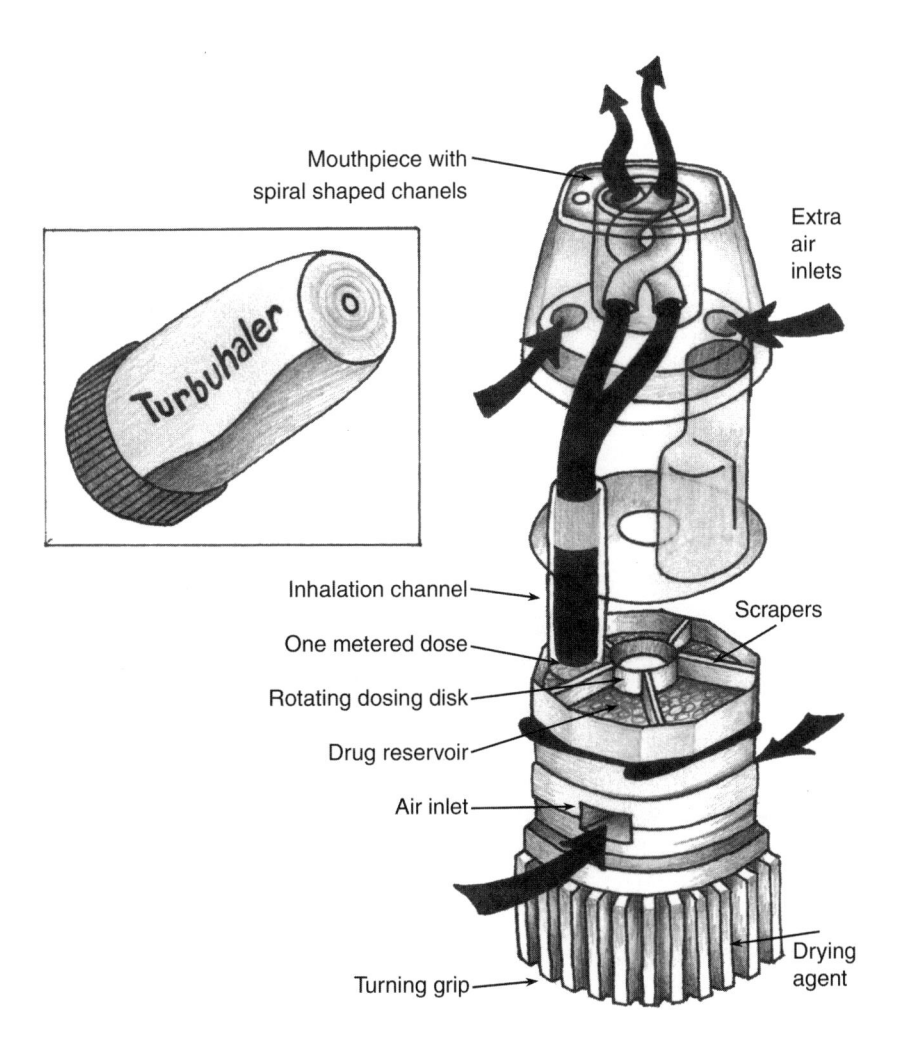

Figure 48.3. A Turbuhaler looks like this.

- Lift the lid of your Diskhaler as far as it will go, then close it again. This gets the medication ready.
- Breathe out.
- Place the mouthpiece gently between you teeth and close your lips around it. Careful not to cover the air holes on the side.
- Breathe in deeply until you've taken a full breath.
- Hold your breath for about 10 seconds, then breathe out slowly.

Always check to see how much medicine is left by looking in the dose counter window. The number you see in this window will tell you how many doses are left.

Diskus

Here are some tips for using your Diskus:

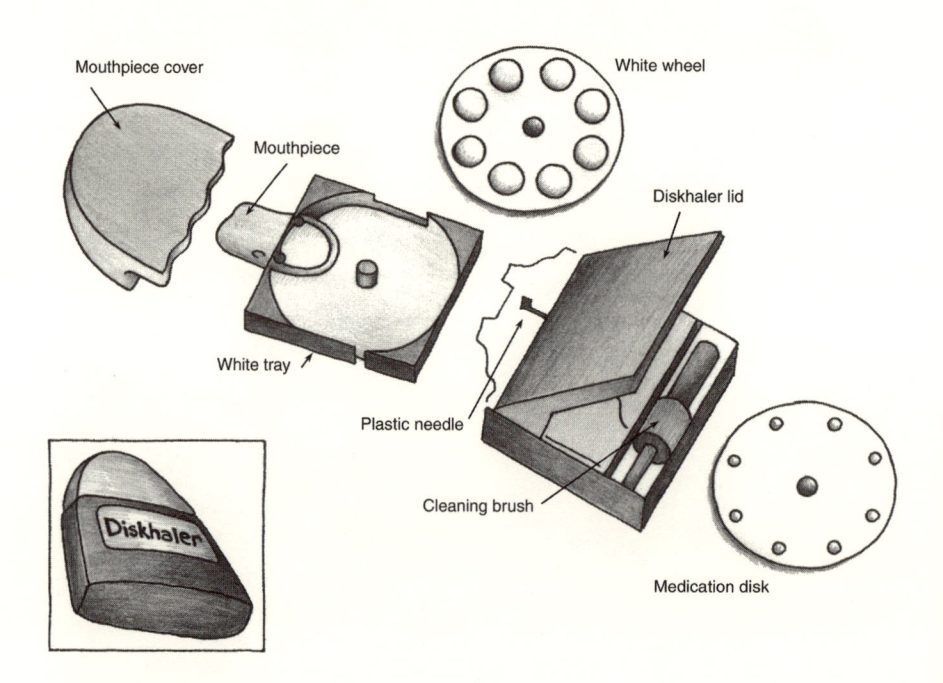

Figure 48.4. A Diskhaler looks like this.

What You Should Know about Medication Delivery Devices

- Open your Diskus by holding it in the palm of your hand, and put the thumb of your other hand on the thumbgrip, then push the thumbgrip until it clicks into place.
- Slide the lever away from you as far as it will go. This gets your medication ready.
- Breathe out away from the device. Don't breathe into the device.

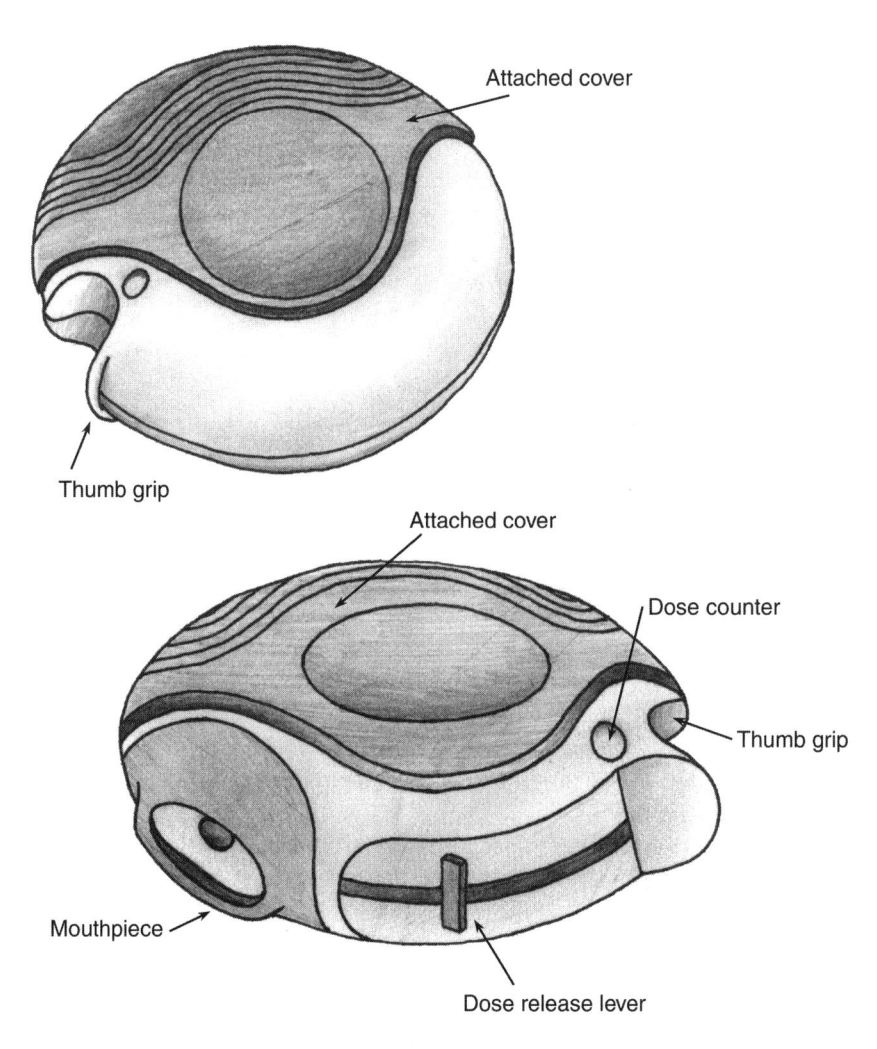

Figure 48.5. A Diskus looks like this.

- Place the mouthpiece gently in your mouth and close your lips around it.
- Breathe in deeply until you've taken a full breath.
- Hold your breath for about 10 seconds, then breathe out slowly.

Always check to see how much medicine is left by looking in the dose counter window. The number you see in this window will tell you how many doses are left.

Nebulizer Treatment and Cleaning

A nebulizer changes liquid medicine into fine droplets (in aerosol or mist form) that are inhaled through a mouthpiece or mask. Nebulizers can be used to deliver bronchodilator (airway-opening) medications such as albuterol, Xopenex, or Pulmicort (steroid).

A nebulizer may be used instead of a metered dose inhaler (MDI). It is powered by a compressed air machine and plugs into an electrical outlet.

Treatment Procedure

1. Place the air compressor on a sturdy surface that will support its weight. Plug the cord from the compressor into a properly grounded (three prong) electrical outlet.
2. Wash your hands with soap and warm water and dry completely with a clean towel.
3. Carefully measure medications exactly as you have been instructed.
4. Remove the top part of the nebulizer cup.
5. Place your medication in the bottom of the nebulizer cup.
6. Attach the top portion of the nebulizer cup and connect the mouthpiece or face mask to the cup.
7. Connect the tubing to both the aerosol compressor and nebulizer cup.
8. Turn on the compressor with the on/off switch. Once you turn on the compressor, you should see a light mist coming from the back of the tube opposite the mouthpiece.
9. Sit or hold child up straight.

What You Should Know about Medication Delivery Devices

10. If you are using a mask, position it comfortably and securely on your child's face.
11. If you are using a mouth piece, place it between your teeth and seal your lips around it.
12. Take slow, deep breaths through your mouth. If possible, hold each breath for 2–3 seconds before breathing out. This allows the medication to settle into the airways.
13. Continue the treatment until the medication is gone.
14. If you become dizzy or feel "jittery," stop the treatment and rest for about 5 minutes. Then continue the treatment, but try to breathe more slowly. If these symptoms continue with future treatments, inform your health care provider.
15. Turn off the compressor.
16. Take several deep breaths and cough. Continue coughing and try to clear any secretions you may have in your lungs. Cough the secretions into a tissue and dispose of it properly.
17. Wash your hands with warm water and soap and dry them with a clean towel.

Care of Nebulizer

Cleaning and disinfecting your equipment is simple, yet very important. Cleaning should be done in a dust- and smoke-free area away from open windows. Here is how to clean your equipment:

1. After each treatment, rinse the nebulizer cup with warm water, shake off excess water and let it air dry.
2. At the end of each day, the nebulizer cup and mask or mouthpiece should be washed in warm, soapy water using a mild detergent, rinsed thoroughly and allowed to air dry. The Pari reusable nebulizer is dishwasher safe, run through cycle on top rack only in a small parts basket.

Note: There is no need to clean the tubing that connects the nebulizer to the air compressor. Do not put these parts in the dishwasher.

Nebulizer Compressor Care

1. Cover the compressor with a clean cloth when not in use. Keep it clean by wiping it with a clean, damp cloth as needed.

2. Do not put the air compressor on the floor either for treatments or for storage.

3. Check the air compressor's filter as directed. Replace or clean according to the directions from your equipment supplier.

4. Always have an extra nebulizer cup and mask or mouthpiece in case you need it.

5. Medications should be stored in a cool, dry place. Check them often. If they have changed color or formed crystals, throw them away and replace them with new ones.

Important: Unplug the compressor before cleaning it.

Chapter 49

Anti-IgE Therapy: A New Class of Asthma Medication

To understand anti-IgE therapy and its role in treating allergies and asthma, it is first important to understand the relationship between allergies and the body's immune system.

IgE antibodies are key players in allergic reactions. IgE antibodies prompt other cells (mast and basophil cells, among others) to begin the complex chain reaction that culminates in allergy and asthma symptoms such as coughing, sneezing, watery eyes, and shortness of breath.

Traditionally, allergies and allergy-induced asthma are managed using medications that treat IgE-mediated symptoms once they have already begun in the body. While each treatment has its use, none of the available therapies provides a preventive measure against the binding of IgE to mast cells.

A novel, more targeted approach to the treatment of allergies and allergy-induced asthma is called anti-IgE therapy. This new class of medications holds great promise for people with moderate-to-severe allergies and asthma because it is specifically designed to block IgE from initiating the allergic response, potentially preventing the onset of symptoms before they start.

The first medication in this class, called Xolair® (omalizumab), has been approved by the U.S. Food and Drug Administration (FDA) for

---

"Anti-IgE Therapy: A Revolutionary Approach to Controlling Allergy and Asthma," by William E. Berger, MD, May 2004. Reprinted courtesy of Allergy & Asthma Network Mothers of Asthmatics (AANMA), 800-878-4403, www.breatherville.org, © 2004.

the treatment of moderate-to-severe persistent asthma in patients age 12 and older whose symptoms do not respond to standard treatment.

Xolair® is the first biologic treatment that targets allergic asthma. "Biologic" means it uses genetically engineered mammalian proteins, rather than chemicals. Physicians say it breaks the "allergy cascade" — the chain of events that lead to asthma. Specifically, it stops the allergic reaction before it begins, by attaching itself to IgE antibodies and preventing them from causing the allergic reactions that set off asthma symptoms.

Xolair is not a medicine you swallow or inhale; it is an injection given two to four times a month. The effects last as long as you continue the injections. For some of those who have taken it, Xolair offers a way to control allergies and asthma when other options have not worked.

Candidates for Xolair must be 12 years of age or older with moderate-to-severe allergic asthma triggered by year-round allergens in the air as confirmed by a doctor using a skin or blood test, whose symptoms persist even when using inhaled corticosteroids. Frequently, such patients will have the following characteristics:

- daily asthma symptoms
- need for a bronchodilator every day
- two or more times a week when asthma symptoms worsen, either quickly or gradually
- asthma symptoms that disturb sleep one or more nights a week
- Below-normal peak flow meter readings (less than 80%)

Researchers are testing Xolair in patients, both children and adult, who have food and pollen allergies, but the product is not yet approved for treating these disorders.

Despite its potential, it's important to note that anti-IgE therapy is not a cure for asthma or allergies, and that in some cases other medications may still be needed. Additionally, while many people who have taken Xolair have been exposed to allergens without experiencing symptoms, it is advised that people still continue to maintain their allergen avoidance program.

Chapter 50

Can Asthma Be Treated with Acupuncture?

You've probably heard about it through word of mouth—that someone knows someone who turned to acupuncture for relief from chronic asthma symptoms. Even the National Institutes of Health issued a consensus statement in 1997 that concluded that acupuncture was useful as an adjunct (add-on) treatment for a number of physical complaints, including asthma. But does it work? What do we know about acupuncture for the treatment of asthma?

Acupuncture Basics

Acupuncture is a component of traditional Chinese medicine (TCM), a body of knowledge that dates back several thousand years. According to TCM, acupuncture works by pricking the body with tiny needles in strategic locations to balance the flow of the body's chi (pronounced "chee"). Chi is a life force that flows through the body. In a healthy state, chi is responsible for the balance of the universal forces of yin and yang in the body. It encompasses not only the physical aspects of life, but also mental, emotional, and spiritual aspects. People who practice various forms of TCM believe that illness is a symptom of an imbalance of yin and yang. They believe that manipulating or stimulating the flow of chi within a person's body can restore a balance, leading the individual back to good health.

"East Meets West: Treating Asthma with Acupuncture," by Gretchen W. Cook, from *Asthma Magazine*, January/February 2003. Reprinted by permission from Elsevier.

In the body, chi is said to flow through various channels that do not correspond to the circulatory or lymphatic systems but rather a separate system of channels called meridians. Along the meridians there are various acupuncture points—anywhere from 700 to over 2,000, depending on the type of acupuncture.

There are a variety of forms of acupuncture, each using specialized techniques or tools. The use of small needles is what we think of as acupuncture, but there are other, less invasive methods, such as acupressure.

If all this sounds like another language, in a way, it is. TCM operates on a vastly different understanding of illness, health, and how the body operates. The truth is that western medicine cannot yet explain quite how TCM works. Scientists are struggling to study these practices, such as acupuncture, and to understand them within a framework of scientific study and empirical evidence. There is much left to learn about acupuncture.

What Science Says

According to Robert E. Fromm, Jr., MD, clinical associate professor at Baylor College of Medicine, when scientists ask, "Does acupuncture work?" the answer is a disappointing "We don't know."

"Acupuncture has been around since 2,000 B.C.," says Fromm. "And there are certainly people who feel they benefit from acupuncture treatments. But right now, no one can definitively prove that it really works."

"The data vary according to the publication," says Joseph Varon, MD, clinical associate professor at the University of Texas Health Science Center in Houston. "There have been many studies that have reported the effectiveness of acupuncture in asthma and many others that have not. In a recent issue of *Chest*, clinicians in Israel looked at this issue in a well-designed study, showing no difference [in the symptoms] of patients who received acupuncture."

In the United States there are certain protocols for medical research that must be followed to ensure "good science." These things include double-blind studies, where neither the patient nor the researcher knows who is getting a real treatment and who is getting a sham or fake treatment. In this situation, data can be gathered without biases influencing the results. Ideally, such studies can be repeated by other scientists with the same results.

In explaining the issues surrounding research into acupuncture, Fromm also refers to the results of the study reported in the May 2002

Can Asthma Be Treated with Acupuncture?

issue of *Chest*. The issue included a double-blind study involving a small group of patients with asthma. Care was taken to ensure the patients were similar in their asthma condition and overall health. "In this study, acupuncture did not seem to provide a benefit to asthma patients," says Fromm. "Granted, it was a small study group, and the study patients did not have acute asthma, but it remains that the data collected failed to demonstrate any benefit of acupuncture therapy."

Reviews of multiple studies of acupuncture therapy present a mixed bag of results, with little objective data supporting acupuncture, and many studies flawed in their design when contrasted to western medical research methods. The problem in applying western research to eastern medicine may be as much cultural as scientific. According to Dr. Youngran Chung of the Department of Pediatrics at Loyola University Health Systems, one problem is that acupuncture is so well established in China that it is not considered a novel or experimental approach. "One reason you find so few good studies is that in China they have been using acupuncture routinely for centuries. Because doctors there have such a solid positive experience with it, it hasn't been subject to review," says Chung. "There aren't the questions there, as there are in the United States."

One problem with studies of acupuncture in western countries is their poor quality. "Most acupuncture practitioners are in private practice—not an academic setting," says Chung. "So when they do conduct studies, they are often poorly designed by traditional standards. For a western scientist, this renders the study results suspect or unusable."

Another problem with applying western study standards to acupuncture is the great variability in the practice of it. "When I read the results of a study, I want to know how many pressure points were used and which ones," says Chung. "Some studies report use of very few points: sometimes only one. I have a problem with that. If the acupuncture is not done well, then the results are not meaningful."

Acupuncture is also "customized" for each patient. "Just as you have different kinds of asthma, there are different ways of doing acupuncture," says Chung. Among people with asthma, there are different types—from exercise-induced asthma to asthma episodes triggered by airborne allergens. Even stress plays a role in asthma exacerbations. "A good acupuncture practitioner takes a complete history to determine lifestyle and other factors at play and then devises a custom regimen for each patient. So if you had a double-blind study where all the patients received the exact same acupuncture treatment, it may well be that the one treatment is not appropriate for all the patients. It is very difficult to design a study that controls for so many variables."

Use of Acupuncture in the U.S.

Even among those in the medical community who don't believe there is a scientific basis for using acupuncture to treat asthma, many do not discourage its use. Fromm points out that acupuncture doesn't seem to do any harm, despite the lack of hard evidence that it is effective in treating asthma. Of course, there are general health precautions to be heeded, such as making sure the needles are treated hygienically. "If a patient of mine were to ask about trying acupuncture to treat a chronic condition such as asthma, I'd say, 'By all means, go ahead.' There are no indications that it does any harm, so my stance would be to encourage the patient to try it," says Fromm. "Acupuncture does involve one-on-one contact with a practitioner who conducts an interview and takes a medical history. It may be that there are therapeutic benefits for some patients just in having that caregiver attention."

The concept that the patient's belief in a therapy may be as beneficial as the therapy itself is called the "placebo effect." Can this play a role in asthma treatment? "Absolutely," says Varon. "Remember that many things—including psychological issues—trigger asthma attacks, and clearly the placebo effect, in my experience, can help some of these patients."

Chung believes that acupuncture has much more of a direct impact on improving asthma. "I see patients with chronic asthma," she says, "and I have successfully used acupuncture to reduce asthma symptoms. The type of treatments I do are more long term for chronic asthma. It might take a long time of therapy—several visits over several months or more, to see any major changes. What I have seen in the patients I've treated is that they have fewer episodes of asthma—fewer breakthroughs of asthma symptoms. So my approach is a preventive-type treatment. And I can report positive results."

Though these results are anecdotal (not proven by scientific study), there are many acupuncturists and patients who believe in such benefits.

Complementary, Not Alternative

Both Fromm and Chung are in agreement on one point: that acupuncture should be tried only as a complement to traditional treatments for asthma.

"I always use acupuncture as an adjunctive treatment, as a supplemental treatment to the medicines they're already on," Chung says. "This is an attempt to improve their condition, which may lead to a reduction in their conventional medicines. I would not treat an acute asthmatic with acupuncture alone. I would make sure that they're getting what they need in terms of traditional medicines—their controller medicines and long-acting anti-inflammatories or inhaled steroids. If they experience an improvement, only then would I consider a reduction in medicines in the asthma management plan."

Fromm recommends a similar approach. "I'd want the patient to seek acupuncture in concert with the traditional physician," says Fromm. "Then, based upon how the patient is doing, adjustments to the medicines can be made."

The Cost

A visit to an acupuncturist will typically cost $60 or more. Initial visits may be more costly because these visits may be longer if the patient's medical history and lifestyle information are documented.

When it comes to paying for acupuncture therapy, patients may find that they have to cover a significant portion—sometimes all—of the cost themselves. While insurers are beginning to cover some of the costs of complementary treatments, acupuncture is not as widely covered as some others, such as chiropractic treatment. It is best to investigate the coverage your health plan offers before beginning treatment. You will then be able to decide if this type of additional therapy will fit into your family's budget.

The Future of Acupuncture

Even with scientific data inconclusive, thousands of people with asthma claim to benefit from acupuncture treatments. Given this conflicting information, what does the future hold?

"Collaboration," says Chung. "In the future there will be better collaboration between acupuncturists and medical researchers."

"Down the road there will be more investigations," Fromm agrees. "Then maybe we can say affirmatively, 'There is a subset of the population that benefits from acupuncture. Here's how and why.'"

Until such a time, however, practitioners will certainly continue to use this treatment method, and it will be up to patients to judge its benefits personally.

In addition to being a component of TCM, acupuncture also fits into the definition of complementary medicine (sometimes also called alternative medicine). This is that area of medicine that employs nontraditional approaches, including herbal and homeopathic medicines, hypnosis, relaxation training, and massage.

Recent surveys of Americans have shown that complementary medicine is gaining acceptance among patients and primary care providers alike. In one study, more than 40% of adults reported using it in some form or another. Furthermore, many health insurance companies now routinely cover many forms of it. In one recent survey of California physicians, 30% of the responding primary care providers reported using or recommending complementary medicine to their patients.

Part Five

Special Concerns about Asthma Management in Children

Chapter 51

The Art of Treating Childhood Asthma

A Common Story

It is a typical scene as I walk into the examination room. There on the exam table sits Roger, a 7-year-old young man with whom I am all too familiar.

Roger is doing what he usually does when I see him in my office: struggling to breathe. As I watch his chest heave up and down, I am struck by his loud wheezing and the exhausted face of his mother, who has been up all night with him. As you might guess, Roger is a frequent visitor both to my office and to the Emergency Room. He has been hospitalized several times. Despite what I think is good management on my part, Roger does not seem to get well.

Upon my persistent questioning, I find that his mom really hasn't been giving him his medicine regularly, despite my instructions. Whenever he does get well, she stops it, because she doesn't want him on medicine all the time.

The above story represents many of the difficult problems in treating asthma in children. Despite a growing understanding of the disease in the medical community, and the development of many new treatments, asthma continues to take a heavy toll on the health of millions of children.

"Treatment Of Childhood Asthma," by Herschel Lessin, MD, © 2004 Healthology, Inc. All rights reserved. Additional information is available at www.healthology.com.

The Basis of Asthma Treatment

Before I can tell you about the specifics of treating childhood asthma, you must learn a few basics about the disease.

There are really two parts to an asthma attack. The first, called the early phase, begins in minutes and can last for hours. It is caused by a clamping down of the muscles that surround the airways. When these muscles contract, they narrow the breathing tubes, making it harder to move air in and out of the lungs. This process is called bronchospasm. The second part of the attack is called the late phase. It begins in hours and can last for weeks. The cause of the late phase is the over-reaction of the "defense systems" in the lungs. When triggered, these defense systems call up an immune system response causing inflammation.

Special cells in the lungs, called mast cells, release chemicals that call up this inflammatory response. One such chemical, histamine, makes the lining of the lungs leak, just like it does to lining of the nose in hay fever.

Another set of chemicals, called leukotrienes, call in more white blood cells, even when they are not really needed. So many of these inflammatory chemicals are released into your airways—already made smaller by bronchospasm—that they get clogged up with mucus plugs, fluids, and cellular debris. The end result is further narrowing of the breathing tubes and increasing difficulty breathing. What's more, there is increasing evidence that all of this inflammation may cause permanent changes in the structure of the airways, making them more prone to future illness. Therefore, managing the inflammatory response at a young age takes on even greater importance.

The take-home message of this rather complex process is that asthma is an inflammatory disease. If one treats only the first part, the bronchospasm, and does not adequately treat the inflammation, then treatment will not be as effective. Inflammation is a slow and chronic process, and its presence may not be all that obvious once bronchospasm goes away. Its treatment must be a long and continuous process. It is quite natural to resist giving children medicine when symptoms are not obvious. Many parents and many doctors fall into this trap. As you will see later, it is absolutely critical to treat the inflammation in order to get asthma under control.

Classification of Asthma

The treatment of your child's asthma depends also on how severely the disease affects your child. Asthma is classified into four categories:

The Art of Treating Childhood Asthma

- **Severe persistent asthma:** This type of asthma is not hard to diagnose. These are the kids who are in the hospital frequently and in the ER or the doctor's office all the time. They have very frightening episodes and often need intense medical support. They are rarely clear and their activities are often limited despite frequent use of several medicines.

- **Moderate persistent asthma:** Children with moderate persistent asthma can also experience symptoms that are quite frightening. They have occasional severe episodes that require hospitalization and ER visits and often do not clear between episodes. They require daily use of medications.

- **Mild persistent asthma:** Children with mild persistent asthma are children that may once in a while have a frightening episode. They have prolonged periods of coughing and do not always clear between episodes. They use inhaled medications more than twice weekly but not every day.

- **Mild intermittent asthma:** These kids have occasional episodes that are usually not severe. They clear completely between episodes and use inhaled medicines less than twice weekly.

It is important to realize that the classification may change depending on the time of year. Children whose asthma symptoms are triggered by viral infections may be sick all winter and clear the rest of the year. Children triggered by pollens will have problems in the spring and fall. The treatment intensity can, therefore, change from season to season. A few unfortunate kids are sick all year round.

The most important point to make is that all children with persistent asthma of any type need daily use of anti-inflammatory medications even when they appear to be clear. It is also important to note that, in children who have seasonal variations in their asthma, the medications and their dosing may vary.

Creating an Effective Treatment Plan

Parents hate to give children medicine. Most children hate to take medicine. My philosophy about medicine is that you should use as little as possible, but as much as you need. People like to ignore that last part. You must use all the medicine necessary to get a good outcome. But if your doctor is just writing prescriptions, you are not getting everything that you need, because the treatment of childhood asthma involves much more than medicines.

The first step is education of the patient and parent. Asthma is a complex disease process, which the patient and his family must understand in order to cooperate with the often-confusing treatments that are prescribed.

Education: Education takes time, a commodity that is often in short supply in a busy pediatrician's office. In my opinion, all asthmatics need to have at least one long (45 min–1 hour) visit devoted solely to patient education and decision making. Many insurance companies will cover a home health nurse for this type of education as well.

Environmental control: The second step is called environmental control. There are many things in our environment that are known to make asthma worse. Every effort must be given to reducing the potential "allergic burden" in the household, particularly in the child's room. There are many resources available at your doctor's office and on the internet that discuss how to "dust proof" a room.

Many asthma patients are allergic to dust, and removing its sources is very important. These include stuffed animals, heavy drapes, plants, and heavy carpets, all of which collect dust. Dust proof covers can be obtained for mattresses and pillows. Bedding should be washed in hot water weekly to kill dust mites. There are chemical carpet treatments to control mites if removal is not an option. Special filters can be placed on forced air heating systems.

Additional triggers: In addition, exposure to toxins must be minimized. Most importantly, no one is allowed to smoke in the house and preferably not at all, since smoke on clothing can be enough to cause symptoms in a sensitive child. Also, pets are not a good idea for the child with asthma, particularly cats which are very "asthmagenic". Chemical fumes from perfumes and paints should be minimized. There are also steps to reduce mold in the household. If you can reduce the allergens in the house, it is less likely that other irritants, such as viral infections, will actually trigger an attack.

Monitor symptoms: Teaching parents how to monitor the severity of symptoms is another step in asthma control. This is only useful for children able to cooperate with the use of a peak flow meter. This is a device that measures how much air your child can blow out when he tries his hardest. The peak flow meter gives you a number that indicates how obstructed the airflow is, and therefore how severe the

The Art of Treating Childhood Asthma

asthma is at that moment. A child must be at least five years old to use a peak flow meter. There are known "normals" for children based on their height, and these numbers can be obtained from your pediatrician. Knowing your child's peak flow value can be very helpful in answering questions like: "How sick is she?" and, "How did she do when we changed her medicine?"

Proper equipment: Lastly, there is the matter of proper equipment. Not only must you have the equipment, you must take it out of the closet and use it. We already mentioned the invaluable peak flow meter. There are two other devices that are usually necessary: a spacing chamber for the inhaler, and a nebulizer:

- *Spacing chamber:* Many asthma medicines come in the form of inhalers. Children are not very adept with inhalers. Much of the medicine is lost in the air and is not actually inhaled into the lungs. Everyone (including adult asthmatics) should use a spacing chamber with inhalers. This is a tube with a one-way valve into which you put the inhaler. The inhaler is then puffed into the tube, which has a mouthpiece or mask at the other end. The child breathes the contents of the tube after the puff. Studies have shown that this device vastly increases the amount of medicine that actually gets into the lungs, where it needs to go to do its work.

- *Nebulizer:* Another useful device is called a nebulizer. This is a compressed air generator that makes a 'mist' of the medicines. Studies have shown that delivering medicine with this device is most effective in getting the medicine where it needs to be: the lungs. This is the device that is used in most doctor's offices and emergency rooms.

Medicines for Asthma

The following is a brief outline of the various types of medications that can be used to treat childhood asthma.

Beta Agonists: These are the most commonly prescribed asthma drugs in children. The most widely used of the beta agonists is albuterol, sold under a number of trade names such as Ventolin and Proventil. These drugs work by stimulating beta receptors on the surface of the muscles surrounding the airways. When these receptors are stimulated, they send signals to the muscle to relax, thereby easing the bronchospasm during the early phase of asthma. This will help asthma symptoms, but do little to control the underlying inflammation. Beta receptors exist in other parts of the body and when stimulated can cause side effects, most notably hyperactivity, increased heart rate, and jitteriness. These medicines can be administered in a several ways, including orally, by injection, inhaler, or in a nebulizer.

Theophylline: This is one of the oldest drugs used to treat asthma. While still widely used in adults, it is not as frequently used in children any more. Its method of action is still not entirely known, but it is used primarily to relieve symptoms, not control inflammation. It has a lot of side effects. When first taken, this drug may make a child feel jittery or nauseous. If too much medication is used, it can cause heart palpitations, insomnia, agitation, or vomiting, and blood levels must be monitored to insure safe use of the medication. Theophylline is administered orally or intravenously.

Mast cell stabilizers: This class of drugs is very useful. They prevent mast cells from calling up the inflammatory response and thus are very effective in preventing inflammation. They are not useful in an acute attack since they do not actually relieve symptoms, but instead help control the underlying inflammatory process. The most commonly used of these drugs are cromolyn and nedocromil, sold under the brand names of Intal and Tilade. These medicines are available by inhaler or nebulizer only. They have extremely few side effects.

Leukotriene inhibitors: This is a new class of drugs and has just recently come into use. These drugs inhibit the inflammatory effects of leukotrienes. They help control the inflammatory response in asthma and are taken orally. Trade names include Singulair and Accolate. The medications have some side effects and are not helpful in relieving immediate symptoms.

Steroids: Steroids are the most potent anti-inflammatory agents known. Taken orally, they are very effective in the relief of all asthma symptoms as well as in the relief of inflammation. Unfortunately, oral steroids such as prednisone, dexamethasone, and others can have severe side effects, particularly when used for more than one week at a time. If used for extended periods, they may result in a number of unfortunate side effects, including poor wound healing and stunted growth. They are most useful for short "bursts" of treatment to improve

The Art of Treating Childhood Asthma

the condition of the patient. Fortunately, steroids have been developed that can be used in an inhaler. These can be given chronically with excellent results and much fewer side effects. Close monitoring is essential when using this class of medications.

Monoclonal Antibodies: Monoclonal antibodies are also finding their way into the management of asthma. Omalizumab (Xolair®) was approved by the FDA in 2003 for patients who are inadequately controlled on the current regimen of corticosteroids and bronchodilators. This medication is indicated only for patients 12 years and up, with a positive skin test, who have moderate to severe uncontrolled asthma. Omalizumab works by blocking the IgE antibody from attaching to some of the inflammatory cells, such as mast cells and basophils, thereby reducing the symptoms of asthma.

Some of the major concerns of this new approach to treating asthma is the growing concern of malignancy and sever allergic reaction known as anaphylaxis. The other major drawback is the fact that it is currently only available in an injectable form. Thus it is important to consult with the doctor regarding such precautions.

The Art of Treating Asthma

As you can probably see by now, there are a lot of things to consider when deciding on asthma treatment. The first thing to understand is the difference between a symptom-reliever drug and a controller drug. Think about ear infections. You can use Tylenol to treat the symptoms, pain and fever, but it does nothing to treat the underlying problem. The same is true in asthma. You can use beta agonists like albuterol to treat the symptoms, but since asthma is an inflammatory disease, you very often must use something to control the inflammation.

Symptom relievers can be given on an as-needed basis when symptoms such as wheezing and cough are present. They can be stopped when the symptoms go away. Controller medicines, such as the anti-inflammatory drugs, must be given on a regular basis, day in and day out, even when there are no symptoms. I see far too many parents who stop all of their child's medicines the moment the symptoms disappear, leaving the chronic ongoing inflammation free to progress without opposition. This will increase the frequency and severity of the child's asthma symptoms, and could possibly cause irreversible changes in the lungs. Consistency in using daily controller medication is essential.

The use of controller drugs is mandatory for all but the mild intermittent asthma patient. That is why proper classification and review by the physician is so important. It is also why education is so important. You, as parents, must understand why the medication must be continued, even when your child appears to be better.

Conclusion

Treating asthma is an art. There are many different drugs to use, and they can be administered in a number of ways: orally, by inhaler, by nebulizer, by injection, or into the vein. They can be given some of the time or all of the time. The treatment of asthma becomes an art when you and your child's doctor craft an individualized treatment plan based on the history of your child's illness and all the considerations described above. The success of this plan for your child depends on your doctor's recognition of the fact that asthma is an inflammatory disease, on your recognition of the level of your child's sickness, and on how well you and your child comply with the treatment plan. Without more educated partnerships between parent and doctor, pediatricians like me will continue to see too many patients like Roger, struggling to breathe.

Chapter 52

Your Child's Cough: Is It Asthma?

Your daughter seems to be coming down with the "bug" that is going around, so you put her to bed half an hour early. After some grumbling, she finally falls asleep, and you tackle the dishes, catch up on a little reading, then head off to bed yourself. But at 3:30 A.M., you wake up to a burst of loud coughing. What should you do?

Coughs are one of the most frequent symptoms of childhood illness, and although they can sound awful at times, they usually are not a symptom of anything dangerous. Actually, coughing is a healthy reflex that helps clear the airways in the throat and chest. Occasionally, though, coughs can be cause for a visit to your child's doctor. If you learn to recognize certain types of coughs, you will know how to handle them and when you should seek medical help.

Types of Coughs and What They Mean

"Barking" Cough: These coughs are usually caused by croup, an inflammation of the larynx (voice box) and trachea (windpipe) brought on by allergies, change in temperature at night, or most commonly a viral upper respiratory infection. When a young child's airway becomes inflamed, it may swell around the vocal cords, making it harder to

---

"Your Child's Cough" was provided by KidsHealth, one of the largest resources online for medically reviewed health information written for parents, kids, and teens. For more articles like this one, visit www.KidsHealth.org, or www.TeensHealth.org. © 2001 The Nemours Center for Children's Health Media, a division of The Nemours Foundation.

breathe. Children younger than 3 years of age have croup most often because their windpipes are narrow—some children have it practically every time they have a respiratory illness.

Croup can occur suddenly in the middle of the night, which can be frightening for both you and your child. Although most cases can be managed at home, if you suspect your child has croup, call your child's doctor to determine whether your child needs to visit him or her.

"Whooping" Cough: The "whooping" sound actually occurs after the cough, when the child tries to take in a deep breath after a round of several coughs in a row.

If your child makes a "whooping" noise (which actually sounds like "hoop") after severe bouts of rapid coughing, it is most likely a symptom of pertussis (whooping cough)—particularly if your child has not received her diphtheria/tetanus/pertussis (DTaP) vaccinations.

Infants with pertussis usually do not "whoop" after the prolonged episodes of coughing, but they may not get enough oxygen or they may even stop breathing with this disease. In infants and very young children, pertussis can be deadly, so call your child's doctor right away.

Cough with Wheezing: When coughing is accompanied by a wheezing sound as your child exhales (breathes out), it is a sign that something may be partially blocking the lower airway. This might be caused by swelling from a respiratory infection (such as bronchiolitis or pneumonia), asthma, or an object stuck in her airway. Call your child's doctor unless your child has this problem often and you have medicine, such as an inhaler or nebulizer, with instructions on how to use the medicine for home treatment of your child's asthma. If the cough and wheezing do not improve with medication, call your child's doctor.

Stridor: Although wheezing usually during exhalation, stridor (pronounced: stry-door) is noisy, harsh breathing (some doctors describe it as a coarse, musical sound) that's heard when a child inhales (breathes in). Most often, it's caused by swelling of the upper airway, usually from viral croup. However, it's sometimes caused by a more serious infection called epiglottitis or a foreign object stuck in the child's airway. If your child has stridor, call your child's doctor immediately.

Sudden Cough: When a child suddenly starts coughing, it may mean she has swallowed some food or liquid "the wrong way" (into

Your Child's Cough: Is It Asthma?

the airway) or something (a bit of food, vomit, or perhaps even a small toy or coin) is caught in her throat or airway. Coughing helps clear the airway and may even continue for a minute or so simply because the throat or airway is irritated. But if the coughing does not seem to improve or your child has trouble breathing, call your child's doctor. Do not try to clear the throat with your finger because you might push the obstruction even farther down the windpipe.

Nighttime Cough: Lots of coughs get worse at night because the congestion in a child's nose and sinuses drains down the throat and causes irritation while the child lies in bed. This is only a problem if your child is unable to sleep. Asthma can also trigger nighttime coughs because the airways tend to be more sensitive and become more irritable at night.

Daytime Cough: Allergies, asthma, colds, and other respiratory infections are the usual culprits. Cold air or activity can make these coughs worse, and they often subside at night or when the child is resting. You should make sure that nothing in your house, like air freshener, pets, or smoke, is making your child cough.

Cough with a Cold: Because most colds are accompanied by a cough, it's perfectly normal for your child to develop either a wet or dry cough when she has a cold. The cough usually lasts about a week, often after all other symptoms of the cold have disappeared.

Cough with a Fever: If your child has a cough, mild fever, and runny nose, chances are she has a simple cold. But coughs with a fever of 102 degrees Fahrenheit (39 degrees Celsius) or higher can mean pneumonia, particularly if your child is listless and breathing fast. In this case, call your child's doctor immediately.

Cough with Vomiting: Children often cough so much that it triggers their gag reflex, making them throw up. Usually, this is not cause for alarm unless the vomiting persists. Also, if your child has a cough with a cold or an asthma flare-up, she may throw up if lots of mucus drains into her stomach and causes nausea.

Persistent Cough: Coughs caused by colds can last weeks, even up to 3 weeks, especially if your child has one cold right after another. Asthma, allergies, or a chronic infection in the sinuses or breathing passages might also be responsible for long-term coughs. If your child's cough lasts for more than a month, you should schedule a visit with your child's doctor.

Coughs in Young Infants: Coughing can wear out babies younger than 6 months, so keep a close eye on any cough your infant develops. These infants are also the population that is most at risk for complications from respiratory syncytial virus (RSV), which is most common in the winter. RSV causes colds and ear infections in older children and adults, but in young babies, it can cause bronchiolitis and pneumonia and lead to severe respiratory problems. The disease starts out like a normal cold but becomes worse until the child has wheezing, a cough, and difficulty breathing. Some children may have to be admitted to the hospital to receive oxygen and fluids.

When to Call Your Child's Doctor

Most childhood coughs are nothing to be concerned about. However, in some instances you should consult a doctor, just to be safe. Call your child's doctor if your child:

- has trouble breathing or is working hard to breathe;
- has a blue or dusky color to the lips, face, or tongue;
- has a high fever (particularly in a young infant or in the absence of congestion or a runny nose; contact your child's doctor for any fever in an infant younger than 3 months of age);
- is an infant (3 months old or younger) who has been coughing for more than a few hours;
- makes a "whooping" sound when she breathes after coughing;
- is coughing up blood (if your child has had a nosebleed recently, this usually is not a problem);
- has stridor when inhaling;
- has wheezing when exhaling (unless you already have home asthma management instructions from your child's doctor);
- is listless or cranky.

Professional Treatment

One of the best ways to diagnose a cough is listening. Your child's doctor will determine how to treat your child based in part on what the cough sounds like.

Your Child's Cough: Is It Asthma?

Because the majority of respiratory illnesses are caused by viruses, doctors do not prescribe antibiotics for many coughs. If bacterial pneumonia or another bacterial infection is suspected, your child's doctor will probably prescribe antibiotics.

Unless your child's cough is keeping her from getting adequate sleep, cough medicines are usually unnecessary. These medicines, both prescription and over-the-counter (OTC), may have unpleasant side effects and can even be dangerous for infants and young children. It's usually best to just let the illness run its course.

Pneumonia, pertussis, RSV, and serious cases of croup may require hospitalization. Usually this is just for close observation and to make sure your child gets enough fluids, but sometimes, if your child is having a hard time breathing, oxygen may be given. A baby with croup may be placed in a "croup tent," a little plastic oxygen tent. A water mist is continuously sprayed into the tent to provide humidification to soothe the baby's irritated airway.

Home Treatment

Home treatments should never take the place of consulting your child's doctor for any of the conditions listed above, but there are several things you can do at home to make your child more comfortable when she has an annoying cough.

- If your child has asthma, make sure you have received asthma-management instructions from your child's doctor. Monitor your child's progress carefully during a flare-up and give asthma medicines according to the doctor's instructions.

- If your child wakes up with a "barking" or "croupy" cough in the middle of the night, take her into the bathroom, close the door, and let the shower run on hot for several minutes. After the room steams up, sit on the bathroom floor with your child for about 20 minutes. The steam should help your child breathe more easily. Try reading a book together to keep your child occupied.

- A cool-mist humidifier in your child's room might help her sleep through the night.

- Cool beverages like juice can be soothing; avoid carbonated or citrus drinks, however, because carbonation and citric acid can be painful on raw areas.

- You should not give your child (especially a baby or toddler) OTC cough medicine without specific instructions to do so from your child's doctor. Many of these medicines suppress coughs, but respiratory illnesses sometimes produce a lot of secretions and coughing helps clear them out of the airway. If the cough were suppressed with medicine, it could actually be harmful to your child. In some instances, these medicines have even caused dangerous side effects when given to infants or very young children. In addition, the guidelines for OTC doses for children are often derived from adult guidelines (not formulated specifically for small children), so the medicine may not work exactly as intended.

- Cough drops, which are fine for older children, are a choking hazard for young children. It's best to leave decisions about your child's medicine to your child's doctor.

Chapter 53

Monitoring Your Child's Asthma

Monitoring means "keeping track of the situation." Monitoring your child's asthma is as important as driving with your eyes open—it lets you avoid mishaps along the way. This chapter discusses asthma monitoring.

Your doctor, obviously, will monitor your child's asthma. He or she will do this by asking about how your child's been doing and by checking your child over. If your child is old enough, your doctor may order pulmonary function tests (or PFTs), which measure how well air is getting in and out of your child's lungs. Your doctor will also give you advice on how to monitor your child's asthma between doctor's appointments. In general, there are two ways to monitor asthma at home:

- monitoring your child's symptoms
- monitoring how well your child's lungs are working, by using a home pulmonary function test device, called a peak flow meter

Monitoring Your Child's Asthma Symptoms

Monitoring your child's asthma symptoms is an effective, "low-tech" way of keeping track of how your child's asthma is doing.

"Monitoring My Child's Asthma," © 2000 Children's Hospital of Eastern Ontario; reprinted with permission. Reviewed by David A. Cooke, M.D., January 2006.

What is good asthma control?

When your child's asthma is well-controlled, he or she will have few (if any) asthma attacks. In addition, your child:

- should rarely (if ever) have a nighttime cough;
- should rarely (if ever) wake up at night because of coughing or shortness of breath;
- should be able to exercise about as long as other children, with little (if any) cough, wheezing, chest tightness, or trouble breathing;
- should handle "colds" as well as other children.

What are the signs of worsening asthma control?

- cough at night
- waking up at night because of coughing or chest tightness
- increased cough, wheezing, and/or trouble breathing with exercise, or reduced ability to exercise because of asthma
- cough or wheeze at rest (reading, watching TV, etc.)

What are the signs of a severe asthma attack?

- severe shortness of breath, rapid or shallow breathing, labored breathing, and/or sucking in of the skin between the ribs or at the base of the neck
- blueness—anywhere
- severe cough or wheezing that returns within 4 hours after a treatment with the child's reliever medication.
- inability to speak in full sentences
- sleepiness due to asthma
- fainting because of an asthma attack

If your child is needing treatments with his/her reliever medication every 4 hours (or more often than your doctor recommends) OR your child has signs of a severe asthma attack, you should have your child assessed by a doctor. You should also see, or talk to, a doctor, if you are worried about your child's asthma.

Monitoring Your Child's Asthma

Monitoring Using a Peak Flow Meter

A peak flow meter lets you keep track of your child's asthma using an easy-to-read, simple machine. The American National Heart, Lung, and Blood Institute recommends peak flow monitoring as part of a home asthma management program, designed to control asthma symptoms, prevent sudden, severe asthma episodes, and maintain a normal activity level. Peak flow meters cannot be used reliably in children under 4 years of age. It is also difficult to obtain reliable results with a peak flow meter in many children between 4 and 6 years of age. By the age of 7 years, most children can, with instruction, use a peak flow meter well.

If you use a peak flow meter, you should record the results in a diary card, or on a calendar. After a few weeks, you will be able to find out your child's personal best peak flow reading. Your doctor can use this number when he creates an Asthma Action Plan for your child. Ideally, your child should check his peak flows in the morning, at night, and whenever he/she or you are wondering whether he/she might be having an asthma attack. It is recommended that whenever peak flows are checked, the child should repeat the measurement three times, and you should use the best measurement for your assessment and for record-keeping. You may even want to record the peak flow readings in a computer spreadsheet, which should let you make graphs to track trends, and perhaps even calculate statistics.

Peak flow meters, like All-Seasons Radials, don't last forever. In most peak flow meters, the little needle (that slides up to give you a reading) eventually loosens, making the meter's readings a bit too generous. After a couple years of regular use, you should check your peak flow meter against a hospital's, or buy a new one.

When a doctor prescribes a peak flow meter, he/she usually will provide you with a written Asthma Action Plan to go with it. The Action Plan is usually based on the stoplight scheme. This will allow you to guide therapy, and judge the importance of changes in your child's peak flow meter readings. In addition to checking where readings lie within your Action Plan, you should look for trends—are the peak flows gradually going up after you start a new treatment, or are they gradually going down (for example, in the spring as the trees start to blossom).

Green Zone: Peak flow reading is between 80–100% of your child's personal best. This is the "All Clear" Zone—your child should continue his or her usual treatments.

Yellow Zone: Peak flow reading is between 50–79% of your child's personal best. This is the "Caution" Zone—your child's asthma may be getting worse. You should change your child's treatment, as recommended by your doctor.

Red Zone: Peak flow reading is less than 50% of your child's personal best. This is an asthma emergency. You should take a reliever medication, as recommended by your doctor. Your doctor may recommend that you then call him/her right away. You should see a doctor or go to the hospital right away if your child is struggling to breath, has blue lips or fingers, has a peak flow still in the Red Zone 30 minutes later, or 6 hours later, your child's peak flow is still less than 70% of his/her personal best, despite additional treatment with his/her reliever medication.

The Alternative Zone

Some recent research has suggested that children's peak flow meter readings may not drop as much during an asthma attack as the traditional stoplight scheme would suggest. Your doctor may recommend an alternative stoplight system, similar to the one given below:

Green Zone: Peak flow reading is between 80–100% of your child's personal best. This is the "All Clear" Zone—your child should continue his or her usual treatments.

Yellow Zone: Peak flow reading is between 70–79% of your child's personal best. This is the "Caution" Zone—your child's asthma may be getting worse. You should change your child's treatment, as recommended by your doctor.

Red Zone: Peak flow reading is less than 70% of your child's personal best. This is an asthma emergency. You should take a reliever medication, as recommended by your doctor. Your doctor may recommend that you then call him/her right away. You should see a doctor or go to the hospital right away if your child is struggling to breath, has blue lips or fingers, has a peak flow still in the Red Zone 30 minutes later, or 6 hours later, your child's peak flow is still less than 75% of his/her personal best, despite additional treatment with his/her reliever medication.

How Doctors Determine the Level of Asthma Control

The treatment of asthma involves reducing exposure to irritants and substances the child with asthma is allergic to, and the use of

Monitoring Your Child's Asthma

medication. The purpose of treating asthma is to achieve good asthma control. The Canadian Asthma Consensus Guidelines give precise definitions of asthma control, for Canadian doctors to use. Table 53.1 gives the definitions of good, and adequate, asthma control, as described in the current Canadian Asthma Consensus Guidelines used by Canadian physicians. If your child's asthma doesn't seem adequately controlled, you should inform your child's doctor, and you should discuss, with your doctor, what you can do to control your child's asthma better.

Table 53.1. Determining Level of Asthma Control

	Good Control	Adequate Control
Daytime Symptoms	None	Less than 3 days per week
Night-time Symptoms	None	Less than 1 night per week
Physical Activity	Normal	Normal
Use of short-acting bronchodilator	None*	Less than 3 doses per week*
Absences from school or work	None	None
Asthma Attacks	None	Mild and Infrequent
Peak Flow Readings	Normal	90% of personal best
Peak Flow Variability (highest number in 2 weeks—lowest number than 10% in 2 weeks, divided by highest number in 2 weeks, multiplied by 100)	Less	Less than 15%
Pulmonary Function Test (at the doctor's office)	Normal	90% of personal best

*apart from before exercise

Adapted from the *Canadian Respiratory Journal* 1996, Volume 3, Number 2.

Complementary (Alternative) Therapies for Asthma

Conventional asthma therapy can improve asthma control and prevent potentially dangerous asthma attacks in virtually all children with asthma. While some families may wish to consider alternative treatments, it must be emphasized that these treatments, when used, should be used in addition to conventional therapy, rather than instead of conventional therapy, to avoid the possibility of a severe asthma attack.

Massage therapy (stroking and kneading motions of the face, head, neck, and shoulders, arms and hands, and legs, feet, and back), for 20 minute sessions, taught by a trained massage therapist, has been shown, in a carefully performed medical research study, to reduce anxiety in children 4–14 years of age, improve pulmonary function in children 4–8 years of age, and, possibly improve pulmonary function in children 9–14 years of age.

A carefully performed study of chiropractic manipulation showed no benefit when added to conventional medical therapy in children with asthma.

Some herbal remedies for asthma contain compounds closely related to medications commonly used in the treatment of asthma. Tea contains caffeine, which is closely related to theophylline, a mild bronchodilator. Ma huang (ephedra)[1] is related to beta-2 agonist relievers (bronchodilators). However, as dosages may not be standardized or may vary, there is no discernible advantage to their use over conventional drug preparations.

Many other alternative therapies for asthma are being promoted. In general, these treatments have not been carefully evaluated for their efficacy, and their potential side effects are often unknown. Some of these therapies rely on non-conventional "allergy testing." Conventional allergy tests usually apply extracts of substances which commonly cause allergies to skin which has been pricked with a needle, or, less often, is injected with a needle into the skin. The results of these tests have been shown to be closely related to allergy-causing antibodies against these substances. Non-conventional "allergy tests," using electrical, magnetic, or other methods, have not been shown to be related to antibodies, and their clinical significance has not been demonstrated. If your child is having allergy tests performed by someone who is not a trained allergist, you should ask whether your child is getting a conventional allergy test or a non-conventional allergy test.

Note

1. Dietary supplements that contain ephedra have been banned in the United States since April 2004. The U.S. Food and Drug Administration (FDA) banned the products after it determined that ephedra posed an unreasonable risk to those who used it. Source: "Sales of Supplements Containing Ephedrine Alkaloids (Ephedra) Prohibited," FDA, April 2004.

Chapter 54

Warning Signs that May Precede an Asthma Flare-Up

Be Aware of Your Child's Warning Signs

Often your child may show warning signs before an asthma flare-up. Warning signs are clues that your child's asthma may be getting worse.

A very young child may not be able to tell you how he or she feels. So you may have to watch a younger child more closely to find out if something is wrong.

Learn your child's warning signs and catch an attack before it gets worse. While warning signs differ from child to child, parents report some common signs. Think about the last time your child had an asthma attack. It may have been preceded by warning signs such as these:

- coughed at night
- had a cold or the flu
- had a fever
- had a stuffy or runny nose
- had a tickle in the throat
- sneezed and had watery eyes
- acted very restless

Excerpted from "Help Your Child Gain Control Over Asthma," U.S. Environmental Protection Agency (EPA), November 2004. For more information about asthma from the EPA visit http://www.epa.gov/asthma.

- face was pale
- had dark circles under the eyes
- had tightness in the chest
- seemed to feel weak or tired
- seemed to have a headache

There may also have been other signs that you noticed. Be sure to review these warning signs with your child's doctor.

Emergency Warning Signs

There are times when you need to take your child to the hospital or urgent care right away. Ask your child's doctor what emergency signs to look for to help you know when your child is having a medical emergency with asthma.

Some parents know their child is having a medical emergency with asthma if he or she:

- is breathing in a different way—faster, or slower, or more shallow than usual;
- is coughing or wheezing and can't stop;
- has bluish fingernails or lips.

Help Your Child Have Fewer Asthma Attacks

- You've taken a great first step. You're reading this information and learning more about asthma.
- Become aware of your child's warning signs that asthma is getting worse. Learn the emergency warning signs of an asthma attack.
- Ask questions. Work with your child's doctor to come up with an asthma action plan that works for your child and your family.
- Follow the action plan. Make sure all the people who care for your child know about the plan and how to follow it.

Chapter 55

Control Your Child's Asthma Triggers

Learn What May Trigger Your Child's Asthma

Triggers are the things that can start your child's asthma attack or make it worse. Your child may have just one trigger or you may find that several things act as triggers.

- For some kids, being around pets or dust can trigger asthma.
- Some kids find their asthma gets worse from cigarette smoke.
- For other kids, running and playing may bring on an asthma attack.

Be sure to work with the doctor to identify your child's asthma triggers.

Once you know what triggers your child's asthma, it is important to take steps to control these triggers. Remembering to smoke outside or keeping pests out of your home means taking action every day. The more these habits are part of your daily life, the less chance there is your child will have an asthma attack.

Take Steps to Control Asthma

First: Think about when your child's asthma got worse. Was your child near someone who was smoking? Playing with a friend's dog? Outside when the air pollution level was high?

Excerpted from "Help Your Child Gain Control Over Asthma," U.S. Environmental Protection Agency (EPA), November 2004. For more information about asthma from the EPA visit http://www.epa.gov/asthma.

Next: Try to identify the triggers that make your child's asthma worse.

Finally: Work with your child's doctor to learn ways to:

- Keep your child away from triggers when possible;
- Remove the triggers from your home, school, or daycare.

When you remove triggers from your home or keep your child away from triggers outdoors, you help your child stay healthy and have fewer asthma attacks.

Common Asthma Triggers

Secondhand Smoke: Secondhand smoke is the smoke from a cigarette, cigar, or pipe, and the smoke exhaled by a smoker. What can you do?

- Don't let anyone smoke near your child.
- If you smoke—until you can quit, don't smoke in your home or car.

Pledge to make your home and car smoke-free by calling 866-SMOKE-FREE (866-766-5337).

Dust Mites: Dust mites are tiny bugs that are too small to see. They live in things like sheets, blankets, pillows, mattresses, soft furniture, carpets, and your child's stuffed toys. What can you do?

- Wash bedding in hot water once a week. Dry completely.
- Use dust proof covers on pillows and mattresses.
- Vacuum carpets and furniture every week.
- Choose stuffed toys that you can wash.
- Wash stuffed toys in hot water. Dry completely before your child plays with the toy.

Pets: Pets are any animals in your home, such as cats and dogs. What can you do?

- Find another home for your cat or dog.
- Keep pets outside if possible.

Control Your Child's Asthma Triggers

- If you have to have a pet inside, keep it out of your child's bedroom.
- Keep pets off of your furniture.
- Vacuum carpets and furniture when your child is not around.

Cockroaches ("roaches" or other "pests"): Look for cockroaches in areas with food and water such as your kitchen and bathroom or areas where you store paper bags, cardboard boxes, or newspapers such as your basement. What can you do?

- Keep counters, sinks, tables, and floors clean and free of clutter. Clean dishes, crumbs, and spills right away.
- Store food in airtight containers.
- Seal cracks or openings around or inside cabinets.
- Use roach baits or traps instead of sprays.
- Cover trash cans.

Mold: Mold grows in damp places such as kitchens, bathrooms, and basements. What can you do?

- If you see mold on hard surfaces, clean it up with soap and water. Let the area dry completely.
- Use exhaust fans or open a window in the bathroom and kitchen when showering, cooking, or washing dishes.
- Fix water leaks as soon as possible to keep mold from growing.
- Dry damp or wet things completely within one to two days to keep mold from growing.

Nitrogen Dioxide: Nitrogen dioxide is a gas that can bother your eyes, nose, and throat. It may also cause shortness of breath. This gas can come from appliances inside your home that burn fuels such as gas, kerosene, and wood. Appliances that burn fuels are sometimes called fuel-burning appliances. What can you do?

- If possible, use fuel-burning appliances that are vented to the outside. Always follow the maker's instructions on how to use these appliances.
- *Gas cooking stoves:* If you have an exhaust fan in the kitchen, use it when you cook. Never use the stove to keep you warm or heat your house.

- *Unvented kerosene or gas space heaters:* Use the proper fuel and keep the heater adjusted the right way. Open a window slightly or use an exhaust fan when you are using the heater.

- *Wood stoves:* Make sure the stove doors are tight fitting. Follow the maker's instructions for starting, burning, and putting out the fire.

- *Fireplaces:* Always open the chimney flue before you build a fire.

Outdoor Air Pollution: Small particles and ozone come from things like exhaust from cars and factories, smoke, and road dust. Watch for the Air Quality Index (AQI) during your local weather report. The AQI is a tool that offers you clear information every day on whether air quality in your area could be a health worry. The AQI uses colors to show how much pollution is in the air. Green and yellow mean air pollution levels are low. Orange, red, or purple mean pollution is at levels that may make asthma worse. What can you do?

When the AQI reports unhealthy levels (orange, red, or purple):

- Have your child play outdoors at times when the air quality is better. In the summer, this may be in the morning.

- Limit outdoor games that involve running hard for a long time.

- Pay attention to your child's asthma warning signs. If you start to see signs, limit outdoor activity. Be sure to talk about this with your child's doctor.

Chemical Irritants: Chemical irritants found in some products in your house may make your child's asthma worse. Your child's asthma may be worse around scented or unscented products, including cleaners, paints, adhesives, pesticides, cosmetics, or air fresheners.

If you find that your child's asthma gets worse when you use a certain product, consider trying different products. If you must use a product, then you should:

- Make sure your child is not around.

- Open windows or doors, or use an exhaust fan.

Remember to always follow the instructions on the label.

Chapter 56

If Your Child Has Asthma, Can You Keep Your Pet?

Only about 10% of the general population has pet allergies, but at least 30% of people with asthma are allergic to animals. So if your child has asthma, it's a good idea to consider whether your pet could be producing allergens that are triggering asthma symptoms.

Contrary to popular belief, your animal's fur probably isn't the culprit. But animal dander (skin flakes), saliva, urine, and feathers can cause allergic reactions. Though pet hair itself isn't the problem, an animal's fur can collect dust mites, pollen, mold, and other allergens. And any animal that lives in a cage (from birds to gerbils) will produce droppings that can attract mold and dust mites.

You may hear people say that certain breeds of dogs or cats, particularly those that don't shed, don't trigger their asthma, but all warm-blooded animals give off these allergens and are capable of causing an allergic reaction.

If you're wondering whether your child is allergic to your pet, it might be a good idea to have him or her tested for allergies. If your child turns out to be allergic to your pet, you'll have to decide whether you'll keep it or find a new home for the animal. The best course is to remove the pet from your home, though this isn't usually the easiest

---

"If My Child Has Asthma, Can We Keep Our Pet?" was provided by KidsHealth, one of the largest resources online for medically reviewed health information written for parents, kids, and teens. For more articles like this one, visit www.KidsHealth.org, or www.TeensHealth.org. © 2004 The Nemours Center for Children's Health Media, a division of The Nemours Foundation.

or happiest solution. Your child, other kids in the family, and even adults in the family may have a tough time with this decision.

In some cases, your child's doctor may say that it's OK to keep your pet if your child receives medicine or allergy shots. If you go this route, you'll also want to take measures at home to limit your child's exposure to the animal, such as keeping the pet out of your child's bedroom and play areas. Hard as this is to enforce, try to teach your child not to hug or kiss the animal. Vacuum and dust regularly and avoid rugs and wall-to-wall carpeting, especially in your child's room.

Unfortunately, such measures may not be enough—because animal allergens are airborne, heating and ventilation systems will spread allergens throughout the house, even if the pet is confined to one room. Keeping the pet in the yard may not be a total solution either because some allergens will eventually be carried in on clothing.

If you decide to keep your pet, it might also be a good idea to:

- Buy an air cleaner. HEPA (high efficiency particulate air) air cleaners can really help, especially for cat allergies. Vacuums are available with HEPA filters as well.

- Keep your child away from the cat's litter box, and place the box away from air vents.

- Have someone other than your child wash and brush your pet every week (this is advisable for cats as well as dogs).

- Encourage everyone in the family to wash their hands after playing with your pet.

- Keep your pet out of the child's bedroom and away from rugs and upholstered furniture. You may need to shut the doors to certain rooms or use baby safety gates to keep cats and dogs out.

If you have a bird, gerbil, or other small caged animal, keep the cage in a room other than your child's bedroom. Make sure the pet stays in its cage at all times, and clean the cage daily—without your child's assistance. You'll also want to let your child's teacher know about your child's allergies if there's a caged pet in the classroom.

If you do decide to find another home for your pet, be sure to talk to your child about his or her feelings. You'll want to assure your child it's not his or her "fault"—and make sure siblings don't blame the child. Losing a pet, even if it is only to another home, may be difficult for everyone in the family. If your child has his or her heart set on a

If Your Child Has Asthma, Can You Keep Your Pet?

new pet, your best bets are a turtle, lizard, snake, or fish. (But be cautious because certain reptiles carry *Salmonella* bacteria.)

Remember, too, that even if you remove the pet from your home, you may not see improvements in your child's asthma symptoms for a while. After a pet is removed from the home, it can take up to six months to reduce the allergen levels to those of a home without pets. Even if the pet is removed, your child may still need to use the asthma or allergy medications that he or she used previously.

When your child is invited to a house with a pet, he or she should take any prescription allergy medicine before going and should (as always) bring along his or her asthma rescue medication as well.

Chapter 57

When to Seek Emergency Care for a Child with Asthma

If your child has asthma, one of your main goals may be to avoid trips to the emergency room (ER) for breathing problems. That makes perfect sense, but it's also important to know when going to the ER is the right choice.

You'll do a better job of making that decision if you discuss this issue with your child's doctor before your child has a severe flare-up. After discussing it, your instructions should be spelled out in your child's asthma action plan. The plan should list peak flow meter readings or specific symptoms that will serve as your cue to go to the ER. If your child is old enough, he or she should know about these important cues as well.

Some general signs that indicate you should seek help very quickly by getting to an ER or calling an ambulance include:

- if there are changes in your child's color, like bluish or gray lips and fingernails;
- if your child is having trouble talking;
- if you can see the areas between your child's ribs and at the base of the neck pull in as he or she inhales (these are called retractions);

"When to Go to the ER if Your Child Has Asthma," was provided by KidsHealth, one of the largest resources online for medically reviewed health information written for parents, kids, and teens. For more articles like this one, visit www.KidsHealth.org, or www.TeensHealth.org. © 2004 The Nemours Center for Children's Health Media, a division of The Nemours Foundation.

- if your child uses his or her rescue medications repeatedly but the flare-up symptoms don't go away after 5 or 10 minutes or they return again quickly;
- if your child's peak flow reading falls below 50% and doesn't improve with medication.

Going to the ER

Some advance planning can make trips to the ER less stressful for you and your child. Here are some ways you can make it a little easier:

- Know the location of your closest emergency room. If there's a children's hospital ER nearby, use that one and have the address and phone number for it readily accessible (it can be written on your child's action plan).
- If you have other children, try to make arrangements with a relative or other caregiver who can care for them in an emergency situation. But don't let the lack of a babysitter delay your trip to the ER. Someone can always come to the hospital and pick up your other children.
- Take along a copy of your child's asthma action plan or a note with the names and dosages of any medications your child is taking, so that you can inform the medical staff at the emergency room.

Preventing ER Trips

Well-managed asthma is rarely life threatening. People who have died from asthma usually haven't taken their medications as prescribed and have a history of repeated severe asthma flare-ups and emergency care. If you and your child take asthma seriously and work to manage it, you can reduce the chances that your child will need to go to the emergency room.

Here are some steps to take:

Follow your child's asthma action plan: It's important to monitor your child's asthma using a written plan your child's doctor has helped you create. This plan will outline your child's day-to-day treatment, list symptoms to watch for, and give detailed, step-by-step instructions to follow when your child has a flare-up.

Help your child avoid triggers: Your child's doctor should be able to help you identify the triggers that can cause asthma flare-ups.

When to Seek Emergency Care for a Child with Asthma

These may include animals, dust mites, mold, tobacco smoke, cold air, exercise, and infections.

Make sure your child takes his or her controller medications: Your child should take these medications as prescribed by the doctor, even when he or she is feeling fine. Skipping controller medications can cause the lungs to become more inflamed, which can lead to a decrease in lung function. (This can happen without your child even experiencing any symptoms). It also puts the child at risk for more frequent and severe flare-ups.

Keep rescue medications with your child: Many kids must go to the emergency room simply because they didn't have their rescue medications handy. Your child should have his or her rescue medication accessible at all times.

Make your child a partner in his or her asthma management: As soon as your child is old enough, make sure he or she understands the asthma action plan and the importance of following it. Some children with asthma, especially teens, resist taking controller medications and rely instead on their rescue medications to help them on an as-needed basis. This is never a good idea and will increase your child's chances of needing emergency care.

Know the early signs of a flare-up: Every child's asthma is different. Some children cough only at night, but others have flare-ups whenever they get a cold or exercise outside. Get to know your child's asthma and pay attention to what happens before he or she has a flare-up, so that you know the early warning signs. These signs may not definitively mean that a flare-up will happen, but they can help you to plan ahead.

A peak flow meter is an extremely useful tool in helping to determine if your child might be getting ready for a flare-up. Your doctor can give you specific number ranges to look for.

Other early warning signs of a flare-up may include:

- coughing, even if your child has no cold
- tightness in the chest
- throat clearing
- rapid or irregular breathing
- inability to stand or sit still

- unusual fatigue
- restless sleep

Maintain good communication with your child's doctor: Be sure to call him or her at the early sign of a flare-up if you have any concerns. Being proactive means you may keep your child's symptoms from worsening and can make a trip to the doctor's office instead of the emergency room.

Chapter 58

Emotional Problems in Young People with Asthma

According to the Centers for Disease Control and Prevention, more than 6 million kids and teens under age 18 in the United States have asthma, a chronic respiratory condition. Pediatric health care providers have become increasingly concerned about the emotional impact that asthma has on adolescent patients, so researchers from Johns Hopkins University in Baltimore, Maryland, investigated the effects of asthma symptoms on the emotions of teens.

A group of 185 11- to 17-year-old adolescents who'd been diagnosed with asthma and were enrolled in managed health care organizations completed comprehensive surveys about the effect their asthma had had on their everyday life. The teens and their parents answered questions about overall health, symptoms of asthma, the effect of asthma on day-to-day functioning, how often doctor and emergency department visits were needed for asthma, and how much they participated in their own asthma care. The teens also answered questions designed to assess their self-esteem and noted whether they felt moody, nervous, or irritable. Teens also reported whether they felt frustrated, uncomfortable, frightened, worried, angry, irritable, or different or left out because of their asthma diagnosis.

"Emotional Problems Common in Teens With Asthma" was provided by TeensHealth, one of the largest resources online for medically reviewed health information written for parents, kids, and teens. For more articles like this one, visit www.TeensHealth.org, or www.KidsHealth.org. © 2004 The Nemours Center for Children's Health Media, a division of The Nemours Foundation.

Many of the teens in this study had needed health care visits for asthma in recent months. Ten percent of the teens had been hospitalized, 41% had visited the emergency department, and 77% had visited the doctor for worsening asthma in the 12 months prior to the time of the survey. In addition, in the four weeks prior to the survey, 30% of students had missed at least one day of school. More than half of the students were classified as having moderate or severe asthma.

In addition to the physical problems that many teens had with asthma, the condition seemed to have had a significant impact on emotional quality of life, too. Seventy-five percent of parents said that they'd worried about their child's emotional health during the four weeks prior to the survey. And over the same time period, 45% of teens said they'd felt depressed or blue, 24% had episodes of crying a lot, and 48% had felt nervous or uptight. The worse a teen's emotional health, the more likely that he or she had experienced worsening asthma symptoms and more days of missed school and asthma-related doctor visits.

What This Means to You

Feelings of depression, nervousness, and episodes of crying are common in teens with asthma, and teens who have more emotional symptoms tend to have more physical asthma symptoms, according to the results of this study. In addition to working with your child's doctor to develop an asthma treatment plan that will help your child control his or her physical symptoms, talk to your child's doctor about how to address the emotional concerns of teens with asthma, like dealing with asthma symptoms at school and fitting in with their peer group.

Source: Sande O. Okelo, MD; Albert W. Wu, MD, MPH; Jerry A. Krishnan, MD; Cynthia S. Rand, PhD; Elizabeth A. Skinner, MSW; Gregory B. Diette, MD, MHS; *Journal of Pediatrics*, October 2004.

Chapter 59

Is Your Child-Care Setting or School Asthma Friendly?

How Asthma-Friendly Is Your Child-Care Setting?

Children with asthma need proper support in child-care settings to keep their asthma under control and be fully active. Use the questions below to find out how well your child-care setting assists children with asthma:

1. Is the child-care setting free of tobacco smoke at all times?
2. Is there good ventilation in the child-care setting? Are allergens and irritants that can make asthma worse reduced or eliminated? Are any of the following present:
   - cockroaches
   - dust mites (commonly found in humid climates in pillows, carpets, upholstery, and stuffed toys)
   - mold
   - pets with fur or feathers
   - strong odors or fumes from art and craft supplies, pesticides, paint, perfumes, air fresheners, and cleaning chemicals

---

This chapter includes text from the following publications of the National Heart, Lung, and Blood Institute's National Asthma Education and Prevention Program: "How Asthma-Friendly Is your Child-Care Setting," 2000; "How Asthma-Friendly Is Your School?" 1999; and "National Asthma Education and Prevention Program Resolution on Asthma Management at School," 2002. Reviewed by David A. Cooke, M.D., January 2006.

3. Is there a medical or nursing consultant available to help child-care staff write policy and guidelines for managing medications in the child-care setting, reducing allergens and irritants, promoting safe physical activities, and planning field trips for students with asthma?

4. Are child-care staff prepared to give medications as prescribed by each child's physician and authorized by each child's parent? May children carry their own asthma medicines when appropriate? Is there someone available to supervise children while taking asthma medicines and monitor correct inhaler use?

5. Is there a written, individualized emergency plan for each child in case of a severe asthma episode (attack)? Does the plan make clear what action to take? Whom to call? When to call?

6. Does a nurse, respiratory therapist, or other knowledgeable person teach child-care staff about asthma, asthma management plans, reducing allergens and irritants, and asthma medicines? Does someone teach all the children about asthma and how to help a classmate who has it?

7. Does the child-care provider help children with asthma participate safely in physical activities? For example, are children encouraged to be active? Can children take or be given their medicine before exercise? Are modified or alternative activities when medically necessary?

If the answer to any question is "no," children in your child-care setting may be facing obstacles to controlling their asthma. Uncontrolled asthma can hinder a child's attendance, participation, and progress in school. Child-care staff, health professionals, and parents can work together to remove obstacles and promote children's health and development.

How Asthma-Friendly Is Your School?

Children with asthma need proper support at school to keep their asthma under control and be fully active. Use the questions below to find out how well your school assists children with asthma:

1. Is your school free of tobacco smoke all of the time, including during school-sponsored events?

Is Your Child-Care Setting or School Asthma Friendly?

2. Does the school maintain good indoor air quality? Does it reduce or eliminate allergens and irritants that can make asthma worse? Allergens and irritants include pets with fur or feathers, mold, dust mites (for example, in carpets and upholstery), cockroaches, and strong odors or fumes from such products as pesticides, paint, perfumes, and cleaning chemicals.

3. Is there a school nurse in your school all day, every day? If not, is a nurse regularly available to the school to help write plans and give guidance for students with asthma about medicines, physical education, and field trips?

4. Can children take medicines at school as recommended by their doctor and parents? May children carry their own asthma medicines?

5. Does your school have an emergency plan for taking care of a child with a severe asthma episode (attack)? Is it made clear what to do? Who to call? When to call?

6. Does someone teach school staff about asthma, asthma management plans, and asthma medicines? Does someone teach all students about asthma and how to help a classmate who has it?

7. Do students have good options for fully and safely participating in physical education class and recess? For example, do students have access to their medicine before exercise? Can they choose modified or alternative activities when medically necessary?

If the answer to any question is no, students may be facing obstacles to asthma control. Asthma out of control can hinder a student's attendance, participation, and progress in school. School staff, health professionals, and parents can work together to remove obstacles and to promote students' health and education.

National Asthma Education and Prevention Program Resolution on Asthma Management at School

Asthma affects nearly 5 million children in the United States—about one child in every 14. This chronic lung disease causes unnecessary restriction of childhood activities and is a leading cause of school absenteeism. Asthma is controllable, however. With proper treatment and support, children with asthma can lead fully active lives.

The National Asthma Education and Prevention Program (NAEPP) believes that schools should adopt policies for the management of asthma that encourage the active participation of students in the self-management of their condition and allow for the most consistent, active participation in all school activities. These policies should allow:

- A smoke-free environment for all school activities.

- Access to health services supervised by a school nurse. These services should include identification of students with asthma; a written asthma management plan for each student with asthma; appropriate medical equipment; and the support of an adult, as appropriate, to evaluate, monitor, and report on the administration of medication to the parent/guardian and/or health provider.

- A written medication policy that allows safe, reliable, and prompt access to medications in the least restrictive way during all school-related activities and self-managed administration of medication (including consideration of allowing students to carry and self-administer medications) consistent with the needs of the individual child and the safety of others.

- A school-wide emergency plan for handling severe exacerbations of asthma.

- Staff development for all school personnel on school medication policies, emergency procedures, and procedures for communicating health concerns about students.

- Development of a supportive and healthy environment that respects the abilities and needs of each student with asthma.

Chapter 60

Combatting Frequent School Absenteeism in Children with Asthma

Plan for Attendance

For most students, missing a few days of the school year is no big deal. However, for children with a chronic health condition, frequent absenteeism becomes a major problem that compounds itself with each passing school year.

Students with asthma and allergies may miss school due to medical appointments, preventive evaluations, or treatments, as well as illness. Therefore, teachers and parents should establish plans for keeping up with daily classroom assignments at the beginning of the school year. Students should not be penalized for missing deadlines or failing to attend a sufficient number of school days if illness is the cause.

One aspect of school absenteeism is entirely preventable and almost never considered: children with asthma who are forced to go to the clinic every time a medication is needed. Some children must use medication three or four times a day. A child who leaves the classroom for one dose of medication per day loses an additional 11 days over the course of the school year.

Teaching children how to use medicines properly and permitting them to carry inhaled medications throughout the day will eliminate

---

This chapter includes "Plan for Attendance," an undated fact sheet reprinted courtesy of Allergy & Asthma Network Mothers of Asthmatics (AANMA), 800-878-4403, www.breatherville.org. "Students with Chronic Illnesses: Guidance for Families, Schools, and Students," is a fact sheet produced by the National Heart, Lung, and Blood Institute, 2002.

this problem. Discuss this with school officials and your physician. Also talk with your doctor about medication options. Some medicines require fewer doses per day than others.

When should asthma go to school?

It is often difficult to decide whether your child should go to school or not. The following guidelines are suggested by the Center for Interdisciplinary Research on Immunologic Diseases at Georgetown University, Washington, D.C.

Your child can go to school with these symptoms:

- a stuffy nose, but no wheezing
- mild wheezing that clears after medication
- the ability to do usual daily activities
- no difficulty breathing

Keep your child home with these symptoms:

- evidence of infection, sore throat, or swollen, painful neck glands
- a fever over 100 degrees F, orally; face hot and flushed
- wheezing that continues to be labored one hour after medicine is given
- weakness or tiredness that makes it hard to take part in usual daily activities
- difficulty breathing

Your child's peak flow meter reading can also help you decide. A lower-than-normal reading, coupled with other early warning signals (such as a chronic cough or pale skin color), may be a sign that an asthma attack is imminent. Parents should medicate their children as instructed by the physician and base their decision to send the child to school on the child's response to the medications.

Good communication among the teacher, parent, and child will enable the child to attend school on marginal days. Notify the teacher that your child is in pre-asthma stages but controlled with medications. If possible or indicated, go to the school to check on your child just before the next medication is due. A quick assessment with the peak flow meter and listening to the child's chest will tell you what you need to know.

Some children's asthma is worse in the morning than at midday. This can be a problem with morning kindergarten or preschool programs. Try to arrange for afternoon school for the younger child, and remember that this tendency may improve as the child gets older. Older children with this same problem don't need to miss an entire day of school. A half day at school is better than none at all.

When does a child need help?

The key to keeping kids in school is keeping them healthy. Children with high absentee rates need medical help. Children who can never participate in physical activities need medical help. Children who are frequently in crisis need medical help. These are signs that the asthma or allergy management plan is not working, and parents and teachers should take the time to identify why the child is missing school and unable to participate fully:

- Is the child under the care of an asthma or allergy specialist?
- Is the asthma or allergy management plan written down?
- Are the home and school environments free of allergens and irritants?
- Is the school environment a healthy place for the child to breathe?

If any of the questions above are answered with "no", the child can be expected to miss more school than necessary. If all the questions above are answered with "yes" and the child is still having problems, further investigation by the physician or perhaps a second medical opinion would be helpful. In a small percentage of cases, children struggle with severe illnesses complicated by insufficient immune responses. These children need support, not condemnation, when they miss many school days.

A child who misses too much school can benefit from a tutor. Many school systems provide this service; however, in most cases the child must miss an extraordinary number of school days before being eligible for help. Parents should not hesitate to request special help for their children.

Is home schooling a good solution for a child with asthma?

Choosing not to enroll your child with asthma in school simply because you believe you can control the child's symptoms better at home can create a false sense of security and inhibit the child's ability to manage his own health. Home instruction may be the only alternative for a small minority of children whose physical condition is severe, but it should never be chosen because of poor home or school coping skills or outdated medical management.

Students With Chronic Illnesses: Guidance for Families, Schools, and Students

Chronic illnesses affect at least 10 to 15 percent of American children. Responding to the needs of students with chronic conditions, such as asthma, allergies, diabetes, and epilepsy (also known as seizure disorders), in the school setting requires a comprehensive, coordinated, and systematic approach. Students with chronic health conditions can function to their maximum potential if their needs are met. The benefits to students can include better attendance, improved alertness and physical stamina, fewer symptoms, fewer restrictions on participation in physical activities and special activities, such as field trips, and fewer medical emergencies. Schools can work together with parents, students, health care providers, and the community to provide a safe and supportive educational environment for students with chronic illnesses and to ensure that students with chronic illnesses have the same educational opportunities as do other students.

What are the family's responsibilities?

- Notify the school of the student's health management needs and diagnosis when appropriate. Notify schools as early as possible and whenever the student's health needs change.

- Provide a written description of the student's health needs at school, including authorizations for medication administration and emergency treatment, signed by the student's health care provider.

- Participate in the development of a school plan to implement the student's health needs:
  - Meet with the school team to develop a plan to accommodate the student's needs in all school settings.
  - Authorize appropriate exchange of information between school health program staff and the student's personal health care providers.

- Communicate significant changes in the student's needs or health status promptly to appropriate school staff.

- Provide an adequate supply of student's medication, in pharmacy-labeled containers, and other supplies to the designated school staff, and replace medications and supplies as needed. This supply should remain at school.

- Provide the school a means of contacting you or another responsible person at all times in case of an emergency or medical problem.

- Educate the student to develop age-appropriate self-care skills.

- Promote good general health, personal care, nutrition, and physical activity.

What are the school district's responsibilities?

- Develop and implement district-wide guidelines and protocols applicable to chronic illnesses generally and specific protocols for asthma, allergies, diabetes, epilepsy (seizure disorders), and other common chronic illnesses of students.

- Guidelines should include safe, coordinated practices (as age and skill level appropriate) that enable the student to successfully manage his or her health in the classroom and at all school-related activities.

- Protocols should be consistent with established standards of care for students with chronic illnesses and Federal laws that provide protection to students with disabilities, including ensuring confidentiality of student health care information and appropriate information sharing.

- Protocols should address education of all members of the school environment about chronic illnesses, including a component addressing the promotion of acceptance and the elimination of stigma surrounding chronic illnesses.

- Develop, coordinate, and implement necessary training programs for staff that will be responsible for chronic illness care tasks at school and school-related activities.

- Monitor schools for compliance with chronic illness care protocols.

- Meet with parents, school personnel, and health care providers to address issues of concern about the provision of care to students with chronic illnesses by school district staff.

What are the school's responsibilities?

- Identify students with chronic conditions, and review their health records as submitted by families and health care providers.

- Arrange a meeting to discuss health accommodations and educational aids and services that the student may need and to develop a 504 Plan, Individualized Education Program (IEP), or other school plan, as appropriate. The participants should include the family, student (if appropriate), school health staff, 504/IEP coordinator (as applicable), individuals trained to assist the student, and the teacher who has primary responsibility for the student. Health care provider input may be provided in person or in writing.

- Provide nondiscriminatory opportunities to students with disabilities. Be knowledgeable about and ensure compliance with applicable Federal laws, including Americans with Disabilities Act (ADA), Individuals with Disabilities Education Act (IDEA), Section 504, and Family Educational Rights and Privacy Act of 1974 (FERPA). Be knowledgeable about any State or local laws or district policies that affect the implementation of students' rights under Federal law.

- Clarify the roles and obligations of specific school staff, and provide education and communication systems necessary to ensure that students' health and educational needs are met in a safe and coordinated manner.

- Implement strategies that reduce disruption in the student's school activities, including physical education, recess, offsite events, extracurricular activities, and field trips.

- Communicate with families regularly and as authorized with the student's health care providers.

- Ensure that the student receives prescribed medications in a safe, reliable, and effective manner and has access to needed medication at all times during the school day and at school-related activities.

Combatting Frequent School Absenteeism

- Be prepared to handle health needs and emergencies and to ensure that there is a staff member available who is properly trained to administer medications or other immediate care during the school day and at all school-related activities, regardless of time or location.
- Ensure that all staff who interact with the student on a regular basis receive appropriate guidance and training on routine needs, precautions, and emergency actions.
- Provide appropriate health education to students and staff.
- Provide a safe and healthy school environment.
- Ensure that case management is provided as needed.
- Ensure proper record keeping, including appropriate measures to both protect confidentiality and to share information.
- Promote a supportive learning environment that views students with chronic illnesses the same as other students except to respond to health needs.
- Promote good general health, personal care, nutrition, and physical activity.

What are the student's responsibilities?

- Notify an adult about concerns and needs in managing his or her symptoms or the school environment.
- Participate in the care and management of his or her health as appropriate to his or her developmental level.

Chapter 61

Animals in School: A Concern for Children with Asthma

Anyone who has ever given away a pet knows the emotional pain and the delicate family politics involved. Imagine a parent's dilemma when the animal in question is the school mascot or the hamsters in the classroom science corner.

In spite of sleepless nights and mounting doctor bills, parents are sometimes reluctant to risk alienating their child's teacher and classmates by asking them to give away a classroom pet. Other parents say their children's symptoms go unnoticed and their pleas for cooperation are dismissed. If this sounds familiar, the following advice is for you.

Know the Facts

All warm-blooded animals can cause allergic reactions, including rodents and birds. Animal allergen is in the dander, saliva, and urine. When dry, airborne allergen particles accumulate in carpets, upholstery, and fabrics, and on books, desks, and walls.

Allergen particles land in the eyes and are inhaled into the nose and lungs. On the skin they can cause itchy rashes, eczema, and hives.

"What to Do when Animals in School Make Your Child Sick," by Ellie Goldberg, M.Ed., © 1993, revised 2003. Ellie Goldberg, M.Ed., the founder of Healthy Kids: The Key to Basics, is dedicated to building educational and health partnerships for people with asthma and other chronic health professionals, businesses, organizations and policy makers. Online at www.healthkid.info.

They can cause a range of allergies and illnesses such as allergic rhinitis, asthma, allergic bronchopulmonary aspergillus, hypersensitivity pneumonitis, conjunctivitis, and chronic sinus and ear infections.

Damp or wet surfaces are a breeding ground for molds, mildews, bacteria, and insects especially if cages or other animal areas are not cleaned properly. Sensitive airways can also be affected by the odors from urine, cedar chips, room deodorizers, and disinfectant sprays, and the flea powders or insecticides used to control fleas and ticks.

"Carpets in the room become a trap for animal dander and are a potential reservoir for biological contaminants," says Martin A. Cohen, Sc.D., C.I.H., Senior Scientist for Environmental Health and Engineering, a company that specializes in indoor air quality.

Animal biology labs with independent room ventilation units that exhaust the air to the outside are less likely to cause problems. Cohen knows one school system that houses its animals in a separate building. Some schools allow only turtles, hermit crabs, fish, lizards, or snakes. Others limit animal visits and pet parades to outdoor areas.

Once a furry animal is introduced into a school, removing it does not immediately stop allergy problems. A central ventilating system can contaminate the entire school. Even after thorough cleaning, the allergens persist for months. Vacuuming just stirs up the particles. Steam cleaning and vacuuming with a HEPA (high efficiency particle accumulator) filter may reduce but not totally eliminate the allergens.

Know Your School

Read the school manual. Knowing the district's official position on animals can help you identify your goal. Find out who is responsible for decisions that affect your child.

Start with a letter to the principal. Explain that furry animals undermine your child's health and ability to attend school. If your school principal isn't helpful, go higher.

You can ask the pupil services or special education director how to get consideration for your child's allergies or to influence practices that you feel disadvantage your child.

Is your school ignoring district policy? Contact the superintendent about implementing policies. Is there no policy? Does the policy need updating? (Some old school policies only provide for advance notice of

Animals in School: A Concern for Children with Asthma

animal visits so that allergic students can stay home.) Contact the town's board of education about changing old policies or developing new ones.

Be Pro-Health, Not Anti-Animal

The experts agree, "Environmental control to reduce exposure to indoor allergens is a critical component of asthma management...Avoiding allergen exposure reduces symptoms, the need for medication, and the level of airway hyperresponsiveness." (National Heart Lung Blood Institute, National Asthma Education Program Expert Panel Report: *Guidelines for the Diagnosis and Management of Asthma*, page 65.) In other words, exposure to an animal can make allergic people sick. Avoiding animals helps them get better.

Your physician's letter for the school records should be more than a list of allergies and medications. The letter should read: "Eliminating allergens and irritants at school is a necessary part of Mary's asthma and allergy treatment."

Work with Your School Nurse

Her professional license and practice standards make her your best ally and advocate. Her role is to document student health needs and plan necessary services and adaptations. Your physician's letter is her guide to eliminating your child's allergic triggers and asthma aggravators at school. Where there is no school nurse, contact the health officer at your local board of health who investigates environmental health problems and enforces standards.

Keep track of peak flow trends at home and at school. Good records teach school staff about a child's airway changes and can demonstrate the effect of allergens and irritants in the classroom. If you have an individualized health plan (IHP), be sure it includes peak flow meter and daily symptom dairy.

Provide resources that help the school nurse educate the school community about allergies and to advocate for health and environmental standards that benefit everyone. Many teachers and parents may not be aware that coughing, wheezing, sneezing, shortness of breath, rashes, hives, red, watery eyes, a runny nose, or unusual irritability may be signs of allergy.

To cope with occasional animal visits, your doctor may recommend using cromolyn eye drops and a few puffs of cromolyn sodium (Intal®) to block an allergic reaction. Whether this approach may help your child depends on his current health and the intensity of the exposure.

Someone should stand by prepared to administer the appropriate medication if your child has a severe reaction.

You Are Not Alone

Allergies to animals are common. Talk privately to parents and teachers. Attend Parent-Teacher Association (PTA) and school board meetings. Find others with similar needs and related concerns. You may discover someone unhappy that students don't wash their hands after handling the animals. Someone else may worry that classroom pets aren't being cared for properly. Other allergy, health, or disability concerns may bring people together to work for a healthier, barrier-free school. As a team, share concerns, get input from staff and parents, review standards in other districts, and develop recommendations for your school.

Know Your Rights

In the 1970s, Congress passed laws requiring schools to remove barriers for children who were being left out and left behind. For example, schools districts build ramps to ensure access for staff and students who use wheelchairs. However, schools may not be equally accommodating when a classroom pet is the barrier. A principal in Ohio told a parent to consider home schooling when the school's animals made her daughter sick at kindergarten registration.

"That is rare," comments Dr. Robert Fox, president-elect of the American Association of School Administrators. "The modern trend is to eliminate animals. These days most schools prohibit animals because so many teachers and students are allergic."

Advocate for Your Child

By law, schools must be accessible and safe for all students. If your child is allergic to animals, you have the right to ask the school to prohibit or remove animals that make your child sick.

Some administrators may be unsure what to do when the school environment or staff practices affect someone's health. They may not know that federal law protects students with allergies and asthma. Share the U.S. Department of Education information, "The Civil Rights of Students with Hidden Disabilities under Section 504 of the Rehabilitation Act of 1973," online at http://www.ed.gov/about/offices/list/ocr/docs/hq5269.html).

Animals in School: A Concern for Children with Asthma

If you get no support from the principal or district authorities, contact your state department of education. Tell your story to the Section 504 specialist in the pupil services or law division. You can also call your regional office of the U.S. Department of Education Office for Civil Rights (DOE-OCR) for information and advice. If all else fails, make a formal complaint to OCR that the school is violating your child's right to a free and appropriate public education.

Teachers Have Allergies

Boyd Bosma at the National Education Association's Human and Civil Rights Office advises that "A doctor's statement ought to be sufficient to notify the school that arrangements need to be made. Local districts or state departments of education should have policies, health standards, or guidelines for schools. Teachers protected by collective bargaining should use their grievance procedures for violations of health policies or unhealthful working conditions."

Companion Dogs

Both Section 504 and the Americans with Disabilities Act (ADA) require schools to serve students who have a companion dog or service animal and students with allergies. Before class placements, schedules and other decisions are made, schools must consider all students' needs. A collaborative approach to problem solving can expand the school's options and help avoid potential conflicts.

Chapter 62

Chickenpox and Corticosteroids: Is Your Child at Risk?

Most people think of chickenpox as a common, almost harmless childhood disease. However, children who contract it usually run high fevers and feel ill for several days. Chickenpox appear as tiny, clear, slightly red-based blisters that first appear on the child's trunk. Normally, these blisters form scabs and begin to heal in 3–4 days. In rare instances, chickenpox may pose a more serious threat, even to the healthiest of children. Therefore, all children (with only a few exceptions) should receive the varicella (chickenpox) vaccine.

Children with suppressed immune systems, those suffering from genetic defects in the immune system, acquired immune deficiency syndrome (AIDS), leukemia, or other forms of cancer, often experience severe complications from chickenpox.

Are asthmatic children treated with oral or injected steroids at risk?

Most children on oral steroids will endure their chickenpox without any complications. In rare cases, usually in children receiving prolonged oral or injected steroids, chickenpox may result in serious complications, even death, unless specific treatment is sought.

"Chickenpox and Corticosteroids: Is My Child at Risk?" © 2005 American College of Allergy, Asthma and Immunology. All rights reserved. Reprinted with permission.

Does chickenpox pose an increased risk to a child who receives a steroid burst?

A steroid burst refers to short-term use of oral steroids, usually 5–7 days. A burst is prescribed in an emergency situation when asthma is suddenly worse. Only in rare cases do children receiving long or short-term oral steroids experience complications from chickenpox. You should notify your physician immediately if your child is exposed to chickenpox and becomes infected while on or just after a recent burst.

Do inhaled steroids also pose a risk for children exposed to chickenpox?

No. There is no evidence to suggest that inhaled steroids pose an increased risk for children exposed to chickenpox. Inhaled steroids reduce asthma symptoms and the need for symptomatic medications, such as oral steroids. Less oral steroids mean less risk for severe chickenpox.

May I discontinue my child's steroid therapy to prevent the risk of side effects or danger from chickenpox?

No. Halting prescribed asthma treatment is much more dangerous to the child than the potential risk from chickenpox. Parents of children receiving oral steroids should protect their children by vaccinating them.

How do I prevent my child from getting chickenpox?

Vaccination helps prevent most cases of chickenpox. The only way to completely prevent chickenpox is to be sure your child avoids contact with children that have been infected by chickenpox. This is not possible because children are most contagious 24–48 hours before their rash appears.

Since I can't completely prevent exposure to chickenpox, should my asthmatic child receive the vaccine?

Absolutely, the vaccine is safe and 95% effective. The current guidelines recommend that all children should receive the vaccine. Even in the rare circumstance your vaccinated child develops chickenpox, the disease should be milder and less likely to have severe complications.

Chickenpox and Corticosteroids: Is Your Child at Risk?

How do I know if my child has been exposed to chickenpox?

Exposure is normally a problem only when there is prolonged contact (about 1 hour). When cases of chickenpox are reported at school, find out whether the infected children are in your child's class. If so, your child has been exposed to chickenpox. If your child's playmate, or a playmate's sibling, becomes infected with chickenpox, consider your child significantly exposed.

What should I do once my child has been exposed?

If your child is receiving or has recently received oral or injected steroids, you should immediately notify your physician that your child has been exposed to chickenpox. Otherwise check for signs of fever which usually precedes the rash. Check his trunk daily for signs of the tiny, clear, slightly red-based blisters that signal chickenpox infection. Incubation for chickenpox is 11–21 days, so continue monitoring her for three weeks. Normally, the blisters begin to scab and heal in 3–4 days. In rare instances, when a child is receiving oral steroid treatment, these blisters may fail to scab. This indicates that the infection is not healing normally.

If your child is receiving oral steroids and exposure occurred within 48 hours, your doctor may prescribe an injection of varicella zoster immune globulin (VZIG), an enriched human antibody preparation. VZIG is highly effective in preventing chickenpox, but only if administered promptly. If your child has been taking only inhaled steroids, there should be no problem, and VZIG is not necessary. In addition, acyclovir, an antiviral agent that shortens the course of chickenpox, is now available for the treatment of chickenpox in child with persistent asthma.

What do I if my child is receiving or has recently received oral or injected steroids and becomes infected with chickenpox?

Inform your physician immediately. Do not wait for a problem to develop.

Remember

Steroid use in asthmatic children under a physician's care is safe and effective. Complications due to chickenpox exposure are rare. The key to preventing complications for children receiving oral steroids is to vaccinate them and notify the child's physician as soon as you become aware of chickenpox exposure.

Part Six

Asthma Statistics and Research

Chapter 63

Asthma Prevalence, Health Care Use, and Mortality

Asthma is a chronic respiratory disease characterized by episodes or attacks of inflammation and narrowing of small airways in response to asthma "triggers." Asthma attacks can vary from mild to life-threatening and involve shortness of breath, cough, wheezing, chest pain or tightness, or a combination of these symptoms. Many factors can trigger an asthma attack, including allergens, infections, exercise, abrupt changes in the weather, or exposure to airway irritants, such as tobacco smoke.

The burden from asthma in the United States has increased over the past two decades. This chapter presents the most recent national data on asthma gathered by the National Center for Health Statistics. Estimates for race/ethnicity and gender are age adjusted to the 2000 population standard to allow comparison of rates between groups.

Prevalence, 2002: Lifetime Asthma Diagnosis, Current Asthma, and Asthma Attack Prevalence

Respondents in the National Health Interview Survey are asked if they were ever told by a health professional that they had asthma.

From "Asthma Prevalence, Health Care Use and Mortality, 2002," National Center for Health Statistics, Centers for Disease Control and Prevention (CDC), reviewed May 4, 2005. The complete text of this document, including information about data sources and other references, is available online at http://www.cdc.gov/nchs/products/pubs/pubd/hestats/asthma/asthma.htm.

Asthma Sourcebook, Second Edition

In 2002, 30.8 million people (111 people per 1,000) had ever been diagnosed with asthma during their lifetime (Figure 63.1). Among adults, 106 per 1,000 had a lifetime asthma diagnosis (21.9 million) compared to 122 per 1,000 children 0–17 years (8.9 million). Among all racial and ethnic groups, Puerto Ricans have the highest rate of lifetime asthma (196 per 1,000) and Mexicans the lowest (61 per 1,000). Grouping all Hispanics together masks this difference. Puerto Ricans were almost 80% more likely, and non-Hispanic blacks and American Indians were about 25% more likely to have ever been diagnosed with asthma than non-Hispanic whites. Females were about 7% more likely than males to ever have been diagnosed with asthma, but among children 0–17 years of age, males were more likely to have an asthma diagnosis, 139 per 1,000 versus 104 per 1,000 for females.

Estimates of current asthma prevalence include people who have been diagnosed with asthma by a health professional and who still have asthma. In 2002, 72 people per 1,000 or 20 million people, currently had asthma (Figure 63.2). Rates decreased with age; 83 per 1,000 children 0–17 years (6.1 million children) had asthma compared to 68 per

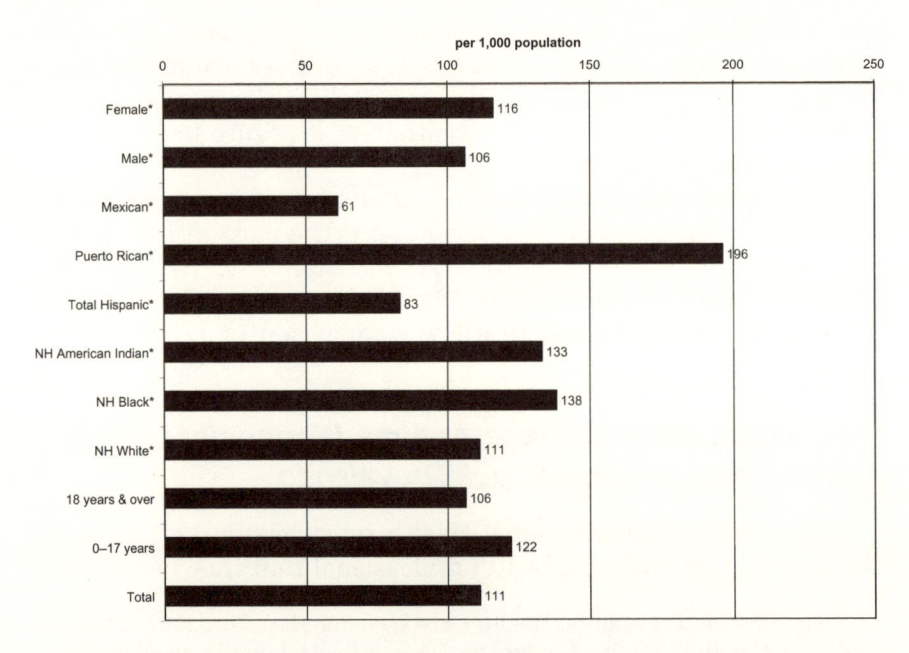

Group	per 1,000 population
Female*	116
Male*	106
Mexican*	61
Puerto Rican*	196
Total Hispanic*	83
NH American Indian*	133
NH Black*	138
NH White*	111
18 years & over	106
0–17 years	122
Total	111

Figure 63.1. Prevalence of lifetime asthma diagnosis, 2002 (Note: *Age adjusted to the 2000 population; Source: CDC/NCHS/National Health Interview Survey).

Asthma Prevalence, Health Care Use, and Mortality

1,000 adults 18 years and over (14 million adults). When race/ethnicity is considered, Puerto Ricans had current asthma prevalence 80% higher than non-Hispanic whites, and non-Hispanic blacks and American Indians had current asthma prevalence 30% higher than non-Hispanic whites. The overall estimate for Hispanics masks the high prevalence among Puerto Ricans. Females had a 30% higher prevalence compared to males. However, this pattern was reversed among children. The current asthma prevalence rate for boys aged 0–17 years (94 per 1,000) was 30% higher than the rate among girls (71 per 1,000).

Asthma attack prevalence, or the number of people who had at least one asthma attack in the previous year, is a crude indicator of how many people have uncontrolled asthma and are at risk for a poor outcome, such as hospitalization. In 2002, 43 people per 1,000 (12 million people) had experienced an asthma attack in the previous year (Figure 63.3). That is, about 60% of the people who had asthma at the time of the survey had an asthma attack in the previous year. Asthma attack prevalence also decreased with age, 58 per 1,000 children 0–17 years (4.2 million children) had an asthma attack in the previous year compared to 37 per 1,000 adults aged 18 years and over (7.7

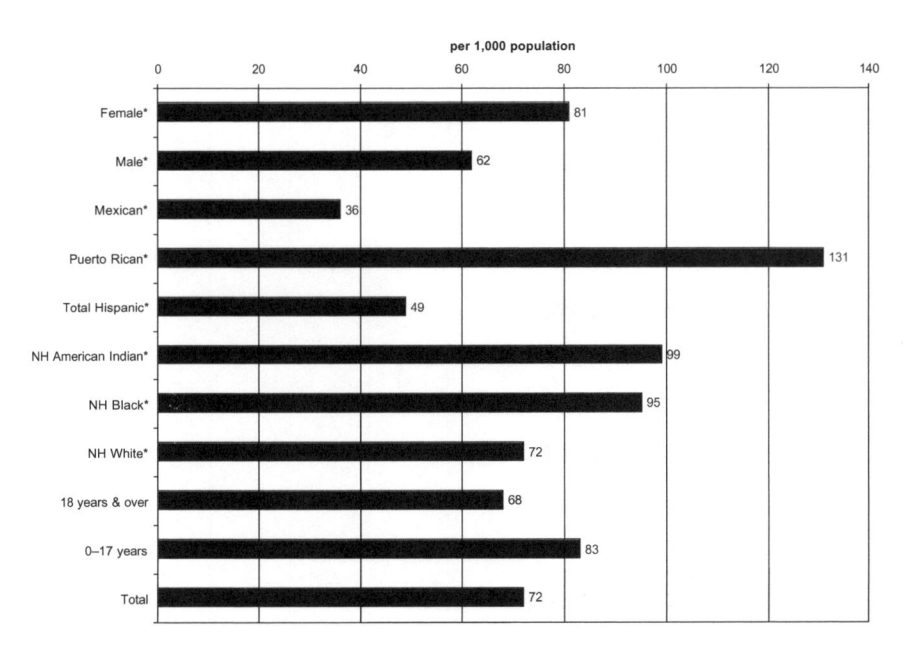

Category	per 1,000 population
Female*	81
Male*	62
Mexican*	36
Puerto Rican*	131
Total Hispanic*	49
NH American Indian*	99
NH Black*	95
NH White*	72
18 years & over	68
0–17 years	83
Total	72

Figure 63.2. Current asthma prevalence, 2002 (Note: *Age adjusted to the 2000 population; Source: CDC/NCHS/National Health Interview Survey).

million adults). Puerto Ricans had the highest asthma attack prevalence, 100% higher than non-Hispanic whites while Non-Hispanic blacks had an asthma attack prevalence about 30% higher and American Indians about 10% higher than non-Hispanic whites. Mexicans had the lowest asthma attack prevalence. Females had about 35% higher prevalence than males. This pattern was reversed among children. The asthma attack prevalence rate for boys aged 0–17 years (68 per 1,000) was 45% higher than the rate among girls (47 per 1,000).

Missed School and Work Days, 2002

Asthma attacks interfere with daily activities, including attending school and going to work. Among those who reported at least one asthma attack in the previous year the following data applied:

- Children 5–17 years of age missed 14.7 million school days due to asthma.

- Adults 18 years of age and over who were currently employed missed 11.8 million work days due to asthma.

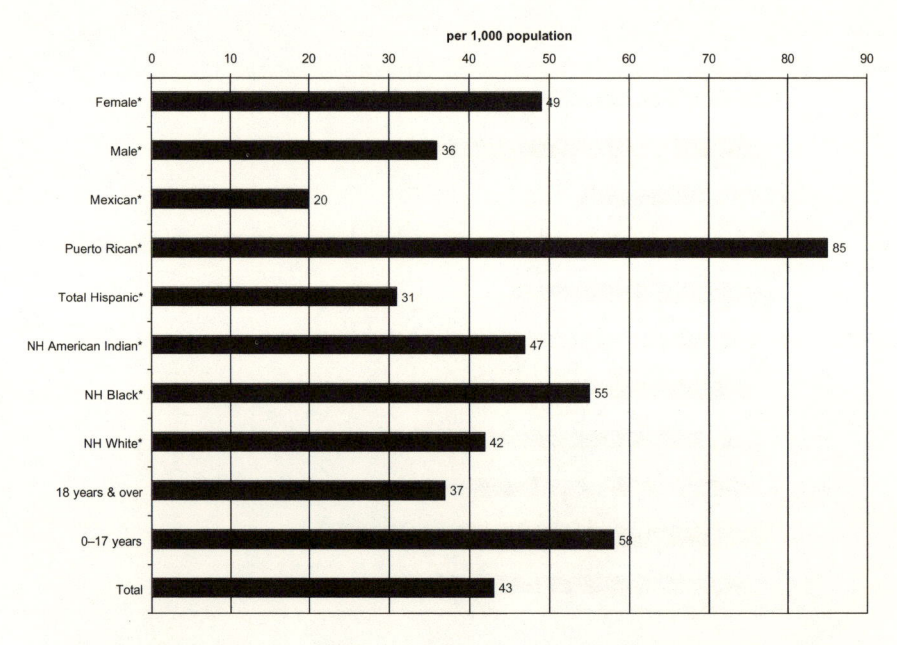

Figure 63.3. *Asthma attack prevalence, 2002 (Note: *Age adjusted to the 2000 population; Source: CDC/NCHS/National Health Interview Survey).*

Asthma Prevalence, Health Care Use, and Mortality

Source: National Health Interview Survey, National Center for Health Statistics, CDC.

Health Care Use, 2002

Health care use for asthma includes outpatient visits to doctors' offices and hospital outpatient departments, visits to hospital emergency departments (EDs), and hospitalizations. Information about Hispanic ethnicity is not consistently available in national health care utilization data, and therefore is not presented. In 2002, there were 13.9 million outpatient asthma visits to private physician offices and hospital outpatient departments, or 492 per 10,000 people (Figure 63.4). Children aged 0–17 years had 5 million visits and an outpatient visit rate of 687 per 10,000 and adults 18 years and older had a rate of 181 per 10,000. In contrast to other asthma measures shown here, blacks had an outpatient visit rate about the same as whites. Females had a 50% higher outpatient visit rate compared to males.

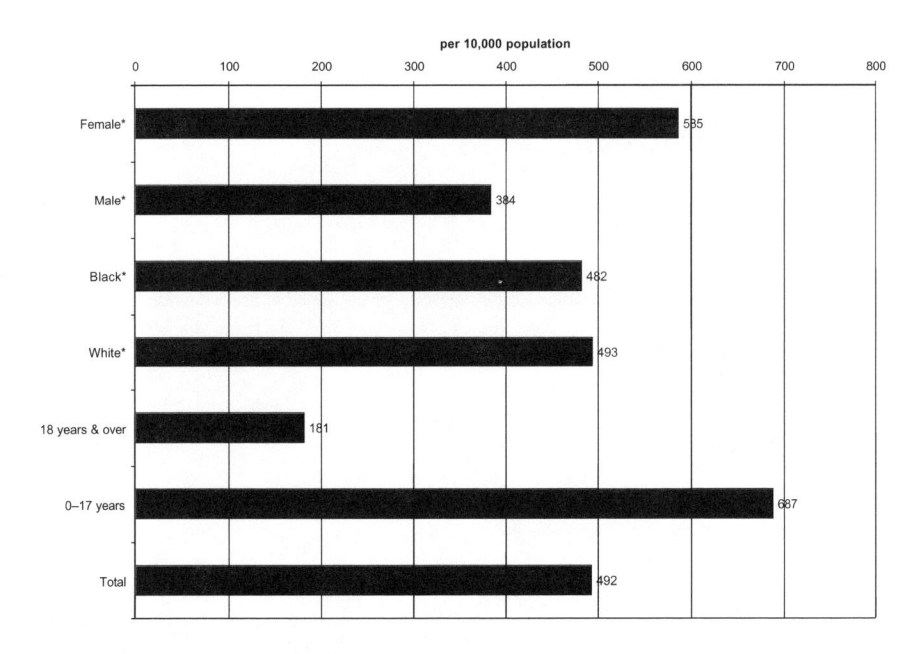

Category	per 10,000 population
Female*	585
Male*	384
Black*	482
White*	493
18 years & over	181
0–17 years	687
Total	492

*Figure 63.4. Asthma Outpatient Visits, 2002 (Note: *Age adjusted to the 2000 population; Source: CDC/NCHS National Ambulatory Medical Care Survey and National Hospital Ambulatory Medical Care Survey).*

Asthma Sourcebook, Second Edition

There were 1.9 million visits to EDs for asthma in 2002, or 67 per 10,000 people (Figure 63.5). Children aged 0–17 years had over 727,000 ED visits, a rate of 100 per 10,000. The ED visit rate was highest among children aged 0–4 years at 162 per 10,000. Adults 18 years and over had 24 ED visits per 10,000. The ED visit rate for blacks was 380% higher than that for whites, and for females, about 6% higher than for males.

There were 484,000 asthma hospitalizations in 2002, or 17 per 10,000 people (Figure 63.6). Among children 0-17 years, there were 196,000 hospitalizations (27 per 10,000). Hospitalizations were highest among children 0–4 years, 59 hospitalizations per 10,000. The asthma hospitalization rate for blacks was 225% higher than for whites. Females had a hospitalization rate about 35% higher than males.

Mortality

In 2002, 4,261 people died from asthma, or 1.5 per 100,000 people (Figure 63.7). Among children, asthma deaths are rare. In 2002, 187

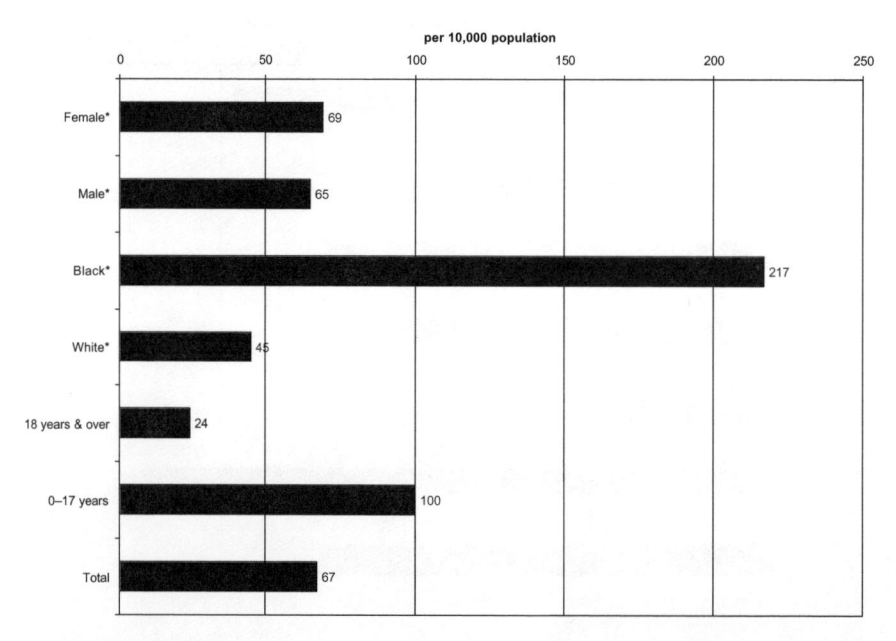

Category	per 10,000 population
Female*	69
Male*	65
Black*	217
White*	45
18 years & over	24
0–17 years	100
Total	67

Figure 63.5. Asthma Emergency Department Visits, 2002 (Note: *Age adjusted to the 2000 population; Source CDC/NCHS National Hospital Ambulatory Medical Care Survey).

Asthma Prevalence, Health Care Use, and Mortality

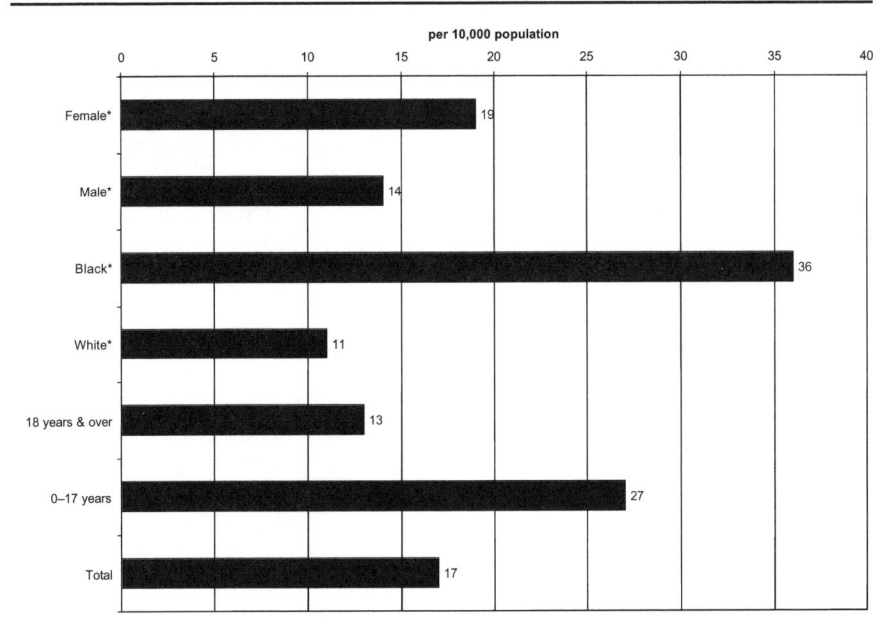

Figure 63.6. Asthma Hospitalizations, 2002 (Note: *Age adjusted to the 2000 population; Source CDC/NCHS National Hospital Discharge Survey).

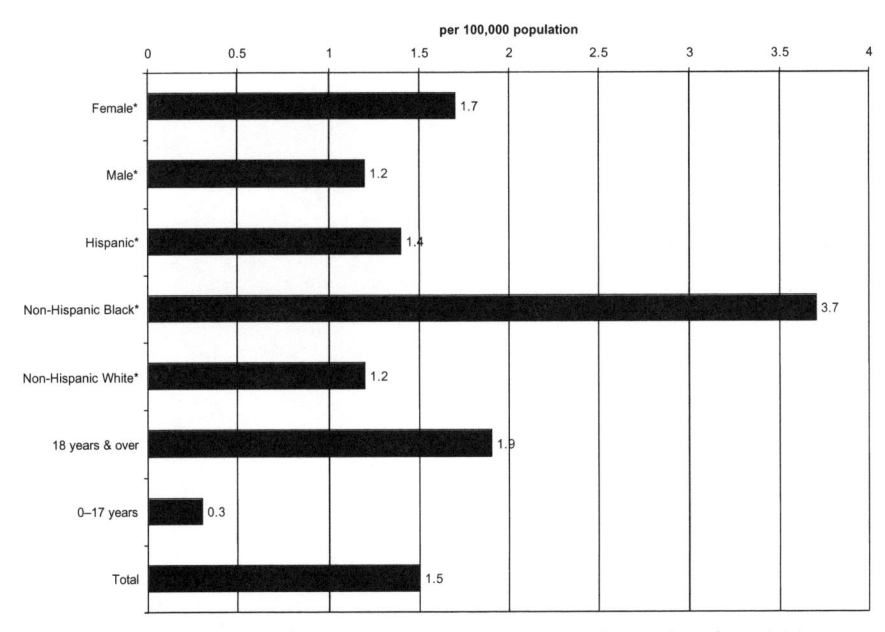

Category	per 10,000 population
Female*	19
Male*	14
Black*	36
White*	11
18 years & over	13
0–17 years	27
Total	17

Figure 63.7. Asthma Deaths, 2002 (Note: *Age adjusted to the 2000 population; Source: CDC/NCHS National Vital Statistics System).

Category	per 100,000 population
Female*	1.7
Male*	1.2
Hispanic*	1.4
Non-Hispanic Black*	3.7
Non-Hispanic White*	1.2
18 years & over	1.9
0–17 years	0.3
Total	1.5

children aged 0–17 years died from asthma, or 0.3 deaths per 100,000 children compared to 1.9 deaths per 100,000 adults aged 18 and over. Non-Hispanic blacks were the most likely to die from asthma, and had an asthma death rate over 200% higher than non-Hispanic whites and 160% higher than Hispanics. National estimates for Hispanic subgroups, such as Puerto Ricans and Mexicans, are not available. Females had an asthma death rate about 40% higher than males.

Chapter 64

Global Burden of Asthma

Summary

- Asthma is one of the most common chronic diseases in the world. It is estimated that around 300 million people in the world currently have asthma. Considerably higher estimates can be obtained with less conservative criteria for the diagnosis of clinical asthma.

- The international patterns of asthma prevalence are not explained by the current knowledge of the causation of asthma. Research into the causation of asthma, and the efficacy of primary and secondary intervention strategies, represent key priority areas in the field of asthma research.

- Asthma has become more common in both children and adults around the world in recent decades. The increase in the prevalence of asthma has been associated with an increase in atopic sensitization, and is paralleled by similar increases in other allergic disorders such as eczema and rhinitis.

Excerpted from "Global Burden of Asthma™," by Matthew Masoli, Denise Fabian, Shaun Holt, and Richard Beasley, developed for the Global Initiative for Asthma (GINA). © 2003 GINA. Reprinted with permission from the Global Initiative for Asthma. The full text of this document, including graphs, maps, and key references, is available online at http://www.ginasthma.com/ReportItem.asp?l1=2&l2=2&intId=95.

- The rate of asthma increases as communities adopt western lifestyles and become urbanized. With the projected increase in the proportion of the world's population that is urban from 45% to 59% in 2025, there is likely to be a marked increase in the number of asthmatics worldwide over the next two decades. It is estimated that there may be an additional 100 million persons with asthma by 2025.

- In many areas of the world persons with asthma do not have access to basic asthma medications or medical care. Increasing the economic wealth and improving the distribution of resources between and within countries represent important priorities to enable better health care to be provided.

- The number of disability-adjusted life years (DALYs) lost due to asthma worldwide has been estimated to be currently about 15 million per year. Worldwide, asthma accounts for around 1% of all DALYs lost, which reflects the high prevalence and severity of asthma. The number of DALYs lost due to asthma is similar to that for diabetes, cirrhosis of the liver, or schizophrenia.

- The burden of asthma in many countries is of sufficient magnitude to warrant its recognition as a priority disorder in government health strategies. Particular resources need to be provided to improve the care of disadvantaged groups with high morbidity, including certain racial groups and those who are poorly educated, live in large cities, or are poor. Resources also need to be provided to address preventable factors, such as air pollution, that trigger exacerbations of asthma.

- It is estimated that asthma accounts for about one in every 250 deaths worldwide. Many of the deaths are preventable, being due to suboptimal long-term medical care and delay in obtaining help during the final attack.

- The economic cost of asthma is considerable both in terms of direct medical costs (such as hospital admissions and cost of pharmaceuticals) and indirect medical costs (such as time lost from work and premature death).

- Until there is a greater understanding of the factors that cause asthma and novel public health and pharmacological measures become available to reduce the prevalence of asthma, the priority is to ensure that cost-effective management approaches which

Global Burden of Asthma

have been proven to reduce morbidity and mortality are available to as many persons as possible with asthma worldwide.

Barriers to Reducing the Burden of Asthma

- Generic barriers including poverty, poor education, and poor infrastructure.
- Environmental barriers including indoor and outdoor air pollution, tobacco smoking, and occupational exposures.
- Low public health priority due to the importance of other respiratory illnesses such as tuberculosis and pneumonia and the lack of data on morbidity and mortality from asthma.
- The lack of symptom-based rather than disease-based approaches to the management of respiratory diseases including asthma.
- Unsustainable generalizations across cultures and health care systems which may make management guidelines developed in high-income countries difficult to implement in low and middle-income countries.
- Inherent barriers in the organization of health care services in terms of the following:
  - geography
  - type of professional responding
  - education and training systems
  - public and private care
  - tendency of care to be "acute" rather than "routine"
- The limited availability and use of medications including the following:
  - omission of basic medications from WHO [World Health Organization] or national essential drug lists
  - poor supply and distribution infrastructure
  - cost
  - cultural attitudes towards drug delivery systems; for example, inhalers
- Patient barriers, such as the following:

- cultural factors
- lack of information
- underuse of self-management
- over-reliance on acute care
- use of alternative unproven therapies

- Inadequate government resources provided for health care including asthma.

- The responsibility of respiratory specialists and related organizations required to care for a wide variety of diseases, which has in some regions resulted in a failure to adequately promote awareness of asthma.

Actions Required to Reduce the Burden of Asthma

- Recognize asthma as an important cause of morbidity, economic cost, and mortality worldwide.

- Measure and monitor the prevalence of asthma, and the morbidity and mortality due to asthma throughout the world.

- Identify and address the economic and political factors which limit the availability of health care.

- Improve accessibility to essential drugs for the management of asthma in low- and middle-income countries.

- Identify and address the environmental factors including indoor and outdoor pollution which affect respiratory morbidity, including that due to asthma.

- Promote and implement anti-tobacco public health policies to reduce tobacco consumption.

- Adapt international asthma guidelines for developing countries to ensure they are practical and realistic in terms of different health care systems. This includes dissemination strategies for their implementation.

- Integrate the Global Initiative for Asthma (GINA) guidelines with other global respiratory guidelines for children and adults. In this respect, there is a requirement to merge the key elements of the different respiratory guidelines into an algorithm for use at the first point of entry of a respiratory patient's contact with health services.

- Promote cost-effective management approaches which have been proven to reduce morbidity and mortality, thereby ensuring optimal treatment is available to as many persons as possible with asthma worldwide.
- Research the causation of asthma, primary and secondary intervention strategies, and management programs including those for use in developing countries.

Chapter 65

Asthma: A Concern for Minority Populations

Overview

Allergic diseases, including asthma, are among the major causes of illness and disability in the United States. Illness and death from asthma have been increasing in this country for the past 15 years and are particularly high among poor, inner-city African-Americans. Although asthma is only slightly more prevalent among minority children than among whites, it accounts for three times the number of deaths. Low socioeconomic status, exposure to urban environmental contaminants, lack of access to medical care, and lack of self-management skills all contribute to the increase in deaths in minority communities.

The National Institute of Allergy and Infectious Diseases (NIAID), a component of the National Institutes of Health (NIH), supports basic, preclinical, and clinical research to prevent, diagnose, and treat infections and immune-mediated illnesses, including asthma and allergies.

Through basic and clinical research, as well as intervention programs, NIAID seeks to improve the diagnosis, treatment, and management of asthma, particularly in the minority populations disproportionately affected by this disease.

National Institute of Allergy and Infectious Diseases (http://niaid.nih.gov), October 2001.

Growing Health Problem

Asthma is a growing health problem in the United States, particularly in inner-city African-American and Latino populations. Asthma is a chronic lung disease characterized by episodes of airflow obstruction. Symptoms of an asthma attack include the following:

- coughing
- wheezing
- shortness of breath
- chest tightness

Asthma occurs in people who are predisposed to develop asthma because of genetic and environmental factors that determine susceptibility. A variety of "triggers" may start or worsen an asthma attack, including the following:

- exposure to allergens
- viral respiratory infections
- airway irritants, such as tobacco smoke and certain environmental pollutants
- exercise

Exposure of susceptible children to some of these triggers in early childhood, notably allergens such as house dust mites or cockroaches, may cause asthma.

Once asthma sufferers learn what conditions prompt their attacks, they can attempt to control their environments and avoid these triggers. Medical treatment with anti-inflammatory agents (especially inhaled steroids) and bronchodilators, however, is usually necessary to prevent and control attacks. With optimal management, people usually can control their asthma. Unfortunately, those living in inner cities cannot always get optimal care. Even currently available treatments do not control severe asthma in some patients, such as children in inner cities.

Asthma: A Health Disparity

NIAID's *Strategic Plan for Addressing Health Disparities* identifies asthma as a key research area. The plan seeks to resolve health disparities by the following:

Asthma: A Concern for Minority Populations

- directing funding for research on diseases known to occur disparately in a population
- identifying environmental, occupational, social, genetic, or biochemical factors that increase susceptibility to infectious and immunologic diseases
- increasing the participation and support of minority scientists interested in research on health disparities, including the number of minority scientists in training
- communicating research developments to the population groups affected by health disparities

The Impact of Asthma

After a decade of steady decline in the 1970s, the prevalence of asthma, hospitalizations for asthma, and death due to asthma each increased during the 1980s and 1990s. Asthma affects an estimated 17 million Americans or 6.4 percent of the U.S. population. Children account for 4.8 million of the nation's asthma sufferers.

Asthma affects slightly more African Americans (5.8 percent) than Americans of European descent (5.1 percent). In 1993, however, blacks were three to four times more likely than whites to be hospitalized for asthma. In 1994, there were 451,000 asthma-related hospitalizations in the United States. Children accounted for 169,000 of these. In 1995, asthma caused more than 1.8 million emergency room visits.

Asthma claims approximately 5,000 lives annually in the United States. Asthma deaths have increased significantly during the past two decades. From 1975 to 1979, the death rate was 8.2 per 100,000 people. That rate jumped from 1993–1995 to 17.9 per 100,000. Particularly alarming, the death rate from asthma for children ages 5 to 14 doubled from 1980 to 1993. African Americans were four to six times more likely than whites to die from asthma. The increasing prevalence of asthma in inner-city children underscores the need for new therapies to prevent asthma and reduce its prevalence.

Poverty, substandard housing that increases exposure to certain indoor allergens, lack of education, inadequate access to health care, and the failure to take appropriate prescribed medicines may all increase the risk of having a severe asthma attack or, more tragically, of dying from asthma.

Uncontrolled asthma also can impose serious limitations on daily life. Asthma is the leading cause of school absenteeism due to chronic illness and the second most important respiratory condition to cause home confinement for adults. Each year, asthma causes more than 18 million days of restricted activity, and millions of visits to physicians' offices and emergency rooms. One study found that children with asthma lose an extra 10 million school days each year. This problem is compounded by an estimated $1 billion in lost productivity for their working parents. Asthma-related health care cost our nation approximately $10.7 billion in 1994, including a direct health care cost of $6.1 billion. Indirect costs, such as lost work days, added up to $4.6 billion.

National Cooperative Inner-City Asthma Studies

To address the special concerns about asthma in the inner city, NIAID launched the first National Cooperative Inner-City Asthma Study in 1991. The primary aim of the study was to find out why asthma disproportionately affects inner-city children and test new treatment and prevention methods. NIAID funds eight inner-city asthma study sites.

- Albert Einstein School of Medicine, New York, NY
- Case Western Reserve University, Cleveland, OH
- Children's Memorial Hospital, Chicago, IL
- Henry Ford Hospital, Detroit, MI
- Howard University, Washington DC
- Johns Hopkins University, Baltimore, MD
- Mt. Sinai Medical Center, New York, NY
- Washington University, St. Louis, MO

Phase I of the first National Cooperative Inner-City Asthma Study (1991–1994) was designed to identify factors associated with severity of asthma in children ages 4–11. This investigation demonstrated that the combination of cockroach exposure and cockroach allergy was a major factor for asthma severity. The study developed and tested a one-year comprehensive educational, behavioral, and environmental intervention.

Phase I enrolled 1,528 children and their families. The study population was 73 percent African American, 20 percent Hispanic, and 7 percent Caucasian. Ninety-three percent of the participants completed the study. Asthma risk factors found to be present in these urban families included the following:

- high levels of indoor allergens, especially cockroach allergen

Asthma: A Concern for Minority Populations

- high levels of tobacco smoking among family members and caretakers
- high indoor levels of nitrogen dioxide, a respiratory irritant produced by inadequately vented stoves and heating appliances

This study provided the most convincing data that cockroach was the major allergen for inner-city children. Low socioeconomic status and African descent were independent risk factors for allergic sensitization to cockroach allergens. Thus, new approaches to reduce exposure to cockroach allergens may be very useful in controlling asthma.

The second phase, completed in February 1996, studied the effectiveness of a comprehensive program to develop improved knowledge about asthma, to promote better asthma self-management skills, and to eliminate or decrease exposure to environmental factors, especially cockroach allergen, associated with increased morbidity from asthma.

More than 1,000 children were enrolled in Phase II of the study. Several sites used a Spanish language program in addition to the standard English language program. These sites employed bilingual counselors and modified the intervention to account for cultural issues unique to a Latino population.

A key component of the Phase II intervention was the use of an "asthma care counselor" whose primary role was to teach and monitor acquisition of asthma self-management skills. This highly successful program reduced by approximately 30 percent major asthma symptoms, hospitalizations, and emergency room visits.

These improvements continued during the second year of the follow-up without the assistance of an asthma counselor, suggesting that the intervention guided the children and their families to acquire self-management skills, which had a long-term benefit to their asthma. This model of asthma intervention in the inner city, if adopted nationwide, could substantially reduce emergency room visits, hospitalizations, and healthcare costs.

In February 2001, based on this scientifically proven intervention, the U.S. Centers for Disease Control and Prevention announced the awarding of 23 grants, totaling $2.9 million, to enable community-based health organizations throughout the United States sites to implement the NIAID model asthma intervention program.

Second Multicenter Study

Based on the success of the first National Cooperative Inner-City Asthma Study, NIAID and the National Institute of Environmental

Health Sciences (NIEHS), another NIH component, initiated a second cooperative multicenter study in 1996. This study recruited nearly 950 children with asthma, ages 4–11, to test the effectiveness of two interventions. One intervention entails a novel communication/physician education system. Information about the children's asthma severity is provided to their primary care physicians, with the intent that this information will optimize the care provided by the physicians.

The other intervention involves educating families about reducing exposure to passive cigarette smoke and to indoor allergens, including cockroach, house dust mite, and mold allergens. Researchers will assess the effectiveness of both interventions by their capacity to reduce the severity of asthma in these children. They also will test protocols for the duration of effectiveness after one year of active intervention is completed. The seven Centers are as follows:

- Albert Einstein School of Medicine, New York, NY
- Boston University, Boston, MA
- Children's Memorial Hospital, Chicago, IL
- Mt. Sinai Medical Center, New York, NY
- University of Arizona Health Sciences Center, Tucson, AZ
- University of Texas Southwestern Medical Center, Dallas, TX
- Odessa Brown Children's Clinic, Seattle, WA

In addition, through support of the U.S. Environmental Protection Agency, an arm of the study will focus on evaluating the effects of indoor and outdoor pollutants on asthma severity.

NIAID Research Centers

NIAID also supports 12 extramural Asthma, Allergic, and Immunologic Diseases Cooperative Research Centers to conduct basic and clinical research on mechanisms of disease and ways to prevent asthma, allergic, and immunologic diseases.

Studies on the Genetic Basis of Asthma

NIAID supports a research program to identify genes associated with allergy and asthma, and to search for related genes in mice. This program was the first to link high IgE levels (high allergic response) to a region of human chromosome 5, near genes for IL-4, and other cytokines.

Chapter 66

Asthma in Children Remains Significantly Out of Control in the U.S.

Findings from one of the nation's largest and most comprehensive surveys about children and asthma to date, Children and Asthma in America, reveal that more than half (54%) of all children with asthma had a severe asthma attack in the past year and more than one quarter (27%) had an asthma attack so bad they thought their life was in danger. The survey results released today underscore the severity of asthma in children in the U.S. and the significant impact the disease has on children and their families.

Presented on behalf of Asthma Action America, the survey findings suggest the U.S. is still falling far short of the national treatment goals established for asthma, and reveal the majority of children with asthma do not have it under control. This places children at potential risk for a variety of consequences including frequent symptoms, missed school, restrictions on activities, emotional distress, hospitalization and even life-threatening asthma attacks. Asthma is one of the most common chronic illnesses among children, with an estimated 5.8 million American children four to 18 years of age currently with the condition.

"These are disturbing findings, especially since asthma is a highly controllable disease," said William Sears M.D., nationally acclaimed

---

"Landmark Survey Reveals Asthma in Children Remains Significantly out of Control in the United States: Asthma Control in Children Falls Far Short of National Treatment Goals," reprinted with permission. © 2005 American Lung Association. For more information about the American Lung Association or to support the work it does, call 1-800-LUNG-USA (1-800-586-4872) or log on to www.lungusa.org.

author, pediatrician and associate clinical professor of pediatrics at the University of California Irvine School of Medicine. "We need to help parents recognize that proper asthma control means children are symptom-free all or most of the time. Parents should talk to their healthcare professional about prevention of asthma symptoms and long-term management so their child does not suffer needlessly."

Asthma Control in Children: Are We Missing The Mark?

In the survey, four out of five respondents reported that their or their child's asthma was well (43%) or completely controlled (35%), yet children missed the mark on nearly every treatment goal established by the National Heart, Lung, and Blood Institute (NHLBI)—part of the National Institutes of Health. A point-by-point comparison shows asthma is not being as well-controlled as it should be.

NHLBI Goals of Therapy

- Minimal or no chronic asthma symptoms (coughing, wheezing, shortness of breath, chest tightness) during the day or night.
- Minimal or no exacerbations (including hospitalization or emergency room visits).
- No limitations on activities; no school/parent's work missed.
- Minimal use of short-acting beta-agonists (rescue inhaler).
- Having a written Asthma Action Plan.
- Visit your healthcare professional to monitor your asthma at least two times per year.

Children and Asthma in America *Survey*

In the past four weeks:

- 2/3 of children (67%) experienced asthma symptoms during the day, during the night or during exercise or exertion.
- Nearly one in five children (19%) experienced daytime symptoms three times a week to daily; almost a quarter (22%) experienced symptoms at least once a week at night.
- 23% have visited the emergency room in the past year.
- 42% reported unscheduled acute care visits in the past year because of asthma.

Asthma in Children Remains Significantly Out of Control

- 54% missed school or daycare in the past year as a result of their asthma, with an average of nearly four days missed.
- 39% of parents of children with asthma missed work in the past year due to their child's condition.
- 62% of children said asthma caused them to limit activities a lot or some.
- Of those who used rescue medications in the past four weeks, nearly half (42%) used them three times a week to daily; nearly one in four (26%) used them daily.
- 54% of children with asthma said they did not have a written Asthma Action Plan.
- 25% of children with asthma had not seen their healthcare professional about their condition in the past year.
- 54% have not had a lung function test in the past 12 months.

Survey Shows Communication Gap between Children and Parents

The *Children and Asthma in America* survey shows a concerning difference between how parents perceive their child's asthma and how children themselves perceive their disease. In fact, when comparing responses of parents and their children with asthma who were 10 to 15 years of age, the survey showed that the majority (71%) of parents and their children disagreed about the child's overall health status. Additionally, 32% of parents and their children disagreed that restrictions on activities was the worse thing about having asthma, 45% disagreed that the child experienced any daytime asthma symptoms in the past four weeks, and 38% disagreed that the child had no asthma symptoms in the same time period. Specifically, over the past four weeks, parents and their children disagreed that the child experienced coughing (46%), shortness of breath (44%), wheezing (40%) and breathing problems (37%).

"It is concerning to see so many parents thinking their child's asthma is under control when many children are experiencing symptoms on a daily basis," said Dr. Sears. "The lack of effective dialogue between parent and child about their asthma could be a major factor in why asthma still remains poorly controlled among America's children. It's important that parents regularly ask their child specific questions about symptoms so they can get an accurate picture of their child's level of asthma control."

More than Half of Those Surveyed Don't Understand Causes of Asthma Symptoms

Asthma is a highly controllable disease when proper prevention and long-term management of the underlying causes are followed. However, the survey reveals widespread misunderstanding about the causes of and treatments for asthma symptoms. The majority admitted they never heard of bronchoconstriction—tightening of the muscles surrounding the airways—(90%) or inflammation—airway-swelling and irritation—(93%)—the two underlying causes of asthma symptoms.

Only 53% of those classified as having severe asthma and 63% of those with moderate asthma reported they or their children took prescription medication for daily maintenance therapy during the past four weeks (like an inhaled corticosteroid). Additionally, 30% of respondents incorrectly named a short-acting beta-agonist (an inhaler used for treating sudden asthma symptoms) as a long-term asthma control medicine. National treatment guidelines recommend daily use of an inhaled corticosteroid as the preferred therapy for people with persistent asthma.

Facilitating Parent/Child Discussions: Helpful Resource Available

To help encourage the dialogue between parents and their child about asthma symptoms, Asthma Action America is offering a free asthma brochure featuring tips from Dr. Sears and the Asthma Control Test™, five questions parents should ask their child to help assess their child's level of asthma control. The brochure and more information about asthma in children are available at www.AsthmaActionAmerica.org or by calling 1-800-377-9575. Survey results can also be found at www.AsthmaInAmerica.com.

About the Survey

Children and Asthma in America was conducted by Schulman, Ronca and Bucuvalas, Inc. (SRBI), a national research firm specializing in health issues. A national sample of 41,433 households was screened to generate households with a child four to 18 years of age with current asthma. The survey included 801 in-depth telephone interviews with parents or caregivers of the designated child with asthma in the household or the child with asthma exclusively if he or she was 16 to 18 years of age. In addition, the survey included interviews with

Asthma in Children Remains Significantly Out of Control

nearly 300 pairs of parents and their children (10 to 15 years old) to provide comparison responses. All interviews were conducted from February to May 2004, and assessed knowledge, attitudes and behavior regarding children and asthma. The maximum expected sampling error associated with a sample of this size would be +/- 3.5 percentage points at the 95% confidence level. The survey was released on behalf of Asthma Action America®, a national asthma education campaign supported by leading organizations committed to improving asthma care in the U.S., and was funded by GlaxoSmithKline. GlaxoSmithKline is a research-based pharmaceutical company and a world leader in respiratory care.

Chapter 67

Studying Strategies to Improve Care for Low-Income Children with Asthma

Introduction

Many children with asthma do not get the care they need, despite the existence of asthma care guidelines and evidence about effective treatments. For example, the appropriate use of controller medications is very important in the treatment of asthma. By helping to reduce the underlying inflammation of the airways in a person with asthma, controller medications diminish asthma symptoms and prevent attacks.

However, among children and adults with persistent asthma, approximately 29 percent are not receiving appropriate controller medications from providers, and some patients are not using the medications appropriately. Among Medicaid-enrolled children with persistent asthma, the underuse of controller medications is widespread, reaching as high as 73 percent. As a result, there are more acute episodes, greater use of emergency rooms and hospitals, and increased treatment costs.

Research has shown that reorganizing the way chronic care is delivered can increase the appropriate use of controller medications among

---

Excerpted from "Chronic Care for Low-Income Children with Asthma: Strategies for Improvement," by Mark W. Stanton, M.A., and Denise Dougherty, Ph.D. (Note: Bernard Friedman, Ph.D., made a significant contribution to this report), *Research in Action*, Issue 18, Agency for Healthcare Qualify and Research, AHRQ Publication No. 05-0073, June 2005. The complete text of this report, including references, is available online at http://www.ahrq.gov/researchchastria/chastria.htm.

children with asthma and have other positive results. Preliminary evidence also suggests that disparities in asthma care can be decreased through the use of strategies sensitive to the needs of racial and ethnic minorities.

Background

Approximately 9 million children (12 percent of children under age 18) have been diagnosed with asthma, according to the 2002 National Health Interview Survey. In 2002, health care costs for children with asthma in the United States totaled more than $6 billion. Hospital stays are usually the most expensive form of medical care, and children age 17 and under are much more likely to be admitted to a hospital for asthma than are adults (27.5 per 10,000 vs. 12.7 per 10,000). In fact, asthma admissions accounted for 7.4 percent (152,000) of all hospital admissions for children and adolescents in 2000. Almost half of hospitalizations for asthma among children are billed to Medicaid.

States are increasingly contracting with Medicaid managed care programs in various forms and giving them the responsibility for providing care to many Medicaid-enrolled children. Managed care, with its emphasis on the organization and coordination of care, has increased expectations about the quality of care that can be provided for those with asthma and other chronic conditions. At the same time, another feature of managed care, fixed prepaid budgets, has raised questions about the ability of these organizations to deliver on their promise.

Data on Asthma Care Show Gaps in Quality

Asthma care guidelines and evidence about effective treatments are available. The National Asthma Education and Prevention Program (NAEPP) Expert Panel issued its revised *Guidelines for Diagnosis and Management of Asthma (EPR-2)* in 1997 and an Update in 2002. However, many children with asthma do not get the care they need.

In addition, even when providers deliver appropriate care, children may not be using controller medications correctly because their parents do not understand the purpose of the medication. According to the 2004 survey on the quality of care in commercial managed care plans from the National Committee for Quality Assurance, about 29 percent of children and adults (ages 5–56) with persistent asthma are not receiving inhaled corticosteroids to control their condition.

The problem of underuse was even more serious among children with persistent asthma enrolled in Medicaid managed care, according to researchers from the Asthma Care Quality Assessment (ACQA) Study. In 1999, these children experienced a very high rate (73 percent) of underuse of controller therapy, with 49 percent of parents reporting no controller use and 24 percent reporting less than daily use.

A related issue is the significant racial/ethnic disparities in asthma status and home management practices. For example, African-American and Hispanic children with similar insurance and sociodemographic characteristics have more severe asthma than white children based on number of symptom days, school days missed, and health status scores. Also, compared to white children, in 1999 African-American and Hispanic children were 31 percent and 42 percent less likely, respectively, to be using controller medications (including inhaled corticosteroids). Finally, African-American children are about three times as likely to be admitted to a hospital for asthma as white children.

Successful Asthma Management

Successful management of asthma has four basic components:

- reducing or controlling exposure to environmental triggers
- objective monitoring of the condition by patient and provider
- taking appropriate medications as indicated
- active involvement of the patient in managing the disease

The last component—patient self-management (and, in the case of children, family management)—is critical to the other three. People with persistent asthma need long-term controller medications. The treatment of choice for the most effective long-term control of asthma is inhaled corticosteroids. This may be supplemented by long-acting beta-agonists in cases of moderate to severe persistent asthma.

Other controller medications include leukotriene modifiers, cromolyn, nedocromil, and theophylline. Long-term controller medications are taken every day, usually over long periods of time, to control chronic symptoms and to prevent asthma episodes or attacks.

Increasing Use of Controller Medications Improves Outcomes

In its systematic review of research on the management of chronic asthma, an Evidence-based Practice Center (EPC) reported that the regular use of inhaled corticosteroids improves long-term outcomes for children with mild to moderate asthma. This systematic review also found that regular use of controller medications reduced hospitalizations. A similar effect was observed in a study conducted among children enrolled in three managed care organizations (MCOs). This study found that children receiving controller medications were only 40 percent as likely to have emergency department visits or hospitalizations compared with children who did not receive such medications.

Specialist and Follow-Up Visits Are Linked to Controller Medication Use

The ACQA study mentioned earlier found that Medicaid-insured children with asthma who received specialist visits or follow-up appointments were more likely to use appropriate controller medications. One possible reason for this is that specialists may be more likely to have systems allowing for more effective patient education. Other reasons are that patients seeing specialists may have more severe disease or be more motivated to follow their physician's guidance.

Patient Education and Self-Management Are Related to Organization of Care

Given the complex and chronic nature of asthma and the importance of routine patient self-management (for example, appropriate use of controller medications, identification of symptoms of an exacerbation, avoidance of environmental triggers), patient education for self-management has been strongly recommended. However, the evidence for specific measures can be unclear.

For example, the EPC report mentioned earlier determined that the evidence on the effectiveness of written asthma treatment plans distributed to the patient was inconclusive. Positive results may depend on how the education is delivered. Patient education is linked to the way in which asthma care is organized within each practice.

The Pediatric Asthma Care Patient Outcomes Research Team (PAC PORT) study used a Planned Care Model to better organize asthma care by combining nurse-mediated organizational change and physician peer leader education. This model was found to be effective in improving asthma care in the primary care setting within managed care.

The Planned Care Model in this study was based on the Chronic Care Model developed by Wagner and colleagues. The core of the Planned Care Model consisted of visits with an asthma nurse trained in the NAEPP guidelines and in self-management support. Part of this training involved learning how to use techniques drawn from motivational interviewing and problem-solving therapy to improve self-management in pediatric chronic illness care. The nurse provided standardized assessments, care planning, coordination with the primary care provider, and self-management tools for the patients and their families.

The peer leader education component consisted of training one pediatrician per practice in asthma guidelines and peer teaching methods. This pediatrician served as an asthma expert who provided support, education, and feedback to other members of the practice related to their asthma management. This component was more effective when combined with the asthma nurse visits. Children receiving care through practices relying on both peer leader education and visits with a trained asthma nurse had 13 fewer symptom-days annually and a 39-percent lower oral steroid burst rate per year relative to usual care. In a follow-up cost-effectiveness study, the researchers found that the additional incremental cost for each of the 13 symptom-free days was $68.17.

Care Is Affected More by Practice Site Than MCO

The ACQA study investigated the extent to which MCOs and their affiliated practice sites consistently used 27 different processes of asthma care. These processes of care included promoting self-management support by teaching spacer technique and strengthening delivery systems by using asthma nurses or other managers.

The policies and practices selected for study were adapted from the Assessment of Chronic Illness Care, a tool for assessing processes of chronic illness care that is based on the Chronic Care Model. These processes have been shown to be associated with high-quality asthma care or in a more general sense, high-quality chronic illness care. Many of them are included as components of quality care in the NAEPP Expert Panel Report mentioned earlier.

Clinicians at 73 practice sites (including community health centers, solo and specialty practices, multispecialty group practices, and academic health centers) completed a survey to assess how frequently their practices were using these processes of asthma care for poor populations. After analyzing the results of the survey, ACQA researchers found that Medicaid MCOs do not consistently influence the processes of asthma care used by their associated practice sites.

The practice sites overall scored well on some processes of care. For example, 84 percent facilitated specialist referral for difficult cases and 90 percent ensured primary care follow-up after an urgent care visit. However, the researchers found wide variability among most processes of care from practice site to practice site.

MCOs appeared to exert a moderate to strong influence on their affiliated practice sites with respect to only five processes of care, three of them related to information systems. For example, a strong relationship was found between MCOs and affiliated practice sites for the use of registries and reports. Two processes of care were strongly related to the MCOs: ensuring primary care follow-up after an urgent care visit and use of asthma nurses or other case managers.

In general, sites were less likely to emphasize processes of care related to self-management support and information systems and more likely to emphasize processes of care related to delivery system design and decision support.

Cultural Competence and Reports to Physicians Can Improve Care

The ACQA researchers also surveyed practice sites to determine the prevalence of certain practices and policies especially associated with quality care for poor and minority children. Their objective was to examine associations between those practices and policies and the quality of care for Medicaid-insured children with asthma.

Cultural and linguistic competence is the ability of health care providers and health care organizations to understand and respond effectively to the cultural and linguistic needs brought by the patient to the health care encounter. Cultural competence policies included:

- recruiting ethnically diverse nurses and providers (71 percent of practices);
- attempts to minimize cultural barriers through printed materials (48 percent);
- offers of cross-cultural or diversity training (39 percent);
- offers to providers of training to develop communication skills (24 percent);
- evaluation of the level of cultural competence among providers (15 percent).

Studying Strategies to Improve Care for Low-Income Children

Also included in the survey were different types of reports to physicians such as:

- lists of asthma patients (15 percent);
- asthma registries to prompt physicians about appropriate medications or services (22 percent);
- reminders about asthma guideline adherence for individual patient encounters (34 percent);
- feedback reports to improve performance in asthma care (30 percent).

The researchers found that both cultural competence practices and the use of reports to physicians were associated with less underuse of controller medications, better asthma physical status at follow-up, and better parent ratings of care. In addition, access to and continuity of care were also associated with better outcomes.

Improving Care

The ACQA study concluded that MCOs participating in Medicaid could play a greater role in improving asthma care processes at practice sites if they placed greater emphasis on improving information systems and self-management support services. In addition to the organizational changes discussed earlier in the Planned Care Model intervention, other interventions to improve professional and patient education and control of environmental asthma triggers might also have positive impacts.

The National Cooperative Inner-City Asthma Study (NCICAS) shows that a multifaceted program that includes social-worker-based asthma education, case management, and home-based interventions to control environmental asthma triggers can reduce asthma symptoms among inner-city children, especially those with more severe asthma. The increase in costs was modest: when compared with usual care, the intervention improved outcomes at an average individual cost of $9.20 per symptom-free day. In this intervention, social workers functioned as case managers.

Self-regulation theory focuses on the ways in which people direct and monitor their activities and emotions in order to attain their goals. Studies found that a two-session interactive seminar for physicians using this theory to assist in altering physician treatment practices resulted in more children being placed on inhaled corticosteroids. This regimen, coupled with physician education in communication and education techniques, resulted in significantly fewer symptoms and fewer follow-up office visits, non-emergency physician office visits, emergency department visits, and hospitalizations in the treatment group compared to controls.

The effects of the physician education persisted over two years, and treatment group physicians expended no more time with their patients than controls. Children of younger single mothers reaped the greatest benefit from the physician education.

A study focused on professional education in public health clinics found that improvements could be obtained only by combining the provision of sufficient equipment and prescription drugs with seminars for providers, all other clinic staff, and administrators. As a result, clinics were able to substantially increase the percentage of patients receiving both inhaled anti-inflammatory and beta-agonist medications over a 2-year period.

Ongoing Research

Other approaches to asthma care improvement for children funded by the Agency for Healthcare Research and Quality (AHRQ), some of which focus on low-income children, are being tested in community health centers and in Head Start programs:

Better Pediatric Outcomes Through Chronic Care: University of Connecticut. Grant No. U18 HS11068-01. This study, focusing on poor, minority, inner-city children with asthma, is developing and testing the use of provider prompts on guideline recommendations at the point of care using affordable information technology. It also provides and tests a family-focused supportive educational intervention delivered by a community health worker.

Managed Care Organization Use of a Pediatric Asthma Management Program: University of Connecticut. Grant No. U18 HS11147. This study, also focusing on inner-city children, tests an asthma management program for its reproducibility, effectiveness in adherence to guidelines, and cost burden on an MCO.

Developing an Asthma Management Model for Head Start Children: Arkansas Children's Hospital, Little Rock. Grant No. U18 HS11062-01. This study is testing a multifaceted case-management model implemented by Head Start personnel for its effects on school absence, acute care utilization, and asthma management practices of children, parents, and staff.

Developing an Asthma APGAR: Olmsted Medical Group. Grant No. R03-HS14476. This project collaborates with rural practice-based research network physicians using participatory action research to modify and validate the asthma APGAR, an asthma severity index developed by the principal investigator. The practice asthma APGAR is used to provide targeted feedback to physicians and practices to guide activities oriented toward translating research into practice.

After assuring face validity, the study will assess the effectiveness of the practice asthma APGAR in helping providers identify gaps in asthma care and develop simple implementable solutions for those gaps. Finally, the researchers will evaluate the potential of spreading use of the tool to other rural practices.

Telephone-Linked Communications for Asthma: Boston Medical Center. Grant No. R01-HS10630-01. The goal of this project is to develop and evaluate an education and monitoring system for children with asthma. TLC-Asthma is a computer-based telecommunications system that will give guidance on asthma management to families and collect information to share with each family's primary care provider on the problems and successes the family is having managing the child's asthma.

Conclusion

Studies show underuse of controller medications among children with asthma and higher rates of negative patient outcomes associated with such underuse. In addition, significant disparities in asthma care exist among minority children. Higher quality asthma care for Medicaid-insured children is associated with practice-site policies to support cultural competence, reports to clinicians, and access and continuity of care. Research also shows that processes of asthma care for children enrolled in Medicaid managed care vary more by practice site than by health plan.

MCOs participating in managed Medicaid could play a greater role in improving asthma care processes at practice sites if they placed greater emphasis on improving information systems and self-management support services. Also, some of the intervention strategies found to be successful in studies could be helpful in improving asthma care. Public and private payers such as state Medicaid programs might want to consider encouraging MCOs and patients to implement one or more of these interventions.

Chapter 68

Asthma Research Highlights from the U.S. Environmental Protection Agency

Foreword

In 2002, the U.S. Environmental Protection Agency (EPA) released its Asthma Research Strategy. Since then, scientists have made significant strides in advancing our understanding of how and why asthma is on the rise and our understanding of what induces and exacerbates the disease. EPA research has focused on three areas: asthma triggers, susceptibility factors, and intervention strategies. This chapter provides an overview of the advances in these areas and highlights studies that are particularly noteworthy because of their contribution to applications that reduce asthma suffered by individuals. This research reflects EPA's commitment to addressing the serious public health threat that is posed by the growing asthma epidemic. While we are proud of the accomplishments of EPA's Asthma Research Program to date, significant uncertainties remain. We need to learn more about the causes and triggers of asthma, as well as how to manage this disease.

From "Asthma Research Results Highlights," U.S. Environmental Protection Agency (www.epa.gov), EPA 600/R-04/161, May 2005. The information in this document has been subjected to review by the U.S. Environmental Protection Agency, Office of Research and Development, and has been approved for publication. Approval does not signify that the contents reflect the views of the Agency, nor does mention of trade names or commercial products constitute endorsement or recommendation for use.

Introduction

Asthma, a chronic respiratory disease characterized by difficult breathing, wheezing, and coughing, is disrupting the lives of an increasing number of Americans. In 2001, more than 20 million Americans had asthma, 6.1 million of which were children. From 1980 to 1994, the proportion of Americans suffering from asthma increased by 75%; in children, the proportion grew by 160%. Asthma also affects some minorities and low-income populations disproportionately.

Because of asthma's increasing incidences, the U.S. government has identified asthma as a top priority for research. *Healthy People 2010*, a guiding document for the Department of Health and Human Services, identified asthma as a "serious and growing health problem" in need of action; and the President's Task Force on Environmental Health and Safety Risks to Children selected asthma as one of four childhood diseases to target. In response, a coalition of U.S. government agencies has launched a cooperative effort to combat asthma. In addition to improving treatment and education for people with asthma, government agencies seek to determine the "how" and "why" of asthma induction (development of new cases) and exacerbation (worsening of existing cases) in order to develop better methods for prevention. Researchers believe that multiple factors are responsible for asthma induction and exacerbation; exposure to environmental factors is a likely contributor. EPA's asthma research focuses on these environmental factors.

Airborne particles and gases, present in different combinations in both indoor and outdoor environments, can exacerbate asthma: they influence the biological processes that trigger asthma attacks and increase the severity of symptoms in people with the disease. EPA researchers are investigating whether exposure to pollutants may also contribute to the initial emergence of asthma in some individuals, especially children. Because allergies can lead to asthma attacks in many people, EPA studies often focus on how environmental factors affect allergic responses.

To incorporate the role of environmental factors into the campaign against asthma, EPA's Office of Research and Development developed a targeted asthma research program outlined by the *2002 Asthma Research Strategy*. Researchers in EPA labs, as well as EPA-funded investigators at universities and other organizations, are currently conducting studies to address three high-priority areas in asthma research. Because some types of air pollution may play greater roles in inducing and exacerbating asthma, the first area focuses on studying these different pollutants and their effects. EPA research focuses primarily on pollutants arising from fuel combustion and bioaerosols, a category that includes indoor molds as well as particles that come from dust mites and cockroaches.

Evidence also suggests that different groups of people tend to have higher risks of either developing asthma or having their symptoms exacerbated because of air pollution. EPA's second area of asthma research deals with susceptibility or factors that increase risk for subgroups of Americans. Because where a person lives in part determines what is in the air he or she breathes, residence history is a priority for research in the susceptibility area. Genetic factors, which may interact with environmental exposures, are also a primary focus.

A third major area of research deals with interventions. Scientists in this area test methods for reducing the risks from environmental factors; for example, by controlling cockroaches and other types of infections, improving indoor air quality, and providing educational opportunities to affected communities. Although this chapter categorizes EPA asthma research into these three areas, many projects and objectives span multiple categories.

This chapter is intended to give the reader an accessible overview of EPA's asthma research program and its accomplishments. Throughout this chapter "Research Highlights" will spotlight EPA research efforts that have made significant contributions to science and real-world applications to improve understanding and associated prevention and treatment strategies of asthma.

Specific Pollutants and Their Ability to Induce or Exacerbate Asthma

EPA's research examines four general types of pollutants: combustion-related products, bioaerosols, air toxics, and pesticides. Research on each pollutant focuses on questions about exposure, effects, and risk management. Exposure questions have to do with what people are actually breathing in—for instance, some studies focus on discovering the relationship between pollution levels inside buildings and outdoor (also known as ambient) levels because measurements are usually taken outside. Effects questions get at the ways the human body responds when exposed to different pollutants. Research on health effects comes from many different fields. For example, epidemiologists might ask whether more people experience asthma exacerbations on days with high levels of a certain pollutant; while molecular biologists might study the chemicals that a lung cell produces when exposed to the same pollutant, providing a biological basis for what the epidemiologist observes. Lastly, questions about risk management aim to improve our ability to prevent negative outcomes, for example, by identifying the source of an asthma trigger so that we may modify the source to reduce levels of the pollutant, irritant, or allergen.

Combustion-Related Products

Burning—whether the fuel is petroleum, coal, tobacco, or a host of other combustibles—releases a mixture of pollutants into the air that includes gases as well as tiny particles. Current EPA studies address the exposures and effects of diesel exhaust, tobacco smoke, and smoke from wildfires, as well as other combustion-related products. Diesel exhaust has come under particular scrutiny. Diesel exhaust now makes up a greater proportion of motor vehicle pollution than in the past, and recent EPA studies indicate that it can exacerbate existing asthma and possibly cause new cases.

One of many challenges in determining the relationship between combustion-related products and asthma is that people breathe in a mixture of different gases and particles. This makes it difficult for scientists to link specific components with biological reactions. Studies show that particulate matter, ozone, and nitrogen dioxide can exacerbate asthma. Researchers are currently working to determine whether these pollutants play a role in the development of asthma. It also seems likely that inhaling a combination of these pollutants may produce a reaction different from the response to any single component.

While acutely smoggy or smoky days may send more asthma sufferers to the emergency room, the role of chronic or low-level exposure also seems to be important. Scientists believe that breathing combustion-related products over time may lead to changes in our immune systems that make people more sensitive to asthma triggers that they encounter every day; for example, molds, pollens, animal dander, or particles rising from dust mites.

Research Highlight: Development of Asthma and Long-Term Ozone Exposure

Regions of southern California have some of the highest levels of ozone and other traffic-related pollutants in the country. EPA has helped support two significant southern California studies that indicate that ground-level ozone can actually contribute to asthma development in otherwise healthy people.

Asthma Research Highlights from the U.S. EPA

EPA epidemiologists conducted research as part of the Adventist Health and Smog Study which collected data from over 3,000 southern California adult Adventists between 1977 and 1992. Interestingly, Adventists provided scientists with a unique opportunity for research because the religious group's dietary and lifestyle habits expose them to fewer everyday risks than the general population. The investigators asked each person whether he or she had ever been diagnosed with asthma, taking special note of individuals who were diagnosed with asthma after the initial 1977 survey. Using information about each subject's home and workplace, the investigators determined how much traffic pollution the individual had been exposed to on a regular basis. Then, they used statistical methods to determine whether long-term exposure to ozone, a widespread pollutant produced when emissions from motor vehicles and other sources react in the atmosphere, could be linked to increased incidence of asthma. Results showed that for adult males, but not females, chronic exposure to ozone is associated with asthma development.

In a second study that EPA supported in conjunction with the California Air Resources Board and the National Institute of Environmental Health Sciences, a team of scientists at the University of Southern California recruited a group of 3,535 school-age children who did not have asthma and followed them for five years. By the end, 265 of the participants had developed asthma. The scientists measured levels of ozone and other traffic-related pollutants in the California communities where the children lived and observed whether the participants played team sports (because outdoor exercise can lead to greater exposures to pollutants when air quality is poor). The results showed that children who play team sports in communities with high-ozone levels were more likely to develop asthma, while children who play sports in low-ozone areas were not at higher risk.

These studies indicate that living in a high-ozone area can put children and adults at greater risk of developing asthma and support the hypothesis that ozone can cause new cases of asthma, not just make symptoms worse for people already suffering from the disease.

—McDonnell et al. 1999, McConnell et al. 2002

Research Highlight: Studies Show That Diesel Exhaust Particles Trigger Asthma Attacks in Animals

An EPA-funded research team at the University of California, Los Angeles, School of Medicine, studied mice to determine whether particles from diesel exhaust alone could trigger asthma attacks. Past studies showed that inhaling diesel exhaust particles in combination with an allergen could make a person much more sensitive to that allergen by activating the person's immune system in a process called adjuvancy. However, although adjuvancy could increase asthma prevalence in the long term, scientists observed asthma flare-ups only hours or minutes after exposure to high concentrations of particles. The University of California, Los Angeles, researchers set out to establish the biological basis for this immediate effect.

The researchers faced the challenge of making a mouse's lungs highly sensitive to pollutants so that they would resemble the lungs of people with asthma, prone to swelling that narrows the airways. Scientists often approach this problem by sensitizing the animals' lungs with an allergen called ovalbumin. The University of California, Los Angeles, team also used a novel approach involving mice bred with a genetic mutation that made their lungs highly sensitive. When exposed to diesel exhaust particles, these mice showed signs of airway inflammation even though they had not been exposed to ovalbumin or any other allergen. Study results support the assertion that diesel exhaust particles alone could trigger asthma flare-ups in mice, and these findings are an important indicator for use in additional asthma research.

As a next step, researchers point to the need to confirm that diesel exhaust particles has similar effects in humans. Related projects at the Southern California Particulate Matter Center and at EPA facilities address the specific processes in the cells that underlie these allergic responses.

—*Hao* et al. *2003*

Research Highlight: Metal Components of Air Pollution and Effects on Asthma

Researchers at EPA's National Health and Environmental Effects Research Laboratory showed that a kind of particulate matter called residual oil fly ash, which arises from oil combustion in power plants, causes immune system changes that make mice more sensitive to dust mite allergens. Because residual oil fly ash is made up of many components, it is unclear which of these cause allergic sensitization.

Evidence suggests that metals such as nickel can exacerbate asthma. Residual oil fly ash often contains nickel as well as the metals vanadium and iron. EPA researchers tested the effects of these metals on mice that commonly develop allergies because some mice—like some human beings—have immune systems that are more likely to react to allergens. They exposed the mice to the metals and "challenged" them by exposing them to dust mite allergen. The results showed that each metal, or a combination of them, could cause the mice to develop a stronger allergy to dust mites.

The sensitization process observed in animal studies may partially explain why some geographic regions have higher rates of asthma. Epidemiologists at the National Research Center for Environment and Health in Munich, Germany, compared two regions in Germany and found that children in Hettstedt, a region with metal-rich air pollution had higher rates of asthma and allergies than those in Zerbst. In collaboration with National Research Center for Environment and Health scientists, investigators from EPA collected samples from air filters in each of these regions. When they exposed allergic mice to these samples, the mice exposed to the metal-rich pollution from Hettstedt had the more severe allergic response. This provides further evidence that the metal components in air pollution increase sensitivity to allergens. EPA scientists are also working to discover the cellular processes involved in allergic sensitization caused by air pollution.

—*Lambert* et al. *2000, Gavett* et al. *2003*

Bioaerosols

Airborne particles originating from dust mites, cockroaches, pets, pollens, bacteria, and household molds can trigger allergic responses and lead to asthma attacks. In addition, research shows that dust mite allergens can cause new cases of asthma, and studies suggest that other bioaerosols may also play a role in asthma induction. Many researchers further speculate that interactions between bioaerosols and other factors, such as combustion-related products or infections including the common cold, can cause or worsen asthma.

A number of research institutions have studied the effects of cockroach allergens on asthma in inner cities. Cockroach allergen is a potent asthma trigger and an important focus for research because roaches are commonly found in inner-city buildings. In addition, EPA scientists and other researchers think that household molds and the damp conditions that foster mold growth may also put residents at great risk of asthma development or exacerbation. Because of the potential importance of mold research and because few other agencies and research organizations have supported research in this area, EPA has made mold, or fungal bioaerosols, a major focus of its asthma research program.

EPA researchers are currently working to identify and describe the many different molds commonly present in household environments. They hope to determine which molds pose the greatest risks to allergic individuals and whether any has the capacity to cause asthma. Identifying the sources of molds, which may grow in damp basements, carpets, dirty air filters, and a number of other places, will also help in developing interventions.

Scientists also intend to determine how much mold a person must inhale in order for it to have an effect. Inhaling just a few particles may sensitize people's lungs, making them more likely to react to future insults. Genetic variations between people may cause their cells to respond differently, perhaps explaining why mold and other allergens cause or exacerbate asthma in some people but not in others. EPA researchers are working to determine the specific ways in which cells and organs respond to molds and other environmental insults.

Research Highlight: Effects of Household Molds on Asthma

Stachybotrys chartarum, a type of black mold or fungus, received media attention recently when its uncontrolled growth rendered several houses uninhabitable. This mold grows on damp walls, is widespread geographically, and has been associated with a range of health problems including asthma. However, few hypotheses about mold exposure, its influence on asthma, or methods for prevention have been tested scientifically. In order to fill these scientific gaps, investigators from multiple EPA research laboratories collaborated to conduct studies aimed at improving understanding and preventing health problems associated with molds like *Stachybotrys*.

EPA researchers exposed mice to samples of *Stachybotrys* taken from homes and looked for immune system responses typical of allergies as well as inflammation and functional changes in the animals' lungs. The results showed that the mold can indeed cause a disease analogous to asthma in mice.

Meanwhile, other EPA scientists have developed sophisticated procedures for identifying *Stachybotrys* and other molds in indoor environments, making it possible to determine which molds are present in a given household. These procedures include methods for rapidly quantifying the amounts of different fungi present in dust, as well as measuring a biomarker that when found in a person's blood indicates exposure to *Stachybotrys*. The mouse and exposure studies set the stage for further research that would help determine that humans are responding to the same allergens as mice and whether these responses can be associated with asthma.

EPA investigators have also been evaluating strategies for preventing mold growth. Strategies include applying antifungal sealants for fiberglass and galvanized steel used in heating and air conditioning systems. Studies show that sealants can reduce mold growth on fiberglass and can completely prevent growth on galvanized steel.

EPA has used a multidisciplinary approach to study *Stachybotrys* and the hazard it creates. EPA researchers are also studying other mold species that may pose a risk in indoor environments.

—Viana et al. 2002, Foarde et al. 2002

Air Toxics

Hazardous air pollutants include 188 chemicals, many of which are respiratory irritants. A diverse array of chemical classes is contained in the hazardous air pollutants list, including several metals which have been previously shown to have a role in the induction and/or exacerbation of asthma. Another chemical class of abundant hazardous air pollutants is carbonyl compounds, including aldehydes and ketones. The sources of carbonyls in the air are varied and include direct emissions from some industrial processes and from the combustion of diesel fuel. Carbonyls can also be derived from complex photochemical transformations of organic chemicals in the troposphere. EPA is investigating the toxicity of the carbonyls derived from the hazardous air pollutants list, along with those found in combustion sources, to determine whether this class of compounds alters cellular processes leading to asthma or an asthma-like condition. These studies are carried out in rodent exposure systems and use isolated lung cells. In terms of exacerbating asthma symptoms, it is known that inhalation of the hazardous air pollutants acetaldehyde by asthmatics can induce bronchoconstriction, while such responses do not occur in normal healthy individuals. This suggests that asthmatics are a sensitive subpopulation. The findings show that at least one carbonyl compound can induce asthmatic symptoms, but it is uncertain whether other carbonyls can cause similar effects. To address that issue, research will also investigate whether all carbonyls are equally potent in inducing effects such as bronchoconstriction or whether different potencies exist. These studies will use data empirically generated in controlled exposure studies as well as structure-activity modeling of the responses. If exposure to different carbonyls results in different potencies, then the chemical structures can be used to explain the reason behind the unequal potencies. This approach will help the Agency pinpoint which carbonyls are the most potent and should be better managed to prevent asthma attacks.

Factors That Make Certain People More Likely to Be Affected by Asthma

Some groups of people are at higher risk of developing asthma or of having environmental factors worsen their asthma. Many of the five factors that EPA identifies as increasing susceptibility to asthma interact with one another. For instance, place of residence and socioeconomic status are linked in many cases. People living in inner-cities are often exposed to a disproportionately high number of environmental risk factors and have a high incidence of asthma. It is also easy to imagine how health status and a person's genetic make-up or health status and activity patterns might be related. However, none of these factors overlaps completely. Income, for example, cannot explain many characteristics of one's home. Consequently, an effort has been made to separate these different risk factors in order to gain a complete understanding of the reasons why different people face different levels of risk.

Residence and Exposure History

If exposure to environmental factors can worsen asthma, people who live, work, or play in areas with a high concentration of allergens, air pollutants, pesticides, or other offending agents are probably at higher risk. The conditions in homes are particularly important because, on average, people spend 70% of their out-of-work time at home.

People inhale a variety of pollutants and allergens commonly present in the air inside their homes and outside in their neighborhoods. EPA studies have focused on people who move into a new neighborhood or a new residence to discover which residential factors influence asthma. After a move, people may be exposed to a different environment of pollutants and allergens and may develop new allergies or respond to changed levels of pollutants. In addition to the outdoor air, factors that can change when a person moves include ventilation, air conditioning, building age, water damage and dampness, indoor combustion sources, and consumer products. By examining changes in residence and exposure history, researchers have been able to identify new hazards and assess the importance of known hazards.

Researchers collect much of their information by surveying people and supplementing surveys by going into the field to make observations and measurements. In order to test more directly whether a person has been exposed to a certain chemical, scientists look for molecules called biomarkers in the person's blood or other biological samples. Biomarkers can simply be a component of the inhaled product that enters the blood stream (an exposure biomarker) or can arise from a more complicated chain of events involving interactions between chemicals and the body's cells (biomarker of early response). As an example, skin test reactivity to common allergens is an excellent biomarker of sensitivity that is much better than attempting to identify allergies through a patient's recall of reactions.

Research Highlight: Air Pollution and Asthma Symptoms in Seattle-Area Children

EPA has the responsibility to protect the most sensitive populations when creating regulations for outdoor air pollutants. Children with asthma constitute a group at greater risk. To gather better information about the effects of air pollution on this group, researchers at the University of Washington's Northwest Research Center for Particulate Pollution and Health studied the relationship between certain air quality measures and asthma symptoms in Seattle-area children.

All of the 133 children, ages 5 to 13 years, who participated in the study were enrolled in the Childhood Asthma Management Program sponsored by the National Heart, Lung, and Blood Institute. Each had mild to moderate asthma. The University of Washington scientists asked participants to keep daily diaries; every morning and evening, participants recorded any asthma symptoms they had experienced. The researchers then compared the diary information with air quality measures, including measures of particulate matter, carbon monoxide, and sulfur dioxide. Using statistical models, the researchers concluded that higher levels of carbon monoxide and particulate matter were associated with greater aggravation of asthma symptoms, increased risk of more severe asthma attacks, and higher use of asthma medication.

Because the specific geography and development in a region can influence air quality, these results depend in part on the distinctive make-up of air pollutants in Seattle. Levels of sulfur dioxide in the region are generally low, so sulfur dioxide does not act as a major asthma trigger in Seattle though it does in other regions where concentrations are higher. Carbon monoxide, on the other hand, is not known to trigger asthma symptoms itself. Scientists believe that monitoring carbon monoxide, one of many products of combustion, indirectly measures the levels of other combustion products that exacerbate asthma, such as nitrogen oxides, ozone, and particulate matter.

Because the make-up of air pollution differs from region to region, conducting studies in various locations provides more complete information about the effects of air pollution on children with asthma. EPA researchers and university scientists supported by EPA are working to gather related information in several U.S. cities, including Detroit, El Paso, and Los Angeles.

—*Yu* et al. *2000, Slaughter* et al. *2003*

Research Highlight: Particulate Matter Levels and Asthma in Inner-City Children

EPA scientists collaborated with scientists at the National Institute of Environmental Health Sciences and the National Institute of Allergy and Infectious Diseases to undertake the Inner-city Asthma Study, an effort focusing on children with asthma in seven U.S. cities.

As a first step in the environmental portion of this study, investigators determined the relationship between indoor and outdoor pollution levels and identified indoor sources of pollutants. The researchers took continuous measurements of particulate matter levels inside 294 homes for two weeks each. They then compared the data for indoor particulate matter levels with measurements for outdoor concentrations and used a questionnaire to relate indoor levels with different activities in the homes. Taking continuous rather than daily measurements of indoor particulate matter allowed the researchers to observe variations in pollution levels throughout the day. For example, researchers observed consistently low levels late at night when people were sleeping and higher levels during mealtimes from cooking and in the evening from smoking.

The research team found that particulate matter concentrations inside the homes of children in the inner-city asthma study tend to be about twice as high as outdoor concentrations. This percentage can vary depending on people's activities and house characteristics. In the study particulate matter from outdoor sources made up approximately 25% of that found indoors; the rest came from indoor sources, including activities such as frying or burning food, burning incense, and especially smoking. Homes of people who smoke have dramatically higher levels of particulate matter. Additionally, the researchers found that indoor particulate matter levels are not substantially different from city to city which makes the science emerging from this study applicable in cities nationwide.

Scientists are currently working on the subsequent steps in this study, which include comparing pollution levels with information about asthma severity to examine the relationship between the two. We observed an association between adverse health effects (missed school days and lower lung function) and combustion products, even in cities where ambient pollution levels are generally low.

—Wallace et al. *2003*

Genetic Susceptibility

Different people respond differently to the same environmental exposures. Scientists believe that a large part of this heterogeneity has a genetic basis. Current EPA studies aim to identify genes that influence asthma susceptibility and to characterize the responses to pollutants and allergens that correspond with these genetic differences.

EPA researchers use various approaches to answer questions about genes and asthma. Using clinical studies, they examine how people with a known genetic make-up respond to controlled amounts of environmental stressors such as ozone. Researchers use these trials to identify which genes may be correlated with differences in responses. EPA researchers use *in vitro* studies—those done in test tubes—to observe the role of different genes in the cells of people with asthma. Scientists also use *in vitro* methods to study the step-by-step processes or mechanisms by which chemicals produce their effects. A third mode of EPA research on genetic susceptibility involves laboratory animals; scientists observe how animals with specific genetic mutations respond to environmental exposures.

Health Status

People with more severe asthma and those who suffer from other heart and lung conditions seem to respond differently to environmental pollutants than healthy individuals. For instance, a small amount of a pollutant may trigger an asthma attack in a person with severe asthma, but it may take a higher dose to affect a healthier individual. In order to better protect the populations at greatest risk, scientists are seeking to understand the interaction between the presence of disease and response to pollutants and allergens. EPA researchers have pursued this question using epidemiological field studies to compare people with different severities of asthma, clinical studies to compare people with asthma and healthy people, and studies involving laboratory animals with characteristics that mimic human diseases.

Research Highlight: Inhaled Pollutants Affect People with Asthma More Severely

To build upon epidemiological evidence showing that people with asthma are more susceptible to air pollution than healthy people, EPA researchers and EPA-supported university scientists studied volunteers in carefully controlled laboratory environments to determine the biological basis for this difference. Though these clinical studies vary with regard to the specific pollutants and outcomes tested, one fact has become clear: study participants who have asthma are more affected than their healthy counterparts.

One group of studies that EPA scientists conducted in cooperation with University of North Carolina researchers examined the effects of ozone. The scientists exposed volunteers to ozone and then tested their ability to exhale air forcefully, a measure commonly used to determine whether a person's lungs are functioning normally. The healthy volunteers responded to ozone with a decreased ability to rapidly exhale; scientists concluded that this response arose because ozone interfered with the healthy subjects' ability to take a deep breath. The subjects with asthma also experienced a decrease in pulmonary function; but for these volunteers, the decrease stemmed from an actual narrowing of the lungs' airways—a much worse situation. In addition, inhaling medication designed to open constricted airways did not effectively combat the airway constriction triggered by ozone. Related research efforts showed that exposure to the pollutant causes the lungs to become inflamed in all subjects. However, scientists observed that the cells causing inflammation differ between people with asthma and healthy people and that the cells that cause inflammation in people with asthma can potentially exacerbate their disease.

In addition to ozone, EPA-funded researchers have also examined the effects of particulate matter on people with and without asthma.

For example, researchers at the University of Rochester found that greater amounts of air pollution particles deposit in the airways of people with mild asthma. The increased particle deposition in the lungs of people with asthma may partially explain why they are more susceptible to some air pollutants.

These studies show that ozone and particulate matter affect people with asthma more severely than healthy people. They help explain the epidemiological evidence by elucidating some of the specific biological mechanisms that underlie this difference. Further research at the cellular and genetic levels will help to explain what causes greater susceptibility in people with asthma.

—Horstman et al. *1995, Peden* et al. *1995, Peden* et al. *1997, Pietropaoli* et al. *2004*

Research Highlight: Exploring the Connections between Genes, Environment, and Asthma

Studies show that people with asthma are more susceptible to many more air pollutants than healthy people are. EPA scientists are trying to determine whether the genetic makeup of people with asthma plays a role in this susceptibility and, if so, which genes and proteins are involved.

Research has shown that certain proteins found attached to white blood cells and floating free in blood and fluid surrounding lung cells are involved in a person's reaction to a common bioaerosol called endotoxin, which comes from bacteria and adheres to many air pollution particles. Although this compound causes inflammation in everyone, people with asthma tend to be more sensitive to endotoxin. This may be because a protein called CD14, which is found on the surface of immune system cells and to which endotoxin binds, is present in higher levels in people with asthma.

In one study, EPA researchers in collaboration with University of North Carolina scientists examined eight healthy people and ten people with asthma in order to investigate the relationship between CD14 and severity of response to endotoxin. They measured levels of certain proteins and cells—those that indicate the level of inflammation—in samples of the participants' sputum collected both before and after the exposure. These experiments showed a correlation between levels of CD14 and the severity of the inflammatory response; when levels of CD14 were high before exposure to endotoxin, the inflammation was more severe. Because levels of CD14 are easily measured, these findings suggest that scientists can predict the severity of a person's response to endotoxin by this simple test.

The gene responsible for producing CD14 protein is present in different variations or alleles. Some of these variations are known to cause a higher concentration of CD14 protein on immune cells. EPA scientists are currently performing studies to determine whether people with asthma who have genetic variations that produce greater amounts of CD14 are more susceptible to pollutants than those with variations that do not affect the level of the protein.

—*Alexis* et al. *2001*

Lifestyle and Activity Levels

Though urban lifestyle seems to be correlated with higher asthma rates, scientists do not know which elements of these lifestyles influence asthma. Low levels of physical activity and increased time spent indoors may be important contributors, especially because urban buildings tend to be constructed in ways that restrict ventilation with outdoor air.

Though a sedentary lifestyle may be a risk factor for asthma and other health problems, exercising outside on bad air quality days can increase exposure to air pollutants. Heavier breathing while practicing an outdoor sport, for example, means that more ozone, particulate matter, and other pollutants enter the active person's lungs.

When small children play outdoors, crawl on the floor, or engage in other normal, child-like behaviors, they can increase their exposure to certain pollutants and allergens. However, these activities are not the only elements placing children at higher risk. There are biological differences between children and adults as well because children's organs and immune systems are still developing. EPA research suggests that environmental exposures can have different, and often more severe, effects on children than on adults.

Socioeconomic Status

The relationship between socioeconomic status and asthma is an important issue in terms of social justice as well as public health. In terms of both prevalence and severity, people with low socioeconomic status are more likely to be affected by asthma. Though outdoor air pollution levels are not as well correlated with socioeconomic status, scientists believe that exposure to indoor air pollutants and allergens may provide a partial explanation. Low socioeconomic status homes and buildings in inner-cities such as Detroit, Baltimore, Los Angeles, and New York City have documented poor indoor air quality. These cities also have high prevalence of asthma. Other factors, such as nutrition, may also be involved. Studies funded by EPA at the University of Southern California involving inner-city children ask whether the amount of vitamin C and other antioxidants can influence asthma.

Interventions to Reduce the Burden of Asthma

Effective actions to prevent environmental factors from inducing or exacerbating asthma must succeed in the context of real-world complexities. In order to have an effect, interventions must incorporate social elements in addition to good science. EPA researchers have been working in regions with high asthma rates, including Detroit, New York, Baltimore, and Los Angeles, to design and test such interventions.

The ideal way to minimize risk from pollutants or allergens is to stop them at their source. Studies that determine which sources produce the most harmful pollutants and how emissions from sources relate to what people actually breathe provide the foundation for interventions. Strategies for addressing these sources include employing new technologies, changing habits, or modifying regulations. Indoors, finding effective ways to manage cockroaches and eliminating tobacco smoke are two interventions with the potential to drastically affect asthma. Other possibilities for improving indoor air quality might include converting to low-emissions building materials and eliminating the dampness that leads to mold growth. Lowering levels of offending pollutants in outdoor air involves reducing emissions from vehicles and industrial facilities.

Beyond targeting sources, air filtration and other secondary measures for controlling air quality present additional strategies for lowering concentrations of pollutants and allergens. An EPA-funded study conducted in Boston public housing found that mattress and pillow covers lower the levels of dust-mite allergens in bedrooms. However, air filtering did not lower levels of particulate matter in homes, and industrial cleaning reduced levels of mouse and cockroach allergens only temporarily. To prove the effectiveness of any intervention method, tests must show that the method not only lowers the concentrations of such agents, but also reduces asthma incidence or exacerbation as a result.

Social aspects are an important area of focus for intervention research. Intervention strategies have been designed for both single-household and community-wide applications. Many have included elements of education in addition to specific actions that aim to reduce allergen levels in homes. Education and community involvement are important because knowing that an action can alleviate asthma only helps if people are motivated to take that action. Home interventions must also be cost-effective in order for people to use them. A team of EPA-funded economists is currently working to determine how much people are willing to pay to avoid the discomfort and inconvenience that asthma imposes—an exercise that will provide guidelines for designing cost-effective prevention methods.

In addition to its research efforts, EPA has launched an asthma education and outreach campaign. The Indoor Environments Division informs Americans about actions they can take to improve indoor air quality. Public health information about outdoor air pollution can be found at www.epa.gov/airnow.

Research Highlight: Controlling Cockroaches in East Harlem

Cockroaches pose a serious risk because allergens from roaches can trigger asthma attacks in people with cockroach allergies. The Inner-City Asthma Study revealed that as many as 68% of inner-city children with asthma are allergic to cockroaches. However, applying chemical pesticides to control roaches can also be risky, especially because this can expose children to harmful chemicals. To address this problem, a group of scientists at the Mount Sinai Children's Environmental Health and Disease Prevention Research Center worked in collaboration with two East Harlem community health organizations to develop a cockroach control program using a method called integrated pest management. Integrated pest management combines nonchemical approaches with education in order to control pests.

The Mount Sinai researchers went to prenatal clinics to recruit two groups of women for the study: a control group and an intervention group. All of the study participants lived in East Harlem. At the outset, about 80% of homes in both groups had cockroaches although the majority of households used pesticides. For six months, the researchers monitored cockroach levels in the homes of both control and intervention group participants; and, for the intervention group only, researchers worked with the participants to institute integrated pest management practices. The interventions included repair services to seal cracks through which roaches enter, training in better sanitation and housekeeping, and minimal application of pesticide gels rather than sprays when necessary. At the end of the six-month period, half of the intervention homes that started out with cockroaches lowered their roach count to zero; in contrast, there was no change for households in the control group. Additionally, integrated pest management methods were no more expensive than traditional methods relying on heavy pesticide application.

These results suggest that integrated pest management can be an effective, less toxic way of controlling cockroaches in urban environments. Because the Mount Sinai study demonstrated the great promise of integrated pest management, researchers at the Columbia University Center of Excellence in Children's Environmental Health and Disease Prevention Research are currently working in collaboration with the New York City Department of Health and the New York City Housing Authority to develop a more expansive study to test the effectiveness of integrated pest management techniques, including measuring the implications for people with asthma.

—*Brenner* et al. *2003*

Conclusion

EPA's asthma research provides the science upon which EPA bases air quality regulations and supports the Agency's public health programs, helping to decrease the incidence of asthma in the U.S. In addition to contributing to the decision-making process at EPA, many of the findings have applications at community and household levels. Methods developed and evaluated by EPA researchers for controlling cockroaches or preventing mold growth may be used by homeowners. Parents may also use information about the risk of playing sports on bad air quality days when planning their children's activities. With its focus on environmental factors of the disease, EPA's research program adds an important component to asthma research pursued by other government agencies and private institutions.

Additional information on EPA's asthma-related publications and resources is available at: www.epa.gov/asthma/ and www.epa.gov/ord.

Future Directions for EPA's Asthma Research Program

Asthma poses a public health challenge that EPA and other government agencies will continue to address. In the future, EPA's asthma research will seek to do the following:

- Improve understanding of who suffers the impacts of environmental exposures on asthma.
  - Define the relationship between exposure to environmental pollutants and the induction of disease in children and severity of asthma in children and adults.
  - Understand gene-environment interaction in asthma induction and exacerbation and determine susceptibility and environmental factors that can be modified to reduce the initiation and severity of asthma.
- Reduce uncertainties in risks assessments for air pollutants that induce or exacerbate asthma.
  - Conduct studies designed to understand the mechanisms by which air pollutants induce or exacerbate asthma.
- Develop new and better strategies to prevent environmentally related asthma induction and exacerbation and to protect the populations at greatest risk.
  - Define the role of molds and other bioaerosols in the induction or exacerbation of asthma, particularly in susceptible populations, as well as their potential synergistic interaction with other pollutants.
  - Develop strategies to remediate risk from exposures to environmental pollutants.

These areas of research will help EPA to continue to protect Americans by providing a sound scientific foundation upon which to base air pollution regulations. In addition, these ongoing efforts will provide information about asthma risk factors and prevention methods that will help consumers, parents, homeowners, and others to make everyday decisions.

References

Alexis, N., M. Eldridge, *et al.* (2001) "CD14-dependent airway neutrophil response to inhaled LPS: Role of atopy." *J Allergy Clin Immunol.* Jan;107(1):31–35.

Brenner, B., S. Markowitz, *et al.* (2003) "Integrated pest management in an urban community: a successful partnership for prevention." *Environ Health Perspect.* 111(13):1649–1653.

Foarde, K.K., D.W. VanOsdell, M.Y. Menetrez. (2001) "Investigation of the potential anti-microbial efficacy of sealants used in HVAC systems." *J Air Waste Manag Assoc.* Aug;51(8):1219–26.

Foarde, K.K. and M.Y. Menetrez. (2002) "Evaluating the potential efficacy of three antifungal sealants of duct liner and galvanized steel as used in HVAC systems." *J Ind Microbiol Biotechnol.* Jul;29(1):38–43.

Gavett, S. H., N. Haykal-Coates, et al. (2003) "Metal composition of ambient PM2.5 influences severity of allergic airways disease in mice." *Environ. Health Perspect.* Sep;111(12):1471–1477.

Hao, M., S. Comier, et al. (2003) "Diesel exhaust particles exert acute effects on airway inflammation and function in murine allergen provocation models." *J Allergy Clin Immunol.* Nov;112(5):905–914.

Horstman, D., B. Ball, et al. (1995) "Comparison of pulmonary responses of asthmatic and nonasthmatic subjects performing light exercise while exposed to a low level of ozone." *Toxicol Ind Health.* Jul-Aug; 11(4):369–385.

Lambert, A., W. Dong, et al. (2000) "Enhanced allergic sensitization by residual oil fly ash particles is mediated by soluble metal constituents." *Toxicol Appl Pharmacol.* May 15;165(1):84–93.

McConnell, R., K. Berhane, et al. (2002) "Asthma in exercising children exposed to ozone: a cohort study." *Lancet.* Feb 2;359(9304):386–91. Erratum in: *Lancet.* 2002 Mar 9;359(9309):896

McDonnell, W. F., D. E. Abbey, et al. (1999) "Long-term ambient ozone concentration and the incidence of asthma in nonsmoking adults: the AHSMOG Study." *Environ Res.* Feb;80(2 Pt 1):110–121.

Peden, D., B. Boehlecke, et al. (1997) "Prolonged acute exposure to 0.16 ppm ozone induces eosinophilic airway inflammation in asthmatic subjects with allergies." *J Allergy Clin Immunol.* Dec;100(6 Pt 1):802–808.

Peden, D.B., R.W. Setzer, R.B. Devlin (1995) "Ozone exposure has both a priming effect on allergen-induced responses and an intrinsic inflammatory action in the nasal airways of perennially allergic asthmatics." *Am J Respir Crit Care Med.* May;151(5):1336–1345.

Pietropaoli A.P., M.W. Frampton, et al. (2004) "Pulmonary function, diffusing capacity, and inflammation in healthy and asthmatic subjects exposed to ultrafine particles." *Inhal Toxicol.* 2004;16 Suppl 1:59–72.

Slaughter, J. C., T. Lumley, *et al*. (2003) "Effects of ambient air pollution on symptom severity and medication use in children with asthma." *Ann Allergy Asthma Immunol.* Oct;91(4):346–53.

Viana, M., N. Coates, *et al*. (2002) "An extract of Stachybotrys chartarum causes allergic asthma-like responses in a BALB/c mouse model." *Toxicol Sci.* Nov;70(1):98–109.

Wallace, L., H. Mitchell, *et al*. (2003) "Particle concentrations in inner-city homes of children with asthma: the effect of smoking, cooking, and outdoor pollution." *Environ Health Perspect.* Jul;111(9):1265–1272.

Yu, O., L. Sheppard, *et al*. (2000) "Effects of ambient air pollution on symptoms of asthma in Seattle area children enrolled in the CAMP study." *Environ Health Perspect.* Dec;108(12):1209–1214.

Chapter 69

Asthma Research Updates from the National Institutes of Health

Enzyme May Play Unexpected Role in Asthma

In a finding that could have important implications for the millions of Americans who suffer from asthma, researchers funded by the National Institute of Allergy and Infectious Diseases (NIAID) have discovered novel sets of genes possibly involved in the disease. Their study has also revealed what the scientists believe is a key role for the enzyme arginase in causing asthmatic symptoms. The research, led by Marc E. Rothenberg, M.D., Ph.D., of Cincinnati Children's Hospital

---

This chapter includes the following press releases from the National Institutes of Health: "Enzyme May Play Unexpected Role in Asthma," June 15, 2003; "Scientists Identify Genes that Regulate Allergic Response to Diesel Fumes," January 2, 2004; "Early Fevers Associated with Lower Allergy Risk Later in Childhood," February 9, 2004; "National Study Shows 82 Percent of U.S. Homes Have Mouse Allergens," June 8, 2004; "Customized Program Reduces Asthma-Related Illness in Inner-City Children," September 8, 2004; "Chronic Sinusitis Sufferers Have Enhanced Immune Responses to Fungi," October 12, 2004; "Genetics Play Role In Response to Most Common Asthma Drug," October 22, 2004; "New Treatment Guidelines for Pregnant Women with Asthma," January 11, 2005; "Cockroach Allergens Have Greatest Impact on Childhood Asthma in Many U.S. Cities," March 8, 2005; "NHLBI Study Suggests Symptom-Driven Therapy May Be Sufficient for Some Adults with Mild Persistent Asthma," April 13, 2005; and "More Than Half the U.S. Population Is Sensitive to One or More Allergens," August 4, 2005. Also included is "Study: Mold in Homes Doubles Risk of Asthma," a press release from the National Institute of Environmental Health Sciences, dated March 1, 2005.

Medical Center, opens the possibility of developing new anti-asthma drugs to block arginase activity.

Asthma is on the rise in the United States and causes at least 5,000 deaths a year. Although the subject of intense study, the condition remains poorly understood at the fundamental level. Dr. Rothenberg and his colleagues used mouse models of asthma along with "gene chip" technology to probe the underpinnings of asthma. "We've identified nearly 300 mouse genes, which we call asthma signature genes, that appear to be involved in asthma pathogenesis," notes Dr. Rothenberg. "This gives us an unprecedented insight into the orchestration of the large number of genes that give rise to asthma."

The findings, published in the June 2003 issue of *Journal of Clinical Investigation*, appear to apply in humans as well, says Dr. Rothenberg. If confirmed through further study, the new knowledge could lead to asthma treatments tailored to an individual patient's disease.

"NIAID has long supported both basic research into asthma and the translation of such basic knowledge into more effective treatment and prevention strategies," says NIAID Director Anthony S. Fauci, M.D. "This finding is an important step towards understanding the pathogenesis of asthma, and it provides new leads to interventions that could reduce the burden of this debilitating and sometimes deadly disease."

In their quest to identify the critical genes involved in asthma, Dr. Rothenberg and his colleagues induced asthma in mice, then analyzed lung tissue with gene chips to see which genes were most active following the attacks. Two strains of asthmatic mice were evaluated following two different methods of asthma induction. A set of 496 genes was activated in the lungs of one mouse strain, while 527 genes "turned on" in the lungs of the second strain. Of these, 291 were same in both groups. The investigators called the shared genes "asthma signature genes."

The large number of genes involved in asthma—more than 6 percent of the mouse genome—came as some surprise, say lead authors Nives Zimmerman, M.D., and Nina King, Ph.D. Even more surprising, according to Dr. Rothenberg, was strong expression of genes involved in amino acid metabolism, in particular the gene encoding the enzyme arginase. Previously, arginase was thought to be limited primarily to the liver, where it helps process the amino acid arginine. "We've learned that arginase is involved in asthma regardless of the specific allergen used to induce the attack," says Dr. Rothenberg.

To learn whether arginase plays a role in human asthma as well, the scientists analyzed fluid and tissue samples from the lungs of asthmatic people and from non-asthmatic control subjects. No arginase was detected in the control samples, but significant amounts were found in the asthmatic lung. Importantly, arginase appears to be the molecule that "kicks off" the chain of action leading ultimately to asthmatic symptoms. Thus, it makes an attractive target for drug intervention. "We hope to come up with a treatment for asthma by targeting arginase," says Dr. Rothenberg.

Reference: Rothenberg, *et al.* Dissection of experimental asthma with DNA microarray analysis identifies arginase in asthma pathogenesis. *The Journal of Clinical Investigation.* 111:1863–74 (2003). doi: 10.1172/JCI200317912.

Scientists Identify Genes That Regulate Allergic Response to Diesel Fumes

The risk of developing respiratory allergies from exposure to diesel emissions depends largely on genetics, according to a study funded by the National Institute of Allergy and Infectious Diseases (NIAID), part of the National Institutes of Health (NIH). Given their findings, researchers estimate that up to 50 percent of the United States population could be in jeopardy of experiencing health problems related to air pollution. The study is published in the January 10, 2004 issue of the British journal *The Lancet*.

"This important study adds to previous data that suggest how modern environmental factors interact with the body's defenses to produce 'airway' diseases considered rare before the advent of industrialized society," says Anthony S. Fauci, M.D., director of NIAID.

"The knowledge provided by this work will help us identify people who are susceptible to the deleterious effects of diesel emissions on the clinical course of asthma and hay fever," says Kenneth Adams, Ph.D., who oversees asthma research funded by NIAID. "It will also help accelerate development of drugs to treat and prevent these diseases."

This study also received support from the National Institute of Environmental Health Sciences, another NIH component.

The authors of the study examined how a family of antioxidant-related genes—*GSTM1, GSTT1* and *GSTP1*—reacts to diesel exhaust particles, a common air pollutant. The body generates antioxidants to detoxify harmful particles and limit the corresponding allergic reaction.

Researchers sampled the DNA of volunteers who are allergic to ragweed to find which forms of the genes they had. The participants were then given doses of ragweed through the nose, followed by either a placebo or quantities of diesel exhaust particles equivalent to breathing the air in Los Angeles, CA, for 40 hours.

The mix of ragweed and diesel exhaust triggered greater allergic responses than ragweed alone. Additionally, the diesel particles caused volunteers who lacked the antioxidant-producing form of the *GSTM1* gene to have significantly greater allergic responses, compared to the other participants. Up to 50 percent of the U.S. population does not have this form of the *GSTM1* gene. Within the group that lacked *GSTM1*, those who had a particular variant of the *GSTP1* gene experienced even greater allergic reactions. Researchers estimate that 15 to 20 percent of the U.S. population falls into this category.

"Diesel emissions can trigger allergic symptoms, but the genetic factors involved in the process are quite complex," says David Diaz-Sanchez, Ph.D., assistant professor in the Division of Immunology and Allergy at the University of California Los Angeles, who co-authored the study with scientists from the University of Southern California. "Our findings suggest that people who lack the genes to make key antioxidants may have difficulty fighting the harmful effects of air pollution."

Dr. Diaz-Sanchez says that he and the other researchers will work to find other genes involved in pollution-related health problems such as asthma, lung cancer and heart disease, with the goal of discovering possible treatments and preventions. "We are focused on investigating ways we can overcome this genetic deficiency," he says. "This may be accomplished by either giving people drugs that replace the role of the genes or by boosting the body's natural defenses."

Reference: F Gilliland *et al.* Effect of glutathione-S-transferase M1 and P1 genotypes on xenobiotic enhancement of allergic responses: randomised, placebo-controlled crossover study. *The Lancet* 363 (9403): 119–25 (2004).

Early Fevers Associated with Lower Allergy Risk Later in Childhood

Infants who experience fevers before their first birthday are less likely to develop allergies by ages six or seven, according to a new study funded by the National Institute of Allergy and Infectious Diseases (NIAID), part of the National Institutes of Health (NIH). The study, published in the *Journal of Allergy and Clinical Immunology*

(February 2004), lends support to the well-known "hygiene hypothesis," which contends that early exposure to infections might protect children against allergic diseases in later years.

"The prevalence of asthma and allergies has increased dramatically worldwide in recent years," says Anthony S. Fauci, M.D., director of NIAID. "This study provides evidence that diminished exposure to early immunological challenges could be one of the reasons for this trend."

"The hygiene hypothesis is widely recognized but largely unproven," says Kenneth Adams, Ph.D., who oversees asthma research funded by NIAID. "The findings of this study strengthen the hypothesis and, after more research, could lead to preventative therapies for asthma and allergies."

The authors of the study followed the medical records of 835 children from birth to age one, documenting any fever-related episodes. Fever was defined as a rectal temperature of 101 degrees Fahrenheit or above. At age six to seven years, more than half of the children were evaluated for their sensitivity to common allergens, such as dust mites, ragweed and cats.

Researchers found that, of the children who did not experience a fever during their first year, 50.0 percent showed allergic sensitivity. Of those who had one fever, 46.7 percent became allergy-prone. The children who suffered two or more fevers in their infancy had greater protection, with only 31.3 percent showing allergic sensitivity by ages six to seven.

In particular, fever-inducing infections involving the eyes, ears, nose or throat appeared to be associated with a lower risk of developing allergies, compared with similar infections that did not result in fevers.

"We didn't expect fever to relate with such a consistent effect," says Christine C. Johnson, Ph.D., M.P.H., senior research epidemiologist of the Henry Ford Health System in Detroit, MI, and one of the co-authors of the study. "It also was interesting that the more fevers an infant had, the less likely it was that he or she would be sensitive to allergies."

Dr. Johnson says that more research is needed to establish if early fevers have a direct effect on allergic development in children. Additionally, she and the other authors are working to determine if early exposure to pets as well as high levels of bacteria could also lower allergy risk. "If we can uncover which environmental factors affect allergic development and why, it may be possible to immunize children against these conditions," she says.

This study also received support from the National Institute of Environmental Health Sciences, another NIH component.

Reference: L Keoki Williams *et al.* The relationship between early fever and allergic sensitization at age 6 to 7 years. *Journal of Allergy and Clinical Immunology* 113(2): 291–296 (2004).

National Study Shows 82 Percent of U.S. Homes Have Mouse Allergens

Scientists at the National Institute of Environmental Health Science (NIEHS), one of the National Institutes of Health (NIH), have found that detectable levels of mouse allergen exist in the majority of U.S. homes. NIEHS researchers analyzed dust samples, asked questions, and examined homes in the first National Survey of Lead and Allergens in Housing, a survey of 831 homes. Allergen levels were studied and related to demographic factors and household characteristics.

82 percent of U.S. homes were found to have mouse allergens. The findings by Cohn *et al.* appear in the June 2004 issue of the *Journal of Allergy and Clinical Immunology*.

The survey was conducted using established sampling techniques to ensure that the surveyed homes were representative of U.S. homes. The homes were sampled from seventy-five randomly selected areas (generally counties or groups of counties) across the entire country. The 831 homes included all regions of the country (northeast, southeast, midwest, southwest, northwest), all housing types, and all settings (urban, suburban, rural).

The selection of homes was controlled to be a representative sample of U.S. homes. For statistics derived from the 831 homes, the contribution from each home was weighted as necessary to ensure that the statistics are representative of the U.S. population.

Dust samples used in the study were collected from kitchen and living room floors, upholstered furniture, beds, and bedroom floors. Kitchen floor concentrations exceed 1.6 micrograms of allergens per gram of dust in about one in five homes (22 percent). The amount of these allergy-triggering particles on the kitchen floor is high enough to be associated with allergies and asthma. Residents of high-rise apartments and mobile homes are at greatest risk, but the allergen is also present in all types of homes.

The NIEHS study, with collaborators at Constella Group, Inc. and the Harvard School of Public Health, characterized mouse allergen prevalence in a representative sample of U.S. homes and assessed risk factors for elevated concentrations. The odds of having elevated concentrations were increased when rodent or cockroach problems were reported.

Exposure to mouse allergen is a known cause of asthma in occupational settings. Until now, exposure to these allergens had not previously been studied in residential environments on a national scale. Clinicians should consider these risk factors when treating allergy and asthma patients.

Customized Program Reduces Asthma-Related Illness in Inner-City Children

A program that reduces allergens and tobacco smoke in the home resulted in fewer asthma-related illnesses in children participating in the intervention than in those who were not, according to a new study sponsored by the National Institutes of Health (NIH). Children taking part in the intervention had 21 fewer days of asthma-related symptoms over the one-year course of intervention.

The study—co-funded by the National Institute of Allergy and Infectious Diseases (NIAID) and the National Institute of Environmental Health Sciences (NIEHS), two NIH institutes—appears in the September 9, 2004 issue of *The New England Journal of Medicine*.

"The burden that childhood asthma places on our society is enormous—accounting for roughly 14 million missed school days each year and $3.2 billion per year in treatment," says Anthony S. Fauci, M.D., director of NIAID. "This important research will provide long-term practical benefits to the millions of children who live with asthma in the form of better quality of life, fewer emergency room visits and hospitalizations and lower healthcare costs."

"These study results are exciting because they show that changes made in the home environment can produce a reduction in symptoms comparable to that achieved with asthma inhalers," notes Kenneth Olden, Ph.D., director of NIEHS.

Asthma, a chronic lung disease characterized by coughing, wheezing and difficulty breathing, affects roughly 20 million Americans. However, children who live in the inner city—in particular African-American and Hispanic children—suffer disproportionately from the disease. Elevated asthma-related illness in this population may stem from exposure to high levels of multiple indoor allergens and tobacco smoke.

More than 900 children ages 5 to 11 with moderate to severe asthma participated in the study. Each participant had to be allergic to at least one common indoor environmental allergen, such as cockroach allergen or mold. The children, most of whom were African American or Hispanic, lived in low-income sections of seven major metropolitan areas—the Bronx, Boston, Chicago, Dallas, New York City, Seattle/Tacoma and Tucson. Once accepted into the study, they were randomly assigned to either the intervention group or a control group.

Based on the child's sensitivity to the selected indoor allergens, investigators designed an individualized environmental intervention, carried out by the child's mother or another caretaker. The intervention focused on educating the family about ways to reduce or eliminate all allergens to which the child was allergic, as well as to reduce exposure to tobacco smoke, and motivating them to pursue these steps. The investigators developed separate interventions tailored to tobacco smoke and to the following allergens—house dust mite, cockroach, pet, rodent and mold.

In addition, families were given specific allergen-reducing measures, such as allergen-impermeable covers for children's bedding and air purifiers with HEPA (high efficiency particulate air) filters, to be placed in key locations within their homes, including the children's bedrooms. Cockroach extermination visits were provided for children who were allergic to cockroach allergens. During the first year of the study, the investigators conducted educational home visits with the families in the intervention group. Throughout the yearlong study and the one-year follow-up, researchers closely monitored all participants' asthma symptoms and home allergen levels.

Children who participated in the intervention had significantly fewer asthma symptoms compared with those in the control group: an average of 21 fewer days of symptoms in the first year and an average of 16 fewer days during the second, or follow-up, year. In addition, the benefits of the intervention occurred rapidly; investigators noted significant reductions in symptoms just two months after the study began.

The levels of cockroach and dust mite allergens in the children's bedrooms in the intervention group were substantially lower than in the control group. Furthermore, the researchers noted a direct correlation between allergen levels and asthma symptoms for the children in the intervention group; the greater the drop in cockroach or house dust mite allergen levels, the greater the reduction in asthma symptoms, suggesting that the allergy-reducing measures—not the educational visits—made the difference.

Most previous environmental intervention studies that have focused on controlling a single allergen or tobacco smoke exclusively, have met with limited success.

"Children with asthma are usually sensitive to more than one allergen," says Daniel Rotrosen, M.D., director of NIAID's Division of

Allergy, Immunology, and Transplantation. "By taking a multifaceted, home-based approach, this new study demonstrates the promising results families can achieve when they incorporate the recommended practices of allergen reduction into their everyday lives."

The Inner City Asthma Study, a cooperative, multicenter study comprising seven centers across the country, is an outgrowth of the National Cooperative Inner-City Asthma Study, which ended in 1996. The principal investigator of the study is Wayne J. Morgan, M.D., University of Arizona College of Medicine, Tucson.

Reference: W Morgan *et al*. Results of a home-based environmental intervention in urban children with asthma-The Inner City Asthma Study. *The New England Journal of Medicine* 351(11): 1068–1080 (2004).

Chronic Sinusitis Sufferers Have Enhanced Immune Responses to Fungi

Scientists supported by the National Institute of Allergy and Infectious Diseases (NIAID), part of the National Institutes of Health, have discovered that people with chronic sinus inflammation have an exaggerated immune response to common airborne fungi. The results of their study appeared online October 12, 2004 in *The Journal of Allergy and Clinical Immunology*.

"This study is the first to show a possible immunologic basis for chronic sinusitis, an important starting point to better understand the etiology of the illness," says Marshall Plaut, M.D., chief of NIAID's allergic mechanisms section. Despite the enormous health impact of chronic sinusitis—nearly 30 million people were diagnosed with sinusitis in 2002, according to U.S. Centers for Disease Control and Prevention, and direct costs of the illness exceed $5.6 billion per year—the condition is very poorly understood, he says.

The researchers, led by Hirohito Kita, M.D., of the Mayo Clinic in Rochester, MN, compared blood samples taken from 18 people diagnosed with chronic sinusitis with blood samples from 15 healthy volunteers. Nasal secretions from the two groups were also examined for the presence of fungal proteins and inflammation-causing immune system molecules.

Airborne microscopic fungi spores abound indoors and out. People may inhale a million or more fungal spores each day, notes Dr. Kita. The mere presence of such fungi in the airways, however, is not enough to cause sinusitis because these spores can be found in the upper respiratory tracts of both sinusitis sufferers and non-sufferers. Indeed, in this study, levels of fungal proteins in nasal secretions were similar in both groups.

The Mayo Clinic scientists looked for evidence that people with sinusitis respond abnormally to these harmless fungi. The investigators exposed immune cells derived from the blood samples to extracts of four common airborne fungi: *Alternaria, Aspergillus, Penicillium* and *Cladosporium*. The cells of chronic sinusitis sufferers released significant amounts of three immune-modulating chemicals, called cytokines, specifically interferon-gamma, interleukin-5 (IL-5) and IL-13. In contrast, cells from healthy volunteers released very little interferon-gamma and no IL-5 or IL-13. The most dramatic responses occurred after exposure to *Alternaria*.

Importantly, says Dr. Kita, the released cytokines represent both major classes of cytokines—interferon-gamma is in the Th1 group and IL-5 and IL-13 are in the Th2 class. This is notable because scientists have thought that allergic reactions involve only Th2 cytokines, Dr. Kita explains. (While chronic sinusitis is not considered to be an allergic disease, people with the condition also often have asthma and allergic rhinitis, giving scientists reason to suspect a link.) The current findings add to an evolving understanding of allergic diseases that suggests symptoms may stem from a combination of Th1 and Th2 cytokines.

The combined effect of excess Th2 and Th1 cytokines released in the presence of fungi may explain a number of chronic sinusitis symptoms, including persistent inflammation of sinus and nasal mucous passages, say the scientists.

Previously, Mayo clinic scientists used intranasal antifungal agents to successfully treat patients with chronic sinusitis. While those studies generated controversy, in part because other researchers were unable to replicate the findings, Dr. Kita says the report supports the rationale of treating chronic sinusitis with antifungals. Clinical trials to further test antifungal therapy for chronic sinusitis are being planned, adds Dr. Kita.

Reference: S-H Shin *et al*. Chronic rhinosinusitis: An enhanced immune response to ubiquitous airborne fungi. *The Journal of Allergy and Clinical Immunology*. Published online Oct. 8, 2004. doi: 10.1016/j.jaci.2004.06.012.

Genetics Play Role in Response to Most Common Asthma Drug

Genes affect how asthma patients respond to albuterol, according to results of a new study of adults with mild asthma. Researchers in

Asthma Research Updates from the National Institutes of Health

the Asthma Clinical Research Network (ACRN) of the National Heart, Lung, and Blood Institute (NHLBI), part of the National Institutes of Health, found that over time, how participants responded to daily doses of inhaled albuterol differed depending on which form of a specific gene they had inherited. While a few weeks of regular use of albuterol improved overall asthma control in individuals with one form of the gene, stopping all use of albuterol eventually improved asthma control in those with another form of the gene. Albuterol is the most commonly used drug for relief of acute asthma symptoms, or "attacks."

The Beta-Adrenergic Response by Genotype (BARGE) trial is the first study of an asthma drug in patients selected according to their genotype, or which forms of a specific gene they have. Published in the October 23–29, 2004 issue of the *Lancet*, the BARGE trial provides important insight as to why albuterol may benefit some people with asthma more than others. The findings could lead to better ways to individualize asthma therapy based on patients' genetic patterns.

"If we can pinpoint which individuals will do better with a certain type of therapy, we can improve their lives more quickly and save them—and the healthcare system—the expense and risk of trying drugs that are less effective for them," comments Dr. Barbara Alving, NHLBI acting director. "This study helps put asthma at the forefront of pharmacogenetics."

Pharmacogenetics is an emerging science that links variations in genotypes to variations in drug responsiveness. Scientists have long known that genes can play a role in how individuals respond to disease and to medications. As drugs move through the body, they interact with thousands of molecules, or proteins. Because genes direct how proteins behave, variations in the structure of a gene can affect how the protein responds to a medication. Many believe that pharmacogenetics will revolutionize health care as it will lead to the development of drugs that target specific molecules more precisely than currently available medications, making them more powerful and less likely to create unwanted side effects.

Asthma drugs are known to vary widely in their effects in different patients. Research suggests that genetics may play a role in these differences.

Albuterol targets the beta-2 adrenergic receptor molecules. As an asthma quick-relief medication, it relaxes the muscles in the airways and quickly opens up the air passages during an asthma attack, when airways are narrowed. BARGE was developed based on observations from earlier studies that suggested that genetic differences in the beta-receptor might play an important role in how patients respond to albuterol.

The BARGE study examined the effects of two forms of the beta-2 adrenergic receptor in patients with mild asthma. The trial paired 78 participants with matching levels of airway function but with different forms of the receptor gene. Researchers compared participants who have two arginine versions of the gene (the arginine genotype) to those with two glycine versions of the gene (the glycine genotype). Albuterol was used daily (two puffs, four times a day) for 16 weeks, and placebo use followed the same timeframe. When participants needed additional symptom relief, they used ipratropium bromide, a different type of quick-relief medication known as an anticholinergic.

While all participants initially responded well to albuterol, after 16 weeks of daily use, those with the arginine genotype had poorer asthma control compared to their matched partners with the glycine genotype. In addition, the arginine participants reported more symptoms, lower FEV1 scores (a measurement of lung function) and more frequent use of quick-relief medication.

Overall, participants with the arginine genotype had improved asthma control when not using albuterol. In contrast, participants with the glycine genotype had better asthma control with albuterol treatment, although not with placebo.

Of the 15 million Americans who have asthma, about one out of six 6 (more than 2 million) have the arginine genotype. Moreover, the arginine genotype is more prevalent in certain ethnic groups, such as African Americans. Currently, tests to determine this genotype are only available in a few research settings.

"Anyone needing regular, daily use of albuterol for asthma control should be considered for a long-term controller medication. Our findings suggest that in patients with the arginine genotype, this will be especially important," said Dr. Elliot Israel of Brigham and Women's Hospital, lead author of the study. "More work is needed to determine how to integrate these findings into clinical practice. In the future, patients with the arginine genotype might even be advised to use an alternate reliever medication."

The National Asthma Education and Prevention Program (NAEPP) recommends quick-relief medication such as inhaled albuterol on an as-needed basis for acute asthma symptoms. Other recommended reliever medications include inhaled anticholinergics and short-acting theophylline. NAEPP clinical guidelines call for a "step-wise" approach to asthma management, in which treatment is adjusted depending on disease severity and symptom frequency. Patients who have symptoms or use quick-relief medication more than a couple of times a week, for example, should add daily long-term control medication such as inhaled corticosteroids or leukotriene modifiers.

"This study highlights one of several variables that plays a role in how a medication will affect an individual," says Dr. James Kiley, director of the NHLBI Division of Lung Diseases. "It also serves as a reminder of how important it is for asthma specialists to regularly assess how their patients are responding to medications so they can modify their drug regimen as needed."

NHLBI established the ACRN in 1993 to conduct multiple, well-designed clinical trials for rapid evaluation of new and existing therapeutic approaches to asthma and to disseminate laboratory and clinical findings to the healthcare community. The ACRN clinical centers that participated in this study are Brigham and Women's Hospital and Harvard Medical School (Boston), Harlem Lung Center and Columbia University (New York City), National Jewish Medical and Research Center (Denver), Thomas Jefferson Medical College (Philadelphia), University of California at San Francisco, and University of Wisconsin (Madison). Two of the clinical centers—the University of California at San Francisco and the University of Wisconsin—also received support from the NIH National Center for Research Resources. The data coordinating center is at Pennsylvania State University College of Medicine.

In a separate study, new ACRN researchers are studying whether similar effects occur with long-acting forms of medication similar to albuterol. These medications, known as long-acting beta-agonists, are increasingly used in concert with inhaled corticosteroids as long-term control medications for patients with moderate or severe asthma.

Note: Albuterol and placebo was provided by Glaxo-SmithKline. Ipratropium bromide was provided by Boehringer Ingelheim Pharmaceuticals, Inc.

Reference: Israel E, Chinchilli VM, Ford JG, *et al.*, for the National Heart, Lung, and Blood Institute's Asthma Clinical Research Network. Genotype Stratified Prospective Cross-over Trial of Regularly Scheduled Albuterol Treatment in Asthma. *Lancet* 2004; 364: 1505–1512.

New Treatment Guidelines for Pregnant Women with Asthma

The National Asthma Education and Prevention Program (NAEPP) is issuing the first new guidelines in more than a decade for managing asthma during pregnancy. The report reflects new medications that have emerged and updates treatment recommendations for pregnant women with asthma based on a systematic review of data on the safety of asthma medications during pregnancy. An executive summary ("Quick Reference") of the guidelines is published in the January 2005 issue of the *Journal of Allergy & Clinical Immunology*.

Poorly controlled asthma can lead to serious medical problems for pregnant women and their fetuses. The guidelines emphasize that controlling asthma during pregnancy is important for the health and well-being of the mother as well as for the healthy development of the fetus. A stepwise approach to asthma care similar to that used in the NAEPP general asthma treatment guidelines for children and non-pregnant adults is recommended. Under this approach, medication is stepped up in intensity if needed, and stepped down when possible, depending on asthma severity. Because asthma severity changes during pregnancy for most women, the guidelines also recommend that clinicians who provide obstetric care monitor asthma severity during prenatal visits of their patients who have asthma.

"The guidelines review the evidence on asthma medications used by pregnant patients," said Barbara Alving, M.D., acting director of the National Heart, Lung, and Blood Institute (NHLBI), which administers the NAEPP. "The evidence is reassuring, and suggests that it is safer to take medications than to have asthma exacerbations. The guidelines should be a useful tool for physicians to develop optimal asthma management plans for pregnant women."

"Simply put, when a pregnant patient has trouble breathing, her fetus also has trouble getting the oxygen it needs," added William W. Busse, M.D., professor of medicine at the University of Wisconsin Medical School, and chair of the NAEPP multidisciplinary expert panel that developed the guidelines. "There are many ways we can help pregnant women control their asthma, and it is imperative that providers and their patients work together to do so."

Asthma affects over 20 million Americans and is one of the most common potentially serious medical conditions to complicate pregnancy. Maternal asthma is associated with increased risk of infant death, preeclampsia (a serious condition marked by high blood pressure, which can cause seizures in the mother or fetus), premature birth, and low-birth weight. These risks are linked to asthma severity—more severe asthma increases risk, while better controlled asthma is tied to decreased risks.

Asthma worsens in approximately 30 percent of women who have mild asthma at the beginning of their pregnancy, according to a recent study by the National Institute of Child Health and Human Development Maternal-Fetal Medicine Units Network and co-funded by NHLBI. The study also found that, conversely, asthma improved in 23 percent of the women who initially had moderate or severe asthma.

"We cannot predict who will worsen during pregnancy, so the new guidelines recommend that pregnant patients with persistent asthma have their asthma checked at least monthly by a healthcare provider," explained Mitchell Dombrowski, M.D., chief of obstetrics and gynecology for St. John Hospital in Detroit, and a member of the NAEPP expert panel. "Clinicians who provide obstetric care should be part of the patient's asthma management team, working with the patient and her asthma care provider to adjust her medications if needed to keep her asthma under control and to lower the risk of complications from asthma for her and her baby."

Key recommendations from the guidelines regarding medications include the following:

- Albuterol, a short-acting inhaled beta2-agonist, should be used as a quick-relief medication to treat asthma symptoms. Pregnant women with asthma should have this medication available at all times.

- Women who have symptoms at least two days a week or two nights a month have persistent asthma and need daily medication for long-term care of their asthma and to prevent exacerbations. Inhaled corticosteroids are the preferred medication to control the underlying inflammation in pregnant women with persistent asthma. The guidelines note that there are more data on the safety of budesonide use during pregnancy than on other inhaled corticosteroids; however, there are no data indicating that other inhaled corticosteroids are unsafe during pregnancy, and other inhaled corticosteroids may be continued if they effectively control a patient's asthma. Alternative daily medications are leukotriene receptor antagonists, cromolyn, or theophylline.

- For patients whose persistent asthma is not well controlled on low doses of inhaled corticosteroids alone, the guidelines recommend either increasing the dose of inhaled corticosteroid or adding another medication—a long-acting beta agonist. The expert panel concluded that data are insufficient to indicate a preference of one option over the other.

- Oral corticosteroids may be required for the treatment of severe asthma. The guidelines note that there are conflicting data regarding the safety of oral corticosteroids during pregnancy; however, severe, uncontrolled asthma poses a definite risk to the mother and fetus; and use of oral corticosteroids may be warranted.

"Several studies have shown that taking inhaled corticosteroids improves lung function during pregnancy and reduces asthma exacerbations—and other large, prospective studies found no relation between taking inhaled corticosteroids and congenital abnormalities or other adverse pregnancy outcomes," said Michael Schatz, M.D., M.S., chief of the Department of Allergy for Kaiser Permanente San Diego Medical Center. Schatz is also a member of the NAEPP expert panel on asthma during pregnancy and author of an editorial accompanying the guidelines report.

The guidelines highlight other important aspects of asthma management during pregnancy, such as identifying and limiting exposure to asthma triggers. Similarly, women with other conditions that can worsen asthma, such as allergic rhinitis, sinusitis, and gastroesophageal reflux, should have those conditions treated as well. Such conditions often become more troublesome during pregnancy.

"As important as medications are for controlling asthma, a pregnant woman can reduce how much medication is needed by identifying and avoiding the factors that make her asthma worse, such as tobacco smoke or allergens like dust mites," added Dr. Schatz.

The NAEPP was established in March 1989 to reduce asthma-related illness and death and to enhance the quality of life of people with asthma. As of January 2005, 40 organizations, including major medical associations, voluntary health organizations, and numerous federal agencies, comprise the NAEPP Coordinating Committee. The NAEPP also coordinates federal asthma-related activities, as designated by Congress through the Children's Health Act of 2000. NAEPP convenes expert panels as needed to ensure that the latest scientific evidence is translated into clinical recommendations to help clinicians provide the best possible asthma care.

Study: Mold in Homes Doubles Risk of Asthma

Exposure to mold and dampness in homes as much as doubles the risk of asthma development in children, according to a study published in the March 2005 issue of the peer-reviewed journal *Environmental Health Perspectives* (*EHP*). Researchers studied 1,984 Finnish children aged one to seven years over a six-year period to see if they developed asthma. Data collection included a baseline survey administered in March 1991, as well as a follow-up survey in March 1997, asking questions about the child's health, parents' health, parent's highest education level, and details of the child's environment including exposure to environmental tobacco smoke and presence of feathery or furry pets.

The study focused particularly on four indicators or moisture or mold in the home, including mold odor, visible mold, visible moisture, and history of water damage. The presence of mold odor proved to be the only significant indicator of asthma development.

A total of 138 children, or 7.2% of the study population, developed asthma during the study period. Having a parent with a history of allergies increased susceptibility in children. Mold odor increased the risk, the study found, independent of parents' medical histories. In fact, children living in homes with mold odor during the initial study period were more than twice as likely to develop asthma in the following six years.

"These findings strengthen evidence that exposure to molds increases the risk of developing asthma in childhood," says lead author Jouni Jaakkola, director of the University of Birmingham's Institute for Occupational and Environmental Medicine. "They also show the importance of heredity—children of parents with asthma have a twofold risk of asthma compared with children of non-asthmatic parents."

Children who were exposed to moisture or mold in the home were also slightly more likely to be exposed to environmental tobacco smoke, to have feathery or furry pets, and to have parents with a lower education level. The study adds to the body of evidence linking asthma with exposure to cigarette smoke.

"This study is important for families everywhere," says Dr. Jim Burkhart, science editor for *EHP*. "Anyone with young children in the home should be aware of the potentially harmful effects of long-term exposure to mold and this potential link to asthma in children."

In addition to Jaakkola, contributing authors included Bing-Fang Hwang of the Environmental Epidemiology Unit at the University of Helsinki in Finland, and Niina Jaakkola of the Department of Health Care Administration at Diwan College of Management in Taiwan. The article is available free of charge at http://ehp.niehs.nih.gov/members/2004/7242/7242.html.

NHLBI Study Suggests Symptom-Driven Therapy May Be Sufficient for Some Adults with Mild Persistent Asthma

Some adults with mild persistent asthma may be able to adequately control their asthma by taking corticosteroids only when needed, instead of taking anti-inflammatory medication daily, according to new results from the Improving Asthma Control Trial (IMPACT). Conducted by the National Heart, Lung, and Blood Institute's (NHLBI) Asthma Clinical Research Network, the one-year, multi-center study found that participants who were treated with corticosteroids intermittently based on symptoms had about the same rate of severe exacerbations and of asthma-related lung function decline as those treated with the standard recommendation of daily long-term control medication.

Asthma is considered mild and persistent when individuals have acute symptoms such as wheezing, coughing, or chest tightness more than twice a week, but not daily, or they have night-time awakenings due to asthma more than two nights a month. The researchers caution that the new findings might not apply to people who have recently developed asthma. In addition, they do not apply to patients with more frequent symptoms or more severe asthma. The results are published in the April 14, 2005 issue of the *New England Journal of Medicine*.

"This study provides evidence of another possible way to treat adults with long-standing mild persistent asthma," stated Elizabeth G. Nabel, MD, director of the NHLBI, part of the National Institutes of Health. "If additional research confirms these findings, then some of these patients may be able to safely treat their asthma with intermittent medication and avoid the added expense and inconvenience of daily therapy. As for all asthma patients, however, individuals should work closely with their healthcare providers to develop and follow the treatment plan that suits them best."

More than 20 million Americans have asthma. For those with mild persistent asthma, guidelines from the National Asthma Education and Prevention Program (NAEPP) currently recommend daily long-term control medication to prevent symptoms and quick-relief medication (inhaled bronchodilator) to treat acute asthma symptoms if they occur.

The recommendation for daily long-term control medication for mild persistent asthma was based largely on clinical trials that showed that anti-inflammatory therapy improves lung function and measures of asthma control. However, participants in these earlier studies had asthma that ranged in severity from mild to moderate, according to the IMPACT authors. The IMPACT study strictly adhered to the guidelines' definition.

James Kiley, PhD, director of the NHLBI Division of Lung Diseases, commented, "By focusing exclusively on mild persistent asthma, the IMPACT study has added to our understanding of possible treatment options for different levels of asthma severity."

Asthma Research Updates from the National Institutes of Health

NAEPP is expected to release updated guidelines in 2006. An expert panel will consider the results of IMPACT and other studies to determine if changes in treatment recommendations for adults with mild persistent asthma are warranted.

IMPACT was designed to identify the best long-term treatment strategy for adults with mild persistent asthma. Researchers compared changes in lung function, frequency and severity of asthma symptoms, and quality-of-life scores in 255 adult patients. Participants were randomly selected to one of three treatment groups. Two groups were assigned to long-term control medication taken twice daily—either an inhaled steroid (budesonide) or a leukotriene modifier (zafirlukast) taken in pill form. The third group received placebo (inactive) medication. All participants were given medications for asthma symptoms—inhaled bronchodilator (albuterol), inhaled corticosteroid (budesonide), and oral corticosteroid (prednisone)—with explicit instructions on when and how to use these treatments depending on the severity and duration of the individual's symptoms.

After one year, changes in lung function and the number of severe attacks did not significantly differ among the three groups. In addition, participants scored similarly on quality-of-life tests regardless of treatment group. Those in the daily inhaled steroid group, however, reported significantly more symptom-free days (equivalent to about 26 additional symptom-free days per year) than participants in the other two treatment groups.

"Although some reports of symptoms differed between those taking budesonide daily and the other participants, these differences were not reflected in the quality-of-life scores," noted Homer Boushey, M.D., Principal Investigator at the University of California San Francisco, and a lead author of the study. "Combined with the fact that there were no significant differences in lung function changes or in the frequency of severe attacks among the treatment groups after a year of treatment, we conclude that, overall, the three treatments had similar clinical effects in this study of mild asthma."

Other reports have noted that many asthma patients do not follow recommendations for daily controller medication. "The results of IMPACT suggest that for some adults with long-standing mild persistent asthma, choosing not to take daily medications might be okay," added Elliot Israel, M.D., Principal Investigator at Brigham and Women's Hospital in Boston and the co-lead author. "But this choice should be made in consultation with the patient's healthcare provider. It's critical that individuals with more severe asthma follow recommendations for daily long-term control medications and that all asthma patients—even those with mild asthma—be aware of signs of worsening asthma and adequately treat their symptoms."

Asthma treatment guidelines also recommend written action plans as part of an overall effort to educate patients in self-management. The plans provide guidance for patients on how to monitor and treat their asthma, including how to recognize when their condition worsens. In general, action plans are based on the patient's symptoms or on "peak flow" measurements of lung function, which can be taken by patients using a hand-held device.

"One of the most important things we did during this study was to work closely with the participants to help them effectively manage their asthma," noted Boushey. "Patients need to know how to recognize asthma symptoms, what to do when symptoms begin, and—perhaps most essential—they must have at hand the means to treat their symptoms quickly."

Clinical centers for the Improving Asthma Control Trial were as follows:

- Brigham and Women's Hospital and Harvard Medical School, Boston, MA
- Columbia Presbyterian Medical Center and Harlem Lung Center, New York, NY
- National Jewish Medical and Research Center, Denver, CO
- University of Wisconsin, Madison
- Thomas Jefferson Medical College, Philadelphia, PA
- University of California, San Francisco

The data coordinating center is at Penn State College of Medicine, Penn State Milton S. Hershey Medical Center, Hershey, PA.

The medications for IMPACT were donated by Astra-Zeneca Pharmaceuticals, headquartered in Wayne, Pennsylvania.

More Than Half the U.S. Population is Sensitive to One or More Allergens

More than fifty percent of the U.S. population tested positive to one or more allergens, according to a large national study. The new findings, based on data from the third National Health and Nutrition Examination Survey (NHANES III), shows that 54.3% of individuals aged 6–59 years old had a positive skin test response to at least one of the ten allergens tested. The highest prevalence rates were for dust mite, rye, ragweed, and cockroach, with about 25% of the population testing positive to each allergen. Peanut allergy was the least common, with 9% of the population reacting positively to that food allergen.

The new findings published in the August 2004 issue of the *Journal of Allergy and Clinical Immunology* were conducted by researchers at the National Institute of Environmental Health Sciences (NIEHS) and the National Institute of Allergy and Infectious Diseases, both components of the National Institutes of Health.

A positive skin test result may mean the individual is more vulnerable to asthma, hay fever, and eczema. "Asthma is one of the world's most significant chronic health conditions," said David A. Schwartz, MD, the NIEHS Director. "Understanding what may account for the rising worldwide asthma rates will allow us to develop more effective prevention and treatment approaches."

NHANES III is a nationally representative survey conducted by the Centers for Disease Control and Prevention between 1988–1994 to determine the health and nutritional status of the U.S. population. Approximately 10,500 individuals participated in the skin testing. During these tests, skin was exposed to allergy-causing substances (allergens) and a positive test was determined by the size of the reaction on the skin. The ten allergens tested include: Dust mite, German cockroach, cat, perennial rye, short ragweed, Bermuda grass, Russian thistle, White oak, *Alternia alternata*, and peanuts.

Researchers also compared skin test responses between NHANES III and the previous survey, NHANES II, conducted from 1976–1980. The prevalence of a positive skin test response was much higher in NHANES III than in NHANES II.

According to the lead author, Samuel J. Arbes, Ph.D. of NIEHS, "An increase in prevalence is consistent with reports from other countries and coincides with an increase in asthma cases during that time." In the U.S., the prevalence of asthma increased 73.9% from 1980 to 1996. However, Dr. Arbes was quick to point out that differences in skin test procedures between the two surveys prevent the authors from definitively concluding that the prevalence of skin test positivity has increased in the U.S. population.

"There is still much we don't understand about why some people become sensitized to allergens and others do not," said Darryl C. Zeldin, MD, senior author on the paper. "Much more research is needed in order for us to understand the complex relationships between exposures to allergens, the development of allergic sensitization, and the onset and exacerbation of allergic diseases such as asthma."

The researchers recently added an allergy component to NHANES 2005–2006. In addition to the other NHANES data collection components, dust samples from the homes of 10,000 individuals are being analyzed for allergens, and blood samples taken from these individuals are being examined for antibodies to those allergens. This new NHANES 2005–2006 allergy component will allow researchers to gain a greater understanding of asthma and the roles that indoor allergens play in asthma and other allergic diseases.

Cockroach Allergens Have Greatest Impact on Childhood Asthma in Many U.S. Cities

New results from a nationwide study on factors that affect asthma in inner-city children show that cockroach allergen appears to worsen asthma symptoms more than either dust mite or pet allergens. This research, funded by the National Institute of Environmental Health Sciences (NIEHS) and the National Institute of Allergy and Infectious Diseases (NIAID), part of the National Institutes of Health, is the first large-scale study to show marked geographic differences in allergen exposure and sensitivity in inner-city children. Most homes in northeastern cities had high levels of cockroach allergens, while those in the south and northwest had dust mite allergen levels in ranges known to exacerbate asthma symptoms.

The study results are published in the March 2005 issue of the *Journal of Allergy and Clinical Immunology*.

"These data confirm that cockroach allergen is the primary contributor to childhood asthma in inner-city home environments," said NIEHS Director Kenneth Olden, Ph.D. "However, general cleaning practices, proven extermination techniques, and consistent maintenance methods can bring these allergen levels under control."

Cockroach allergens come from several sources such as saliva, fecal material, secretions, cast skins, and dead bodies. People can reduce their exposure to cockroach allergen by eating only in the kitchen and dining room, putting non-refrigerated items in plastic containers or sealable bags, and taking out the garbage on a daily basis. Other measures include repairing leaky faucets, frequent vacuuming of carpeted areas and damp-mopping of hard floors and regular cleaning of counter tops and other surfaces.

NIH provided $7.5 million to researchers at the University of Texas Southwestern Medical Center at Dallas and seven other research institutions, including the Data Coordinating Center at Rho, Inc. for the three year study.

Asthma Research Updates from the National Institutes of Health

"We found that a majority of homes in Chicago, New York City and the Bronx had cockroach allergen levels high enough to trigger asthma symptoms, while a majority of homes in Dallas and Seattle had dust mite allergen levels above the asthma symptom threshold," said Dr. Rebecca Gruchalla, associate professor of internal medicine and pediatrics at the University of Texas Southwestern Medical Center and lead author of the study.

"We also discovered that the levels of both of these allergens were influenced by housing type," noted Gruchalla. "Cockroach allergen levels were highest in high-rise apartments, while dust mite concentrations were greatest in detached homes."

While cockroach allergen exposure did produce in increase in asthma symptoms, researchers did not find an increase in asthma symptoms as a result of exposure to dust mite and pet dander. "Children who tested positive for, and were exposed to, cockroach allergen experienced a significant increase in the number of days with cough, wheezing and chest tightness, number of nights with interrupted sleep, number of missed school days, and number of times they had to slow down or discontinue their play activity," said Gruchalla.

While cockroaches are primarily attracted to water sources and food debris, house dust mites, microscopic spider-like creatures that feed on flakes of human skin, reside in bedding, carpets, upholstery, draperies and other "dust traps." Dust mite allergens are proteins that come from the digestive tracks of mites and are found in mite feces.

Researchers tested 937 inner-city children with moderate to severe asthma symptoms. The children, ages 5 to 11, were given skin tests for sensitivity to cockroach and dust mite allergens, pet dander, and mold. Bedroom dust samples were analyzed for the presence of each allergen type.

This study was part of the larger Inner-City Asthma Study, a cooperative multi-center project comprised of seven asthma study centers across the country. The coal of the study was to develop and implement a comprehensive, cost-effective intervention program aimed at reducing asthma incidence among children living in low socioeconomic areas.

Chapter 70

Researchers Find Obesity Is Associated with Asthma

If you need one more compelling reason to put down the donuts and exercise more to drop those extra pounds, you now have it: Researchers are making a strong case for a link between obesity and asthma.

The question is far more than an academic curiosity. The Centers for Disease Control and Prevention (CDC) and many physicians define clinical obesity as have a body mass index (BMI) of 30 or higher. According to the CDC, 63.1 million Americans over the age of 20 are clinically obese. An additional 71.7 million are clinically overweight, which is a BMI rating of 25 to 29.

"Assuming a prevalence of obesity of 30% among U.S. adults and estimates of relative risk ranging from 1.6 to 3.0, [this] suggests that about 15% to 38% of asthma in adults might be caused by obesity and thus might be preventable," says Earl Ford, M.D., of the Centers for Disease Control and Prevention (CDC) in Atlanta.

Children and adolescents are not faring any better in the battle of the bulge. The CDC reports the number of overweight children, ages 6 to 11 years old, increased 376% between 1965 and 2002. During the same years, the number of overweight adolescents, ages 12 to 19 years old, increased by 350%.

Also during this period, dramatic increases have occurred in the rate of asthma in the United States. The CDC reports that 20.3 million

---

"A Weighty Issue for Those with Asthma," by Gregory Alford, from *Asthma Magazine*, July/August 2005. Reprinted by permission from Elsevier.

Asthma Sourcebook, Second Edition

people in the U.S. currently report having asthma, 9 million of them children. The number of people who report having asthma increased 75% from 1980 to 1994.

Current Research Trends

In years past, the assumption was that many asthmatics were obese because their physical limitations caused or contributed to their weight gain. However, recent studies suggest chemical changes in the

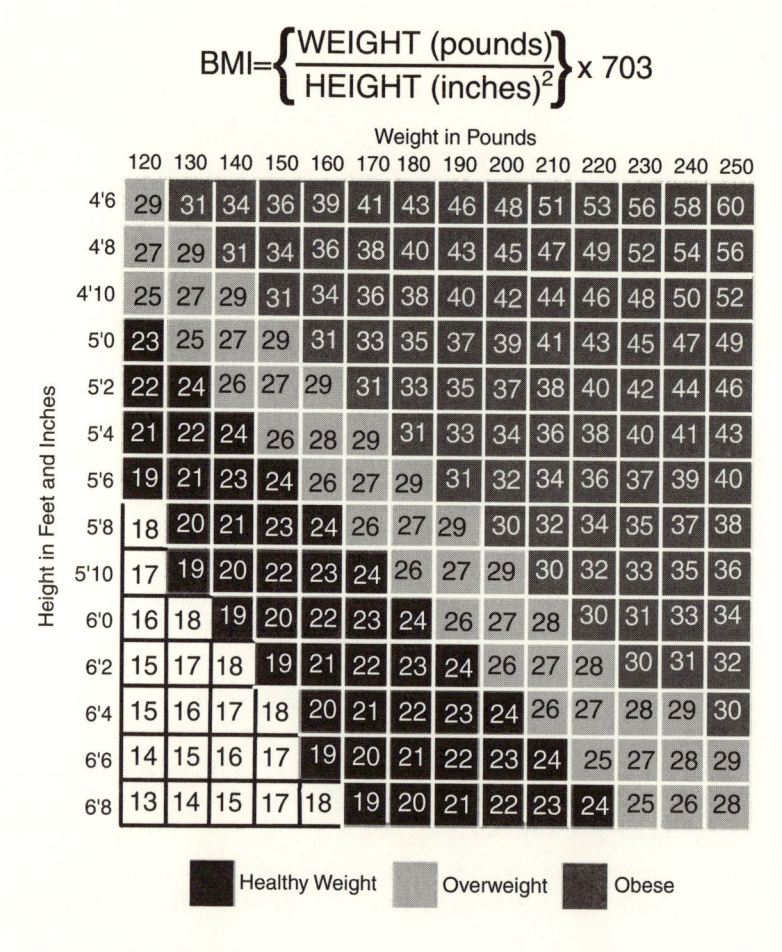

$$BMI = \left\{ \frac{WEIGHT\ (pounds)}{HEIGHT\ (inches)^2} \right\} \times 703$$

Height \ Weight (lbs)	120	130	140	150	160	170	180	190	200	210	220	230	240	250
4'6	29	31	34	36	39	41	43	46	48	51	53	56	58	60
4'8	27	29	31	34	36	38	40	43	45	47	49	52	54	56
4'10	25	27	29	31	34	36	38	40	42	44	46	48	50	52
5'0	23	25	27	29	31	33	35	37	39	41	43	45	47	49
5'2	22	24	26	27	29	31	33	35	37	38	40	42	44	46
5'4	21	22	24	26	28	29	31	33	34	36	38	40	41	43
5'6	19	21	23	24	26	27	29	31	32	34	36	37	39	40
5'8	18	20	21	23	24	26	27	29	30	32	34	35	37	38
5'10	17	19	20	22	23	24	26	27	29	30	32	33	35	36
6'0	16	18	19	20	22	23	24	26	27	28	30	31	33	34
6'2	15	17	18	19	21	22	23	24	26	27	28	30	31	32
6'4	15	16	17	18	20	21	22	23	24	26	27	28	29	30
6'6	14	15	16	17	19	20	21	22	23	24	25	27	28	29
6'8	13	14	15	17	18	19	20	21	22	23	24	25	26	28

■ Healthy Weight   ■ Overweight   ■ Obese

Figure 70.1. BMI Weight Chart for Adults. (Source: Surgeon General's Call to Action to Prevent and Decrease Overweight and Obesity, 2001.)

body caused by obesity may be contributing to the increase in the incidence of asthma. The following are examples of current areas of investigation:

- Increased physical stress caused by excess weight may reduce lung capacity (*J Appl Physiol* 1995;79:1199–1205).

- The obese take additional, shallower breaths than people of normal weight. This increases airway responsiveness to allergens and other asthma triggers, and narrows the airways (*J Appl Physiol* 1983;55:1269–1276).

- Carrying too much body weight causes an increase in the production of certain compounds that result in low-grade inflammation, which increases the risk of asthma, type 2 diabetes, and cardiovascular disease (*J Allergy and Clin Immun* 2005; 115:925–7).

Although researchers are making headway, they still have more questions than answers about the link between obesity and asthma. "Obesity has the capacity to impact lung function in a variety of ways," says Jeffrey Fredberg, professor of bioengineering and physiology at Harvard University in Cambridge, Massachusetts. "None of them are good and all of them are poorly understood. More research is needed to explain the relationship between asthma and obesity."

Obesity's Role in Asthma: What the Research Shows

A plethora of studies show clinically obese children are more likely to be asthmatic than children of average weight. In one study, Loreto G. Sulit, M.D., of Rainbow Babies and Children's Hospital at Case University School of Medicine in Cleveland, led a research team that studied medical records of 788 children from age 8 to 11. They found excess weight resulted in an increase in the rate of not only asthma and wheezing but also sleep-related disorders (*Amer Jour of Resp and Crit Care Med* 2005;171:659–664).

"Compared with those with neither wheeze nor asthma, children with active wheeze had significantly higher BMI and a greater prevalence of obesity," says Dr. Sulit.

At any age, the combination of asthma and obesity also seems to result in more serious asthma attacks. Obese or overweight individuals constitute 75% of people seeking emergency room asthma treatment (*Chest* 2003;124:795–802).

"The incidence of asthma and obesity is increasing worldwide, and asthma is often more severe in the obese," says Christine Ballantyne, M.D., director of the Center for Cardiovascular Disease Prevention at the Methodist DeBakey Heart Center in Houston. "We found that fat tissue inside of the abdomen is an important source of eotaxin, a molecule that is an inflammatory mediator known to play a key role in asthma."

Inflammation is a central feature of asthma. The inflammatory process leads to increased mucus production and sensitivity in the airways of the lungs. Once inflammation is present, the bronchial tubes become sensitive to conditions or factors in the environment. These things act to trigger a constriction or tightening of the airways, causing the classic asthma symptoms of wheezing, chest tightness, and shortness of breath. This is why anti-inflammatory medications such as inhaled corticosteroids are a major part of care plans for those diagnosed with moderate to severe asthma.

Research into the role of inflammation in the disease process is gaining momentum. One current area of interest is how fat tissue plays a role in creating hormones such as leptin that cause low-grade inflammation throughout the body. The clinically obese are known to have higher-than-average leptin levels. Regardless of weight, asthmatics have increased blood levels of leptin, which suggests it plays a role in the disease. In addition, fat tissue also appears to decrease the blood levels of adiponectin, a hormone that has anti-inflammatory properties (*Cur Opin Pharma* 2004;4:281–289).

Losing Weight Can Be an Effective Asthma Treatment

The good news is that losing weight helps the clinically obese breathe more easily. In a randomized controlled study from Finland, 38 people with a BMI of at least 30 treated for moderate asthma with corticosteroids were placed on a strict, supervised diet (*Br Med J* 2000;320:827–832). The average weight loss in the group was about 40 pounds.

"Their lung function improved, there was less obstruction of the airways, and they also found that their quality of life was much better," says Dr. Brita Stenius-Aarniala, professor of Pulmonary Medicine and Allergy at Helsinki University Central Hospital, Helsinki, Finland. "They used less asthma medication, and the group who lost weight, when we followed them for a year, had fewer admissions to hospitals than the group that did not lose weight."

She admits she is not sure why weight loss can lead to such a marked improvement in asthma symptoms. She speculates symptoms

Researchers Find Obesity Is Associated with Asthma

may improve because less weight eases the mechanical load on breathing and less fat on the chest wall reduces compression of the bronchial tubes.

In small studies, people who have lost considerable amounts of weight after undergoing bariatric surgery report that their asthma symptoms improved or disappeared. Dr. Ford of the CDC says there is a need for large, randomized clinical trials on weight loss, including bariatric studies, to yield valuable insights into the obesity-asthma relationship.

"Whether weight-loss programs need to be tailored to patients with asthma deserves consideration," Dr. Ford says. A program of calorie restriction and increased exercise produces the most consistent long-term weight loss. By losing weight this way, asthmatics can increase their level of physical activity and improve their overall health.

"Health care professionals can help to dispel any lingering doubts among most asthmatic patients about their ability to engage in adequate physical activity," Dr. Ford says. "Clearly, many aspects of obesity and asthma deserve further research."

Chapter 71

Researchers Discover Gene that Determines Asthma Susceptibility

Disruption of a single gene, *Nrf2*, plays a critical role in determining the susceptibility to asthma. A research team led by Shyam Biswal, PhD, at the Johns Hopkins Bloomberg School of Public Health found the absence of *Nrf2* exacerbated allergen-mediated asthma in mice models. The study's findings, published in the July 4, 2005, edition of the *Journal of Experimental Medicine*, may hold therapeutic potential for the treatment of human asthma.

Asthma is a complex inflammatory disease of the airway characterized by airway inflammation and hyperreactivity. The incidence of asthma has doubled in the past two decades in the United States, affecting 20 million Americans. Controlling inflammation is a focus of asthma therapy. Inflammation occurs when certain cells migrate into the airways. These "inflammatory" cells release reactive oxygen species (ROS), causing the airway lining to swell and restrict. ROS is thought to cause lung tissue damage as well. ROS levels are normally offset by antioxidants in non-asthmatics. Recently, researchers have been hunting for novel genes that regulate inflammation with the hope of developing them as targets for the next generation of asthma drugs.

"Researchers Discover Gene that Determines Asthma Susceptibility by Regulating Inflammation," July 5, 2005, is reprinted with permission from the Office of Communications and Public Affairs for the Johns Hopkins University Bloomberg School of Public Health. © 2005 The Johns Hopkins University. All rights reserved.

Suspecting that a defect in antioxidant response exacerbates asthma severity, the team of researchers began looking into the genetic factors that might contribute to this deficiency. In 2002, Biswal's lab discovered *Nrf2* acts as a master regulator of the majority of antioxidant pathways and detoxifying enzymes for environmental pollutants. This led researchers to consider the role of *Nrf2* in lung inflammatory diseases caused by exposure to allergens. They found that the absence of the *Nrf2* gene increased migration of inflammatory cells into the airways and caused an enhanced asthmatic response in mice. "*Nrf2* is critical for proper response to allergens in lungs and maintenance of a balance between ROS production. Antioxidant capability regulated by *Nrf2* may be a major determinant of susceptibility to allergen-mediated asthma," says Biswal. "*Nrf2* regulated pathways seem to intervene inflammation at several points."

The findings provide a better understanding of the human body's defense mechanisms to stress, which may hold clues to better control the inflammation process and improve control over asthma and its symptoms. Study coauthor Tirumalai Rangasamy, PhD said that the next step for researchers will be to look for molecular mechanisms of regulation of asthmatic inflammation by *Nrf2* and determine if there are alterations in the response of *Nrf2* gene in asthma-prone humans. Future studies will determine the therapeutic potential of targeting *Nrf2* for treatment of asthma.

"Disruption of *Nrf2* enhances susceptibility to severe airway inflammation and asthma in mice" was written by Tirumalai Rangasamy, Jia Guo, Wayne A. Mitzner, Jessica Roman, Anju Singh, Allison D. Fryer, Masayuki Yamamoto, Thomas W. Kensler, Rubin M. Tuder, Steve N. Georas, and Shyam Biswal.

Chapter 72

Discovery of Gene Clusters Could Lead to New Asthma Treatment Based on Genetic Profiles

Children who suffer from acute asthma attacks share a genetic profile that appears to be unique to these children, according to a new study by researchers at Cincinnati Children's Hospital Medical Center. The discovery opens the door to the possibility of designing treatments specifically tailored to children who suffer from the severest forms of asthma. The findings appear in the February 10, 2005 issue of the *Journal of Allergy and Clinical Immunology*.

The study is based on an Affymetrix "GeneChip" analysis of RNA (ribonucleic acid) isolated from the nasal epithelium of children who have an acute case of asthma or asthma stabilized with medication. The analysis revealed two distinct gene expression profiles in these groups of children, according to Gurjit K. Khurana Hershey, MD, PhD, director of the Center for Translational Research in Asthma and Allergy at Cincinnati Children's and senior author of the study.

"We found that children who were having an acute asthma attack had a gene expression profile that was clearly different from those seen in someone with stable (controlled) asthma. The amazing thing was that the gene expression profiles were consistent across patients, despite the likely differences with respect to the cause of asthma," she said.

"Asthma Gene Clusters Identified," a Pediatric Health News Release. This information is reprinted with permission from the Cincinnati Children's Hospital Medical Center website, http://www.cincinnatichildrens.org. © 2005 Cincinnati Children's Hospital Medical Center. All rights reserved.

Asthma is the most common chronic disease of childhood affecting 20 million Americans, according the Centers for Disease Control and Prevention (CDC). Experts know that environmental factors can lead to asthmatic conditions in children, but they also know that genetics contributes to susceptibility. There are no cures for asthma, but it can be controlled with treatment.

To date, researchers have identified individual genes involved in asthma, but this is the first time that clusters of known genes have been identified as being activated in acute forms of childhood asthma.

Dr. Hershey said the findings open the door to the possibility of developing treatments based on the unique genetic profile of patients. For example, specific therapies for acute asthma could be targeted to genes that are seen in acute, but not stable, asthma. Also, in addition to differentiating between an acute and stable asthma attack, the genetic profile may be useful in identifying an imminent asthma attack.

Researchers examined 54,675 genes. They discovered eight gene clusters in all, consisting of 161 genes. At least one cluster was identified that was comprised of genes active in acute asthma, but not stable asthma. They also identified gene clusters that were active in stable asthma, but not the acute form of the disease.

"Now that we know what genes are turned on during an asthma attack, we will conduct studies to see if this genetic profile can be used to customize care. The current methods of treatment primarily consist of anti-inflammatory drugs, which may not be optimal for acute attacks," Dr. Hershey said.

Previous studies using microarray technology have been conducted using RNA from adults with asthma, but this approach has not been successfully used in human studies involving children with asthma. In pediatrics, it is difficult to obtain tissue in sufficient quantities for analysis, especially during an asthma attack. But because asthma begins in childhood, the genes identified in adults may not reflect genes involved in childhood asthma, she said.

This study exclusively focused on genes associated with epithelial cells. Genes associated with mucosa and underlying cells are likely to be involved as well.

Dr. Hershey is expanding her research in cooperation with the Computational Medicine Center (CMC), a research partnership with Cincinnati Children's and the University of Cincinnati College of Medicine. The center specializes in combining computational resources with medicine and genetics in order to customize care for patients based on the patient's individual genetic makeup.

Discovery of Gene Clusters Could Lead to New Asthma Treatment

"Dr. Hershey's research is a good example of research that we believe will benefit patients, based on the use of novel algorithms and analysis from computational medicine. In this study, we show that asthma is controlled by two different genetic profiles. Now, in computational medicine, we will combine all of our clinical knowledge of disease with information from genetic and genomic data analyses. This, in turn, will lead to customized care based on a patient's personal needs," according to Bruce Aronow, PhD, co-director of the CMC and co-author of the study.

"Our ultimate goal is to provide physicians the data they need to prescribe the most effective medications, discover new therapies, and to help prevent disease," he said.

Ultimately, Dr. Hershey's goal would be to identify gene profiles that are expressed during asthma that are exacerbated by different factors, such as exercise, viral infection or allergic triggers. In doing so, physicians will be in a better position to assess and treat a patient's asthma with greater precision.

"As we learn more about disease and how patients respond to treatment, we will eventually be able to develop customized therapy for patients with different gene expression profiles," she said.

Chapter 73

Do Hormonal Cycles Affect Asthma?

We all know that estrogen and progesterone are critical players in a woman's reproductive process. But could these hormones also improve her breathing? According to a recent report published in the March 2004 issue of *Annals of Allergy, Asthma & Immunology*, there is strong evidence that estrogen and progesterone may actually improve lung function and asthma. Conversely, during periods when hormonal levels are lower than average—menstruation and menopause—women with asthma may be at increased risk of asthma attacks.

Below, the report's author, Dr. Catherine L. Haggerty of the University of Pittsburgh, Graduate School of Public Health, offers an explanation for these findings and talks about how this information might help women identify high-risk times for asthma attacks.

Can you describe first the basic premise of your report? What are the effects of hormones on respiratory function?

The report looked at the association between estrogen and progesterone and pulmonary function, and asthma among women.

The data suggests that both estrogen and progesterone may be involved in improving pulmonary function and asthma. So in younger

---

"Do Hormonal Cycles Affect Asthma?" by Erica Heilman, © 2004 Healthology, Inc. All rights reserved. Additional information is available at www.healthology.com.

women, during the premenstrual and menstrual phases when these hormone levels are lower, asthmatics have been found to experience an increase in asthma attacks, increased hospitalization, decreased pulmonary function, and maybe an increased need for medications such as bronchodilators to treat their asthma systems.

Oral contraceptives, which really dampen and smooth out these fluctuations in hormone levels, have been found to improve pulmonary function in some women as well.

Reports of lung function during pregnancy were a bit more mixed. About a third of pregnant women report that their asthma improves during pregnancy. Another third report no change, and the final third report that it actually worsens. But there are other factors that may be affecting pulmonary function in pregnant women such as increase in gastroesophageal reflux and increase in intra-abdominal pressure and all of these things also affect lung function. So it may be that even if estrogen and progesterone have a positive effect, pulmonary function is affected by so many things in pregnancy that that might be the reason for the differences among women.

There is not as much data on menopausal women. I've done some studies on hormone replacement therapy in menopausal women and found that women who take hormone replacement therapy have better pulmonary function and less pulmonary obstruction than women who do not take hormone replacement therapy even after accounting for other factors that may be associated with pulmonary function such as smoking. So even after taking smoking into account, HRT is still associated with better pulmonary function.

Do we know why estrogen and progesterone may improve lung function?

Asthma is characterized by inflammation and narrowing of the airways. This inflammation may occur as a result of a hyperimmunity. So the immune system might be overly revved up. Progesterone has been shown to suppress the immune system and so in that sense it's protective or helpful. It may reduce the increased inflammation that's occurring.

Additionally, both progesterone and estrogen have been found to reduce constriction of the airways and relax the bronchial smooth muscle in the airways. Progesterone is responsible for relaxing uterine smooth muscle—that's its natural function, and it's been found to impart these effects throughout the whole body—so it also works to relax the muscles in the airways.

Do Hormonal Cycles Affect Asthma?

Who may experience worsening asthma symptoms?

Premenstrual women may notice a worsening of asthma symptoms just before and during the menstrual cycle. This is the time when estrogen and progesterone are at their lowest levels, and it's also the time at which they really drop. So certainly women could see if they notice a pattern in asthma related to the menstrual cycle. This could be something they could discuss with their doctor at that time.

Another time to look for changes would be as women move through and into the menopausal period because at this time estrogen and progesterone also rapidly decline.

What is the percentage of women with asthma who have worsening symptoms during their periods?

The majority of the data suggests about a third of the women, but the range is really about a third to a half of women who are specifically asked if they experience worsening of asthma.

Why is this relationship between lung function and hormones important?

Understanding that in a subset of women, asthma may worsen during times of low hormonal levels, we may be able to better predict who is at risk for more frequent asthma attacks, and when. In some women there may be treatment suggestions that could be made based on this information. I don't think at this time we could make any recommendations. But if women discuss these patterns with their doctor, they may find benefit from using oral contraceptives to smooth out the fluctuations in hormonal levels. And there may be therapeutic strategies that could be developed in the future, which takes advantage of this relationship.

Chapter 74

Are All Aerosol Therapy Devices Equally Effective?

New evidence-based guidelines for the selection of aerosol medication devices conclude that health-care providers should avoid basing device selection exclusively on device efficacy. Instead, the choice should be based on other patient-related factors. All aerosolized medication delivery systems are equally effective when used properly. Aerosolized medication is typically used to treat patients with respiratory conditions, such as asthma or chronic obstructive pulmonary disease (COPD).

For the first time, the American College of Chest Physicians (ACCP) and the American College of Allergy, Asthma, and Immunology (ACAAI) have developed joint evidence-based guidelines for the selection of aerosol delivery devices. Published in the January 2005 issue of *CHEST*, the peer-reviewed journal of the ACCP, the guidelines were developed by an international panel of pulmonary experts and provide recommendations on overall device selection and device selection for several commonly encountered clinical settings.

Based on a systematic review of pertinent randomized, controlled trials (RCT), panel members compared metered-dose inhalers (MDIs)

"New Guidelines Conclude All Aerosol Therapy Devices Equally Effective," from the American College of Chest Physician's website (www.chest.org). Reprinted with permission from the American College of Chest Physicians, © 2005. Additional information about asthma and lung health is available in the American College of Chest Physicians patient education guides, online at http://www.chestnet.org/patients/guides/.

with or without spacers/holding chambers, dry powder inhalers, and nebulizers, delivering both bronchodilators (beta2-agonists) and inhaled corticosteroids in order to determine the best recommendations for device selection. To achieve a fair comparison, RCTs were selected only if the same drug was used in the different delivery systems tested. Due to the limited number of published RCTs of inhaled corticosteroids, the majority of the studies reviewed and selected were RCTs of bronchodilators. Overall, guidelines state that aerosolized medication delivery systems, when used with comparable drug doses, provide equivalent efficacy and, therefore, recommend that health-care providers not base device selection exclusively on device efficacy but rather on several criteria, including device availability; cost; convenience; and the patient's age, competence in using the device, and preference.

"The current practice of device selection for the delivery of aerosolized asthma or COPD medication is largely based on the device's effectiveness in delivering the medication to the patient. Although there are advantages and disadvantages associated with each device and medication, when used properly, all aerosol devices can work equally well and can be interchanged," said guidelines chair Myrna B. Dolovich, P.Eng., Associate Clinical Professor Medicine and Radiology, McMaster University, Hamilton, Ontario, Canada. "Health-care providers should choose a device based on the individual characteristics of each patient. If asthma control is not achieved using one delivery device, it may be beneficial for patients to switch to another device after consulting with his or her provider."

Guidelines also incorporate recommendations for device selection in specific clinical settings, including the emergency department, ICU (intensive care unit), and inpatient and outpatient situations. Specific recommendations include the following:

- **Inpatient setting:** Nebulizers and MDIs with spacer/holding chambers are appropriate for use in the inpatient setting.

- **Emergency department setting:** Nebulizers and MDIs with spacer/holding chambers are appropriate for delivery of beta2-agonists in the emergency department.

- **Patients supported by mechanical ventilation:** Careful attention to details of the technique employed for administering medications by MDI or nebulizer to mechanically ventilated patients is critical, since multiple technical factors may have clinically important effects on the efficiency of aerosol delivery.

Are All Aerosol Therapy Devices Equally Effective?

Panel members also strongly recommend that clinicians provide patients with sufficient instruction on the use of their aerosol inhaler in order to maximize asthma control.

"Many health-care providers are confused by the large number of aerosol delivery devices available and have difficulty explaining their correct use to patients," said Professor Dolovich. "Physicians, respiratory therapists, and nurses caring for patients with respiratory diseases should be familiar with issues related to performance and correct use of aerosol delivery devices in order to instruct their patients on proper usage."

"Evidence-based guidelines are based on a comprehensive review of clinical research findings, allowing medical professionals to make the most effective and patient-focused decisions on the diagnosis and treatment of diseases," said Paul A. Kvale, M.D., FCCP, President of the American College of Chest Physicians. "The new evidence-based guidelines for aerosol therapy integrate individual clinical expertise with the best available evidence on respiratory medication and delivery devices. Ultimately, by following these evidence-based guidelines, clinicians will have a more current and consistent approach to selecting aerosol therapy for patients."

"Use of inhaled aerosols has revolutionized the care of obstructive respiratory disease by allowing the selective delivery of optimal concentrations of drugs to the airway without creating the undesirable side effects that might result from systemic administration," said Myron J. Zitt, M.D., President of the American College of Allergy, Asthma and Immunology. "Nonetheless, the caregiver is in a quandary as to which aerosol delivery system is best for his or her patient. The new evidence-based guidelines provide additional criteria for device selection. Regardless of what delivery system is chosen, patient education is essential to assure optimal outcomes."

Chapter 75

Inhaled Steroids and the Risk of Glaucoma

Inhaled Steroids and Asthma

Inhaled steroids are now considered the cornerstone of asthma treatment. The National Institutes of Health released its updated version of the *Expert Panel Report on the Guidelines for the Diagnosis and Treatment of Asthma* in February 1997. This report strongly supports the use of inhaled steroids to reduce and prevent asthma symptoms in people with moderate to severe asthma.

Adverse Side Effects from Inhaled Steroids

The use of high-dose inhaled steroids has reduced the need for long-term oral steroids in many asthma patients. Doctors have known for many years that long-term use of oral steroids (available in tablet or liquid form) has been associated with a greater risk for glaucoma, cataracts, and other side effects, and they regularly monitor for these adverse effects. Because inhaled steroids are given in small doses directly to the airways and are much less available to the rest of the body, they have a much lower risk for systemic side effects than oral steroids. There are a number of preparations available in different strengths that can be prescribed in a range of low to high doses.

© Copyright 2005 National Jewish Medical and Research Center. All rights reserved. For additional information, visit http://asthma.nationaljewish.org/ or call 1-800-222 LUNG.

At this time, there is only limited information on adverse side effects from inhaled steroids, especially with higher doses. However, as with any medicine, there is a concern for the potential of adverse effects. Physicians should identify patients who have a greater risk for side effects and use the lowest dose of medicine needed to control the disease. In addition, a number of asthma medicines are available which may be used to reduce the need for high dose inhaled steroids for many patients.

The Risk of Glaucoma with Inhaled Steroids

There has been a recent report raising concerns about the use of high-dose inhaled steroids and an increased risk of developing ocular hypertension or glaucoma. Ocular hypertension is high pressure within the eye that can possibly result in partial or complete loss of vision. A recent study reviewed patients over 65 years of age who were referred to an eye specialist and included patients who were taking various doses of inhaled steroids, including higher than recommended doses. A high dose inhaled steroid was defined as a daily dose exceeding 1500 mcg per day. This is calculated by taking the dose per inhalation for the specific inhaled steroid and multiplying that by the number of inhalations a person takes per day.

The study showed that patients who were on high-dose inhaled steroids for longer than three months had a higher risk for developing glaucoma. This study points out that caution should be used with long-term use of high-dose inhaled steroids in elderly patients. It is important to note, however, that the risk for glaucoma overall increases with age due to the aging process. The study implies that high-dose inhaled steroids should be used cautiously in patients who already have glaucoma. It is reassuring that this study noted that people who were taking low to moderate doses of inhaled steroids were not at greater risk for glaucoma.

It is important to remember that many people require routine inhaled and occasional oral steroids to control their asthma. Good asthma control is crucial and inhaled steroids play a major role in asthma management. If you are taking a high dose of an inhaled steroid for more than three months, you may benefit by receiving care from or consulting an asthma specialist. An asthma specialist is experienced with the current asthma medicines, how to adjust the dose of these medicines for their best effect and when to monitor for side effects.

Chapter 76

Studying Ways to Improve Asthma Treatment Outcomes

Summary

Asthma, among the most common of chronic diseases, is difficult to manage. Despite dramatic advances in prevention, diagnosis, and clinical treatments, the incidence of the disease has increased significantly in recent years and vast numbers of asthma patients—including a disproportionate number of children—do not receive adequate care to control their disease. As a result, much of the $12.7 billion in annual costs for asthma is spent for expensive emergency care, hospitalizations, and time lost from work—most of which could be avoided.

As asthma specialists, allergists have consistently shown that they can provide effective, economical asthma management.

Scope of the Asthma Epidemic

Asthma is a chronic inflammation of the lung's airways characterized by a chronic cough, shortness of breath, or wheezing. In severe cases the airways contract and the patient cannot get enough air into the lungs. An estimated 17 million Americans, or about 6.4 percent

---

Excerpted from "Asthma Management and the Allergist: Better Outcomes at Lower Cost," edited by Stanley M. Fineman, MD, MBA, and William E. Berger, MD, MBA; © 2002 American College of Allergy, Asthma and Immunology; reprinted with permission. The full text of this document, including references and abstracts of outcome and cost studies, is available online at http://www.acaai.org/NR/rdonlyres/94456F99-4FAC-4CAA-A405-A79EF5F4BC6C/0/BlueBook.pdf.

of the population, have asthma. About 5 million of those affected by the disease are children, and a disproportionate number of the 5,000 people who die of asthma each year are under the age of 18.

Curbing the asthma epidemic, preventing needless suffering and premature deaths, and controlling the runaway costs of treating the disease are top priorities of the nation's health care policy makers and the nation's allergists.

Impact of Asthma

The most recent surveillance survey conducted by the Centers for Disease Control and Prevention (CDC) reports that 26.7 million Americans have been diagnosed by a physician as having asthma at some time in their lives. Of these, 14.6 million said they had asthma or asthma-like symptoms in the year prior to the survey. African Americans are slightly more likely than Caucasians to have asthma, yet the death rate among blacks is nearly three times as high as among whites.

Annually, asthma accounts for approximately:

- 10.8 million physician or outpatient visits;
- 478,000 hospitalizations;
- 2 million emergency room visits; and
- 28 million missed school and work days.

According to the National Institute of Allergy and Infectious Diseases (NIAID), asthma deaths have increased steadily since the 1970s, when asthma accounted for 8.2 deaths per 100,000 population. By 1995, the rate had jumped to nearly 18 deaths per 100,000.

The economic impact of asthma also is substantial. Direct health care expenditures such as physician visits, hospital, and emergency room services, medications and other interventions are estimated to be $7.4 billion. About $3.2 billion of those direct costs are spent on asthma care for children and adolescents under the age of 18. Indirect costs such as decreased worker productivity and days lost from work by adults who have asthma or care for children with asthma, and other losses are an estimated $5.3 billion.

Asthma Treatment Outcomes

With their years of specialty training and clinical experience in asthma management, allergists are more likely than other physicians to know and follow the state-of-the-art treatments that improve outcomes and reduce costs and adhere to practice guidelines that experts agree are the standard of care. This training and expertise also make allergists the experts in identifying offending allergy triggers and educating patients on avoidance tactics—essentials to the proper treatment of the disease since the majority of asthma is allergic asthma.

Numerous clinical studies have concluded that specialists are more likely than non-specialists to manage asthma based on the latest clinical study findings, to identify and institute procedures to reduce allergy triggers for the disease, and to follow consensus guidelines developed by experts in the field. It is well documented that asthma

Table 76.1. Cost of Asthma Care

Direct medical expenditures	Costs in $M
Hospital care	
Hospital inpatient care	$2,054.6
Hospital emergency care	546.3
Hospital outpatient care	722.6
Physician's services	
Physician inpatient care	110.9
Physician office visits	742.7
Prescriptions	3,188.1
All direct expenditures	**$7,365.3**
Indirect costs	
School days lost	$1,107.3
Loss of work (outside employment)	
Men	415.0
Women	1,128.2
Housekeeping	841.7
Mortality	1,813.9
All indirect costs	**$5,306.0**
All costs	**$12,671.3**

Source: Weiss and Sullivan. *J Allergy Clin Immunol* 2001.

care delivered under the supervision of an allergist results in improved outcomes and more effective use of health care resources.

Allergists were instrumental in developing the National Institutes of Health (NIH) Guidelines and other best practice recommendations for the management of asthma. Epidemiologists and clinicians who specialize in allergy and immunology are leaders in clinical research and education to improve understanding of complex disease processes, risk factors, genetic and environmental factors, and the pathophysiologic and immunologic characteristics of different subsets of asthma.

Because of these benefits, many patients, physicians and other providers, as well as many managed care organizations strive to involve allergists in asthma care. When managed aggressively by a specialist, asthma need not be a life-threatening or disabling disease. In most patients, the condition can be controlled so that acute asthma attacks are avoided.

Hospitalizations

In one clinical study, hospital admissions decreased 67 percent and the average length of hospital stay declined 38 percent, from 4 days to 2.5 days, for patients with moderate-to-severe asthma after they were seen by an allergist. In another study, care coordinated through an asthma center by a multispecialty team of experts resulted in an 89 percent decrease in hospital admissions.

Among children studied in East Harlem in New York City, where the asthma mortality and morbidity rates are among the highest in the nation, patients who were not under the care of an allergist in an outpatient intervention program had 2.5 times more hospitalizations than children being cared for by specialists. Another study of patients who required intubation for asthma found that an aggressive program of education, regular outpatient visits with specialists, and access to an emergency call service significantly reduced the number of inpatient hospitalizations.

A similar study of adults with moderate-to-severe asthma documented a 77 percent reduction in hospitalizations in the 12 months after the patients completed a course of outpatient treatment in a comprehensive asthma care center, compared to the rates of hospitalization in the six months prior to starting the program.

Emergency Department Visits

Despite the availability of new therapies and medications that can prevent acute asthma episodes, many patients still require emergency health services to treat uncontrolled exacerbations of the disease. Clinical studies document that emergency department (ED) visits for asthma can be the result of poor disease management. Patients who are cared for by asthma specialists invariably require fewer ED visits. A study of a Kaiser Health Plan in San Diego compared treatment outcomes for patients who came to the ED with acute asthma symptoms. Patients who were referred to specialists experienced 50 percent fewer relapses requiring an ED visit than patients who continued to be treated by a primary care physician.

In one study of individuals with severe asthma, the average annual number of ED visits was 3.45 for each patient enrolled in a specialty allergy clinic, compared to 6.1 visits for patients who were not enrolled. In another study, a 76 percent reduction in ED visits followed comprehensive treatment in a specialty allergy center.

Sick Care Office Visits

Annually in America, about 11 million physician office and outpatient clinic visits are for the treatment of asthma. Supervision of care by an allergist can reduce the number of sick care office visits for asthma patients. A study of patients with moderate-to-severe asthma in a Kaiser Permanente health plan in Denver, for example, found sick care office visits were reduced by 45 percent in patients who received follow-up care by an allergist for at least one year.

Missed Days from Work or School

Aggressive management of asthma by an allergist also can reduce the number of work and school days missed because of asthma, a loss that has an estimated value of $2.6 billion annually. One center reported that its adult patients averaged an estimated 80 percent reduction in missed work days, and children required approximately 65 percent fewer days off from school after receiving care in a multidisciplinary asthma center.

In another study, an asthma management program combined with subspecialty care in the treatment of 50 patients with asthma reduced missed days from work or school from 310 to 73.

Patient Satisfaction and Quality of Life

Patients who receive asthma care from an allergist experience improved emotional and physical well being, and they also are more satisfied with their physician and with the quality of their general medical care.

In a survey of nearly 400 patients treated in a large health maintenance organization, significant quality-of-life improvements were reported by patients treated by allergists, compared to those treated by generalists or in the emergency department. Improvements were seen in the areas of physical functioning, emotion, pain relief, and general health.

In a suburban private practice, patients were surveyed after the initiation of an asthma management program that followed the NIH Guidelines and was supervised by an asthma specialist. The patients reported significant improvements in their ability to participate in activities, their emotional well being, and in the control of asthma symptoms.

Despite all this, some health care plans still today place obstacles in front of patients seeking referral to an asthma specialist, even when referral to a specialist is recommended in the NIH Guidelines and other national consensus recommendations. The result is conservative or sporadic treatment that may cause disease progression, airway remodeling, and permanent damage to the lungs. It also is more likely to increase hospitalizations, emergency room visits and other high-priced interventions, and add to the number of days missed from work or school.

Asthma Treatment Costs

Numerous studies have shown that aggressive management and treatment of asthma by an allergist not only produces better health outcomes, but also can reduce the total costs of the disease. One large, urban specialty asthma center, for example, estimates that specialty care reduces insurance claims for asthma-related services by at least 45 percent to as much as 80 percent.

Former Surgeon General David Satcher has decried the alarming increase in costs. "Families and communities are paying more to treat asthma, while at the same time more people are dying from it," he said.

In a study sponsored by the Asthma and Allergy Foundation of America, a 54 percent increase in the cost of asthma care was documented between 1985 and 1994 while, at the same time, deaths from the disease rose by 41 percent. The increased costs reflect a steep rise in medication costs, yet nine out of 10 prescriptions were for "rescue" medications to manage severe asthma attacks, rather than for inhaled steroids used to prevent such attacks. The study's authors concluded that the results indicated that many patients were not being treated according to established guidelines.

Even when asthma patients attend frequent clinic programs offering intensive specialty services, costs are saved in the long-term by reducing the number of emergency department visits and other acute care interventions. In one center, a savings of $137 per patient per year was realized among patients who made frequent, regular visits to a comprehensive allergy clinic, compared to patients who went less frequently to an emergency room for treatment of acute asthma symptoms. Other research has documented that the services in specialty clinics result in a higher quality of care, including strategies to help patients control their disease and reduce the incidence of acute symptoms that require hospitalization or emergency room services.

Failure to control asthma has a particularly high price: estimates are that more than 80 percent of all resources expended for asthma treatment is used by 20 percent of patients whose disease is not adequately controlled. A study of more than 2,000 asthma patients participating in one managed care plan found that patients evaluated and followed by allergists required less utilization of resources for acute, uncontrolled disease than patients who are never seen by an allergist, or those seen but not actively followed.

Hospitalizations

Asthma is responsible for 478,000 hospital admissions annually, which cost an estimated $2 billion. Patients under the care of allergists are hospitalized less often for asthma symptoms and have shorter lengths of stay, which can lower the cost of inpatient asthma care dramatically.

In a retrospective study of 70 patients with moderate-to-severe asthma, decreased hospitalizations following evaluation by an allergist contributed to an overall savings of $145,500, or $2,100 per patient. In another study of patients requiring intubation for asthma, enrollment in an intervention program supervised by asthma specialists saw per-patient hospital costs reduced 95 percent from $40,253 to $1,926.

Yet another study of 125 patients showed that the number of hospitalizations decreased from 38 to 4, and the costs of inpatient care dropped from $192,926 to $20,308, after the patients were enrolled in a specialty allergy clinic.

Emergency Department Visits

The cost of emergency department visits for asthma is estimated to be $546 million annually. In a study of 207 asthma patients treated by specialists at one midwest asthma center, reductions in hospitalizations and emergency department visits were substantial, representing an annual cost savings of $2,714 per patient—more than $560,000.

Another study reported a fall in emergency department visits from 74 to 17, and cost reductions of $34,706 to $7,973, for 125 patients after they enrolled in a specialty asthma clinic.

Indirect Costs

Lost school days for children and days missed from work for adults with asthma, or those who must stay home to care for children with asthma, are estimated to cost more than $2.6 billion annually. Asthma is a leading cause of missed school days among children, causing an estimated 10 million absences each year. In one survey of adults with asthma prior to enrollment in an asthma management program, a total of 194 days missed from work were reported by 78 patients. Care by an allergist or other asthma specialist has been shown to reduce lost days from work or school by 80 percent or more.

How Allergists Achieve Cost-Effective Outcomes

Asthma patients receive added value when care is managed by an allergist. Specialty training, knowledge, and experience enable the allergist to perform the following services:

- accurately diagnose the disease, its types, subtypes, and severity
- identify the external factors, including allergens that trigger an asthma attack, and provide counseling on how to avoid those triggers
- administer immunotherapy or "allergy shots" for allergic asthma to reduce sensitivity to allergy triggers
- use current best practices to develop and implement an aggressive treatment plan that is tailored specifically to the needs of individual asthma patients
- maintain disease control through detailed, multi-faceted treatment plans that include prevention, aggressive use of appropriate medications and other interventions to prevent asthma symptoms, ongoing patient education, and self-care strategies managed by the patient

Aggressive Asthma Management: The New Standard of Care

Until 1991, it was the consensus of physicians that asthma therapy should be conservative and medications introduced one at a time, with dosage increases only when the condition worsened. Contrasted to this are the latest evidence-based guidelines stipulating that asthma should be diagnosed as early as possible and treated aggressively while it is still mild. Otherwise it may worsen and cause permanent scarring and irreversible remodeling of the lungs' airways.

The disease should be treated with multiple medications, if necessary, to control symptoms as soon as they appear. Allergists, with their extensive experience using these medications, are able to prescribe them properly for the individual patient. Aggressive therapy should be initiated at the onset to establish immediate control of symptoms; it then may be stepped down as the patient's condition improves. An allergy history, physical exam, and skin tests may be needed to identify factors triggering asthma exacerbations. Although the cost of the initial therapy may be high, it is outweighed by significant long-term health benefits and cost savings.

A study of medical treatments for 1,574 patients enrolled in a managed care plan found that the best managers of asthma are specialists who tend to be very aggressive in ordering tests and deploy the most resources in terms of office time and medical procedures. The study found that the costs of care were about the same or less than the care given by non-specialists, and outcomes and disease control were significantly improved for the patients treated by specialists.

New Perspectives on Asthma

As more is learned about asthma, researchers are discovering that the disease is far more complex than previously thought and consists of several subtypes, such as allergic asthma, exercise-induced asthma, asthma related to bacterial or fungal infections, and asthma in the elderly. Each type can have different symptoms or triggers, and each requires a different approach to diagnosis and treatment. Allergists, with extensive experience treating all forms of asthma, understand its complexities and know that it is essential to distinguish among different types. They can assess the severity of each case and develop case-specific treatment plans that have the greatest likelihood of success with individual patients.

Growing Consensus for Specialty Care of Asthma

As asthma management becomes more sophisticated, health care plans are seeking a competitive edge through programs that optimize patient health education, prevention, and aggressive up-front treatment to avoid severe flare-ups of any chronic disease. Programs that reduce participant turnover and enable managed care organizations to provide life-long services are most successful at satisfying patients and reducing costs.

Managed care organizations have an added motivation to optimize asthma management now that the National Committee for Quality Assurance has made the appropriate use of asthma medications a key indicator of managed care quality. Primary care physicians also are demanding a greater say in selecting appropriate treatments and in referring patients to specialists when the disease is severe, atypical, or requires specialized knowledge for optimum management.

The Emerging Role of New Treatments and Preventions

Recent studies have focused on identifying risk factors that contribute to asthma or to the severity of the disease, as well as new approaches to treating or preventing asthma and its symptoms. Here are some examples:

- The majority of people who have asthma have allergic asthma, and the role that allergies play in the disease is gaining ever more attention. The first national Cooperative Inner-City Asthma Study, sponsored by NIAID, identified exposure to cockroaches and cockroach allergy as a major influence of the severity of asthma in inner-city children ages 4 to 11.

- Allergists promote asthma self-management skills to assist people in eliminating or decreasing exposure to asthma "triggers."

- Specialists are more likely than generalists to follow established clinical care guidelines and can provide the most authoritative information to health care providers, families, and other caregivers to optimize prevention and treatment strategies and decrease asthma severity.

- A growing body of clinical research shows that immunotherapy, or "allergy shots," often reduces patients' sensitivity to the allergens that trigger asthma attacks and significantly reduces the severity of the disease.

- Allergists are involved in clinical trials to test other promising techniques, such as the use of monoclonal antibodies to inhibit

Studying Ways to Improve Asthma Treatment Outcomes

the inflammatory process that leads to asthma. Consequently they usually are the first clinicians to become aware of and implement proven new treatments.

When to Refer to an Allergist

The NIH expert panel report recommends that asthma patients be referred to a specialist when they experience following conditions:

- have difficulty achieving or maintaining control of their condition
- have had a life-threatening asthma attack
- are not meeting the goals of asthma therapy after three to six months of treatment or are not responding to current therapy
- have symptoms that are unusual or difficult to diagnose
- have other conditions such as severe hay fever or sinusitis that complicate their asthma or its correct diagnosis
- need additional diagnostic tests to determine the severity of their asthma and what causes its symptoms
- require additional education or guidance in managing any complications of therapy, adhering to their treatment plan, or avoiding asthma triggers
- are candidates for immunotherapy
- have severe, persistent asthma
- require continuous oral high-dose inhaled corticosteroid therapy or have taken more than two bursts of oral corticosteroids in one year

The guidelines also recommend that children under the age of 3 with moderate or severe asthma and children beginning daily, long-term therapy should see an asthma specialist.

The NIH Guidelines for referral to an asthma specialist are in general accord with guidelines developed by the American College of Allergy, Asthma and Immunology (ACAAI), the American Academy of Allergy, Asthma and Immunology (AAAAI) and the Joint Council of Allergy, Asthma and Immunology (JCAAI), and are endorsed by the Allergy-Immunology Subsection of the American Academy of Pediatrics (AAP).

The guidelines of these professional medical societies for the specialty of allergy, asthma, and immunology further state that referral to a specialist is indicated when the following conditions apply:

- the patient's asthma is unstable, or the response to therapy is limited, incomplete or very slow, and poor symptom control interferes with the patient's quality of life
- identification of allergens or other environmental factors which may be triggering the patient's disease is required
- co-existing illnesses or their treatments complicate the management of asthma
- the diagnosis of asthma is in doubt
- there is concern about side effects that have occurred or may occur with asthma medications
- the patient asks for a consultation

Conclusion

A substantial and growing body of published clinical data and other research demonstrate significant discrepancies in outcomes between asthma care that is managed by generalists without specialty training in the complexities of asthma, and disease management under the direction of an allergist who can add significant value to patient care.

An evidence-based review of the literature provides convincing documentation that aggressive management of asthma by a specialist improves outcomes for patients, lowers overall treatment costs for payers, and reduces the indirect costs to society. Specialty care results in fewer hospitalizations and other emergency interventions, fewer missed days from work or school, and significantly enhanced health and quality of life for those who suffer from asthma.

As more is learned about the mechanisms of asthma and new therapies are developed to control the severity and progress of the disease, the allergist will continue to play an important role in improving the health outcomes for patients with asthma.

Chapter 77

Studying the Long-Term Effects of Asthma Therapy

Introduction

Physicians today have a variety of medications to offer children with asthma, but little data documenting the long-term outcomes of any given treatment plan. This is disconcerting to both physicians and parents as they attempt to select the best course of treatment for an affected child, knowing that he/she probably faces years on medication to control the chronic inflammatory processes underlying asthma. For example, treatment with inhaled corticosteroids has been highly recommended as one option for improved control of asthma, but concerns have arisen over adverse effects in children, especially effects on growth. Short-term studies have demonstrated a decrease in growth during the first year on inhaled corticosteroids, but long-term data have been lacking. Other concerns exist as well, including the possibility of cataracts. Balanced against these concerns are the desires to reduce urgent care visits and hospitalizations, to improve or slow the decline of lung function, and to improve quality of life for both child and the family. And, while nedocromil, cromolyn, or a leukotriene inhibitor provide other choices, the same basic question of long-term risk versus benefit still exists for each of them as well.

"Long Term Effects of Asthma Therapy," by Stanley J. Szefler, © Copyright 2005 National Jewish Medical and Research Center. All rights reserved. For additional information, visit http://asthma.nationaljewish.org/ or call 1-800-222 LUNG.

The Childhood Asthma Management Program (CAMP) Study

The Childhood Asthma Management Program (CAMP) was a multicenter, randomized, double-masked clinical trial designed to answer just such questions by determining long-term effects of treatment for mild-to-moderate childhood asthma.[1] Three daily inhaled treatments were compared: (1) budesonide, a glucocorticoid, 200 µg twice daily; (2) nedocromil, a nonsteroidal anti-inflammatory, 8 mg twice daily; and (3) placebo, twice daily. All participants also used albuterol, a short-acting beta-agonist bronchodilator, as needed for symptom control.

1,041 children ages 5 through 12 were enrolled at eight centers between December 1993 and September 1995 and followed from four to six years. Follow-up visits were held two and four months after randomization and at four-month intervals until March through June 1999. The children discontinued study medications at this point and then returned two to four months later for final testing. The study results were summarized in an article in *The New England Journal of Medicine*.[2]

One of the unique features of the CAMP trial is that for the first time a study provides a comprehensive picture of the outcomes of selecting a medication, with key information about clinical impact, changes in pulmonary function, and adverse effects. Clinical indices included urgent care visits and hospitalizations, episode-free days, use of prednisone or albuterol, night-time awakenings, compliance, daily symptom score, and psychologic testing scores. Measures of pulmonary function consisted of FEV1 (forced expiratory volume in one second), FEV1/FVC (forced vital capacity), and methacholine challenge. Indicators of adverse effect comprised changes in actual and projected height; bone density, fractures, and age; development of cataract; and Tanner score.

The three treatment groups had similar baseline characteristics and the same length follow-up (mean = 4.3 years). Typically, the children were first diagnosed with asthma at age three, approximately five years prior to entering the study. Slightly more than half of each group had moderate asthma; the rest had mild asthma. During the six months prior to enrollment, they had used one or more treatment regimens: inhaled corticosteroid (36 to 41% of each study group), cromolyn or nedocromil (38 to 47%), or oral corticosteroid (30 to 39%). They had an average of only 10 symptom-free days per month, needed albuterol several times per week to treat symptoms, and recorded approximately one night-time awakening per month due to asthma. The hospitalization rates were also similar.

The CAMP study compared the results of long-term treatment with budesonide or nedocromil versus placebo. Three areas were evaluated: pulmonary function, clinical outcomes, and adverse effects.

Pulmonary Function: None of the groups demonstrated a long-term effect on FEV1 after administration of bronchodilator, possibly because an irreversible change in lung function may have already occurred in the patients prior to the study. The children had already had asthma for a mean of five years before enrollment, while some studies recommend treatment start within two to three years after onset of disease to minimize changes in lung function. However, airway responsiveness did improve in all groups, with significantly greater improvement in the budesonide-treated group. Nedocromil was similar to placebo in this category.

Clinical Outcomes: Budesonide treatment was associated with a sharp reduction in hospitalization (43% lower), urgent care visits (45% lower), and use of prednisone (43% lower) compared with placebo. Nedocromil use was similar to placebo in rate of hospitalization, although it was associated with a lower rate of urgent care visits (27%) and use of prednisone (16%). Budesonide was also associated with the most improvement in control of asthma, including fewer symptoms, less use of albuterol, more episode-free days, longer times to treatment with prednisone or other nonassigned asthma medication, and number of days on which another asthma medication was prescribed. Nedocromil treatment was similar to placebo in most of these categories, although courses of prednisone were reduced relative to placebo ($p<0.01$), but not as much as with budesonide use. Compliance was similar with budesonide and placebo, but lower in the nedocromil group ($p<0.01$).

Adverse effects: The only significant adverse effect noted was a reduction in rate of growth in the budesonide-treated group, a mean of 1.1 cm difference in height. This reduction in height occurred primarily in the first year of treatment and did not worsen with continued use of budesonide. Nedocromil was not associated with a reduction in height. Other measures, including bone age, projected final height, and Tanner stage, were similar in all three treatment groups at the end of the study. One child in the budesonide group developed a "questionable posterior subcapsular cataract." This study participant had also received beclomethasone, oral prednisone, and intranasal corticosteroids during the study.

Case Study Summary

The following case history will illustrate how this information can be applied in the clinical setting.

David is an 8-year-old male with mild persistent asthma that has been worsening. David reports problems with night-time awakenings (approximately once or twice a month) and asthma symptoms when he plays sports at school. He currently uses his albuterol inhaler almost daily (approximately 8 to 14 puffs per week). A new patient, he recently moved to the area, has had difficulty adjusting to the move, and wants to play sports again "like the other kids." His prior treatment consisted of albuterol inhaler as needed, with occasional visits to the emergency room when the inhaler did not resolve his asthma symptoms. The parents previously refused to consider any type of long-term treatment with a steroid, including inhaled corticosteroids, because they have heard that "steroids are harmful" and that they "stunt growth."

The husband recently transferred here and his wife now has a new job. They are especially concerned with David's health, but also with the constant disruption to family life, loss of sleep, and lost time on the job. His physical exam is normal except for some indications of allergic symptoms, edematous nasal passages with thin secretions, and allergic shiners. His pulmonary function was $FEV1$ 89% predicted with a reversal by 15% with 2 inhalations of albuterol. His $FEV1/FVC$ ratio was 0.83. After performing an exercise challenge in the office, his $FEV1$ decreased by 20% and there were diffuse expiratory wheezes on auscultation after he finished the challenge. This was quickly relieved with 2 inhalations of albuterol.

Questions Arising from the Case

- What options for David's treatment can you recommend to the parents?
- What results do you anticipate for the clinical outcome, pulmonary function, and risk factors for each of these?
- How should you address the parental concerns about the use of inhaled corticosteroids?

Four basic approaches can be suggested for David's treatment.

Studying the Long-Term Effects of Asthma Therapy

1: David could continue with the current treatment plan. However, his asthma is obviously not under good control. The primary reason he is not receiving additional medication is his parents' lack of knowledge about other options, including detailed information on the risks and benefits.

If David were to continue with this approach, the CAMP study results suggest the following outcomes:

- continued symptoms of respiratory distress occurring several times per week and after exercise
- possible need for a course of treatment with prednisone for more significant exacerbations
- some improvement in night-time awakenings and use of albuterol if he is closely monitored and uses the inhaler properly (that is, if his follow-up mimics that of a child enrolled in the clinical trial)
- no significant improvement in episode-days
- no improvement in FEV1
- some improvement in airway responsiveness to methacholine challenge as he grows older
- no increased risk for delayed growth or cataracts

This option offers little clinical or pulmonary improvement and does not address the parents' concerns over disruptions in the family's daily lives. In addition, it puts David at continued risk for breakthrough symptoms, difficulty with exercise, and risk for night-time episodes and emergency care visits. It does not address David's stated desire to play sports, a goal that might help him better comply with a treatment plan.

2: David could receive nedocromil, one of the drugs evaluated in the CAMP study. Nedocromil is an inhaled anti-inflammatory drug for the treatment of asthma that is not a steroid. The children in the CAMP study received 8 mg, twice daily, delivered by four 2-mg actuations of a pressurized metered-dose inhaler. After four to six years of treatment, the study group demonstrated no improvement in FEV1, but this was true for the budesonide and placebo groups as well. Airway responsiveness did improve (ratio 1.8, follow-up: baseline) but the degree of improvement was the same in the placebo group (ratio 1.9), indicating that the nedocromil was not responsible. Unfortunately, similar information about the long-term effects of cromolyn, a nonsteroidal anti-inflammatory agent like nedocromil, is not available to help determine if it is a good alternative. To ensure the most improvement in David's respiratory function, the inhaled corticosteroid budesonide should be considered in place of nedocromil.

Nedocromil treatment would probably improve two important clinical outcomes for David: urgent care visits and the need for prednisone, both of which are major parental concerns about David's illness. However, hospitalizations for asthma will not be any better than just treating symptomatically. Long-term treatment with nedocromil is also unlikely to improve other key aspects of asthma control (compared with placebo treatment), including number of symptoms, night-time awakenings, use of albuterol, number of episode-free days, and number of days on which another asthma medication is needed. This suggests that nedocromil will not satisfactorily address the parents' desire for David's successful treatment to be accompanied by a reduction in disruptions to family life. One potential complication of treatment with nedocromil is its association with reduced adherence to the treatment schedule, usually attributed to the taste of the medication. Therefore, careful monitoring of medication administration will be necessary.

Nedocromil treatment would ease the parental concerns over adverse effects of long-term medication. It is not associated with decreased growth or with other adverse effects over the four to six years of this study.

3: David could be treated with an inhaled corticosteroid such as budesonide, which was evaluated in the CAMP study. Budesonide, an inhaled corticosteroid, appears to give David the best chance for improvements in both respiratory function and clinical outcomes but does carry a risk of a small reduction in growth during the first year of treatment. (Children in the CAMP study received 400 µg budesonide daily with a breath-actuated metered-dose inhaler.) The CAMP study used FEV1 measurement after bronchodilator use as the best indicator of improved lung function and this did not improve with budesonide, nedocromil, or placebo use. Budesonide does offer David the most improvement in airway responsiveness; a three-fold increase over baseline values (significantly greater than that seen with placebo or nedocromil treatment) was noted in the CAMP study. David would likely see the most improvement in a wide variety of clinical outcome measures with budesonide as well. He could expect fewer hospitalizations or urgent care visits, factors that should assist the family's goal for reduced disruptions to daily life. He could expect better asthma control in general, with fewer symptoms, reduced use of his albuterol inhaler, more episode-free days, and less need for treatment with prednisone or other additional asthma medication.

A major concern of his parents, however, is the use of any steroid. They will need additional information explaining the distinction between use of a daily inhaled corticosteroid such as budesonide and use of a systemic drug such as prednisone. The results of the CAMP study should allay their fears about reductions in growth rate, in particular. David can expect a slight reduction in growth during the first year of treatment (approximately 1 cm) and that small change can be demonstrated to the parents with a ruler. Secondly, they should be reassured by the fact that this reduced growth velocity does not continue during subsequent years of treatment. In fact, David can expect to attain his full projected adult height. No other adverse risks were associated with long-term budesonide treatment, which will also greatly reassure the parents that this medication is safe for David to take on a daily basis.

4: David could receive another medication, such as a leukotriene blocker. While clinical studies address the general efficacy of leukotriene inhibitors, no similar data are available addressing long-term effects of four to six years of treatment. David's parents would not have their concerns about long-term safety addressed, nor could they receive valuable information about long-term results for effectiveness of this treatment option. Such information is sorely needed to help both the physician and the parents select the best treatment option for David.

Summary

The selection of the optimal treatment plan for children with mild or moderate asthma can be simplified and enhanced using the results of the CAMP study. This long-term, comprehensive picture of treatment with placebo, nedocromil, or budesonide answers many questions about predicted improvement in respiratory function, changes in clinical outcomes, and risk of adverse effects. These types of data are badly needed for other available and investigational medications as well, as physicians and parents search for the best therapeutic option.

It should be noted that the results of the CAMP study that was conducted at National Jewish Medical and Research Center as one of the eight study centers had a significant impact on the recent revisions made to the National Asthma Education and Prevention Program *Guidelines for the Diagnosis and Management of Asthma*. Largely due to the findings in this study, inhaled steroids are now recognized as the preferred medication for the management of persistent asthma in both children and adults. A detailed discussion of the rationale for this approach was recently summarized in a supplement to the *Journal of Allergy and Clinical Immunology*.[3]

References

1. The Childhood Asthma Management Program Research Group. The Childhood Asthma Management Program (CAMP): design, rationale, and methods. *Control Clin Trials* 1999; 20:91–120.

2. The Childhood Asthma Management Program Research Group. Long-term effects of budesonide or nedocromil in children with asthma. *New Engl J Med* 2000;343:1054–63.

3. National Asthma Education and Prevention Program Expert Panel Report: Guidelines for the Diagnosis and Management of Asthma Update on Selected Topics 2002, *J Allergy Clin Immunol* 110:1A-8A, S141–S219, 2002.

Part Seven

Additional Help and Information

Chapter 78

Asthma-Related Terms

airways: Common term used to describe the passages in the lungs that move air into and out of the body. Sometimes called bronchial tubes, bronchi or respiratory system.[1]

allergen: A substance which causes an allergic response in sensitive individuals. Allergens can be either natural (for example, pollen, dust) or manmade (for example, perfume, cleaning agents).[1]

allergic reaction: Response in sensitive people to specific allergens. An allergic reaction can occur in different parts of the body. Common areas include the skin, the eyes, the respiratory system, and the gastrointestinal tract. Symptoms often include itching, sneezing, runny nose, coughing, wheezing or shortness of breath.[1]

allergic rhinitis: Inflammation of the mucous membranes in the nose that is caused by an allergic reaction.[2]

Terms in this glossary were compiled from several sources which are identified by number. 1. These terms are from "Asthma Essentials: Glossary," © 2005 National Education Association Health Information Network. All Rights Reserved. Reprinted with permission. 2. These terms are excerpted from various publications of the U.S. Environmental Protection Agency (EPA). 3. These terms are from "Asthma Speaker's Kit for Health Care Professionals: Glossary," National Center for Environmental Health, Centers for Disease Control and Prevention (CDC), February 2005. 4. These terms were excerpted from "Microbes: In Sickness and in Health," National Institute of Allergy and Infectious Diseases (NIAID), July 2002. 5. These terms were excerpted from "Airborne Allergens: Something in the Air," NIAID, April 2003.

allergy/allergies: An over reaction by the body's immune system to a specific substance called an allergen. An allergy occurs only in people sensitive to a particular allergen(s).[1]

anaphylactic shock/anaphylaxis: The most severe or extreme type of allergic reaction, creating a potentially life-threatening medical emergency. Most common cause is reaction to a medication. Other causes include insect stings and foods.[1]

antibiotic: A drug used to treat some bacterial diseases.[4]

antibodies: Molecules (also called immunoglobulins) produced by a B cell in response to an antigen. When an antibody attaches to an antigen, it destroys the antigen.[4]

antigen: A substance or molecule that is recognized by the immune system. The molecule can be from a foreign material such as bacteria or viruses.[4]

asthma: A lung disease which is usually ongoing or continuous (chronic). Symptoms include wheezing, coughing, feeling of "tightness" in the chest, difficulty breathing, itching neck, throat, and ears. Symptoms vary greatly from person to person, and usually, individuals with asthma also experience "ups and downs" with symptoms. No cause or cure is yet known. Symptoms can be well managed and stabilized for most people who have asthma. Certain substances or conditions trigger asthma symptoms.[1]

asthma action plan: A document which outlines the treatment approach for an individual asthma patient; developed in consultation with the health care provider, family members, and caregivers. Effective action plans help patients control their asthma and live healthy active lives.[1]

asthma attack: See asthma episode.[1]

asthma episode: A time when asthma symptoms flare up or intensify, requiring immediate adjustments in treatment and medication to get symptoms under control. Asthma episodes may occur suddenly, with few warning signs, or build slowly over a period of hours or even days. Most asthma episodes can be handled by following the student's asthma action plan. Often called "asthma attacks," the more appropriate term is "asthma episode."[1]

Asthma-Related Terms

asthma management: A comprehensive approach to achieving and maintaining control of asthma. It includes patient education to develop a partnership in management, assessing and monitoring severity, avoiding or controlling asthma triggers, establishing plans for medication and management of exacerbations, and regular follow-up care.[3]

asthma management plan: Detailed guidelines for schools to use in working with all students and staff to manage asthma in those students who have it.[1]

atopy: The propensity, usually genetic, for developing IgE-mediated responses to common environmental allergens.[3]

B cells: Small white blood cells crucial to the immune defenses. Also known as B lymphocytes, they come from bone marrow and develop into blood cells called plasma cells, which are the source of antibodies.[4]

bacteria: Microscopic organisms composed of a single cell and lacking a defined nucleus and membrane-enclosed internal compartment.[4]

basophils: White blood cells that contribute to inflammatory reactions.[5]

bronchial tubes: The major airways of the respiratory system that carry air from the trachea (windpipe) to the microscopic air sacs (alveoli) in the lungs.[1]

bronchiole: One of the finer subdivisions of the airways, less than 1 mm in diameter, and having no cartilage in its wall.[2]

bronchitis: An infection or inflammation in the bronchial tubes caused by bacteria, a virus, an allergy or irritating dust and fumes. Typical symptoms may include coughing, wheezing, shortness of breath, chills, fever, fatigue, and excessive phlegm.[1]

bronchodilator: A medication used by many people who have asthma to relax bronchial muscles, and in turn, open up the bronchial tubes.[1]

bronchospasm; bronchoconstriction: The tightening in the airways of the respiratory system that occurs with asthma or allergies. Caused when the muscles around the bronchial tubes contract in response to specific triggers.[1]

bronchus: One of the subdivisions of the trachea serving to convey air to and from the lungs. The trachea divides into right and left main bronchi, which in turn form lobar, segmental, and subsegmental bronchi.[2]

causal factors: Risk factors that sensitize the airways and cause the onset of asthma. The most important of these factors are allergens and chemical sensitizes.[3]

chemical sensitization: Evidence suggests that some people may develop health problems characterized by effects such as dizziness, eye and throat irritation, chest tightness, and nasal congestion that appear whenever they are exposed to certain chemicals. People may react to even trace amounts of chemicals to which they have become "sensitized."[2]

chronic obstructive pulmonary disease (COPD): Refers to chronic lung disorders that result in blocked air flow in the lungs. The two main COPD disorders are emphysema and chronic bronchitis, the most common causes of respiratory failure. Emphysema occurs when the walls between the lung's air sacs become weakened and collapse. Damage from COPD is usually permanent and irreversible.[2]

contributing factors: Risk factors that either augment the likelihood of asthma developing upon exposure to them, or may even increase susceptibility to asthma. These factors including smoking, viral infections, small size at birth, and environmental pollutants.[3]

dander: Scaly or shredded dry skin that comes from animals or bird feathers. Dander may be a cause of an allergic response in susceptible persons.[1]

diesel: A petroleum-based fuel. Diesel exhaust is an important source of particulates and other pollutants that adversely affect human health.[2]

DNA (deoxyribonucleic acid): A complex molecule found in the cell nucleus which contains an organism's genetic information.[4]

dust mites: Tiny insects that are invisible to the naked eye. Every home has dust mites. They feed on human skin flakes and are found in mattresses, pillows, carpets, upholstered furniture, bedcovers, clothes, stuffed toys, and fabric and fabric-covered items. Body parts and feces from dust mites can trigger asthma in individuals with

Asthma-Related Terms

allergic reactions to dust mites, and exposure to dust mites can cause asthma in children who have not previously exhibited asthma symptoms.[2]

environmental control measures: Specific procedures undertaken to remove known allergens or irritants from a designated area.[1]

environmental tobacco smoke: Mixture of smoke exhaled by a smoker and the smoke from the burning end of the smoker's cigarette, pipe, or cigar. Also known as secondhand smoke. Environmental tobacco smoke is an important indoor air pollutant.[2]

Epi-Pen: The trade name, or manufacturer's name, for a device used to deliver epinephrine, a medication used to bring quick relief by improving breathing and heart function in life-threatening medical emergencies.[1]

exacerbation: Any worsening of asthma. Onset can be acute and sudden, or gradual over several days. A correlation between symptoms and peak flow is not necessarily found.[3]

exercise-induced asthma: Asthma symptoms which appear following strenuous exercise. Symptoms may be minimal or severe enough to require emergency treatment. About one in 10 students experience exercise-induced asthma.[1]

forced expiratory volume (FEV): Denotes the volume of gas that is exhaled in a given time interval during the execution of a forced vital capacity. Conventionally, the times used are 0.5, 0.75, or 1 sec, symbolized FEV0.5, FEV0.75, FEV1. These values are often expressed as a percent of the forced vital capacity.[2]

forced inspiratory vital capacity (FIVC): The maximal volume of air inspired with a maximally forced effort from a position of maximal expiration.[2]

forced vital capacity (FVC): Vital capacity performed with a maximally forced expiratory effort.[2]

fungi: Any of a group of parasitic lower plants that lack chlorophyll, including molds and mildews.[2]

genes: Units of genetic material (DNA) that carry the directions a cell uses to perform a specific function.[4]

ground level ozone: Ground-level ozone (smog) is formed by a chemical reaction between volatile organic pollutants (VOCs) and oxides of nitrogen (NOx) in the presence of sunlight. Ozone concentrations can reach unhealthy levels when the weather is hot and sunny with little or no wind. Ozone at the ground level causes adverse effects on lung function and other adverse respiratory effects. It is one of the six "criteria" pollutants for which the U.S. Environmental Protection Agency (EPA) has adopted National Ambient Air Quality Standards.[2]

HEPA: High efficiency particulate arrestance (filters).[2]

hidden ingredients: Some prepared food products contain derivatives or "byproducts" of other foods. These "hidden ingredients" may or may not be shown on the food label.[1]

histamine: A depressor amine derived from the amino acid histidine and found in all body tissues, with the highest concentration in the lung; a powerful stimulant of gastric secretion, a constrictor of bronchial smooth muscle, and a vasodilator that causes a fall in blood pressure.[2]

hypersensitivity diseases: Diseases characterized by allergic responses to pollutants. The hypersensitivity diseases most clearly associated with indoor air quality are asthma, rhinitis, and hypersensitivity pneumonitis. Hypersensitivity pneumonitis is a rare but serious disease that involves progressive lung damage as long as there is exposure to the causative agent.[2]

immune system: A complex network of specialized cells, tissues, and organs that defends the body against attacks by disease-causing microbes.[4]

immunoglobulin: A class of proteins produced in lymph tissue in vertebrates that function as antibodies in the immune response.[2]

indoor air pollutant: Particles and dust, fibers, mists, bioaerosols, and gases or vapors.[2]

induction of asthma: The process of lung sensitization and respiratory inflammation resulting in increased difficulty with breathing; it can be caused by a variety of external stimuli (for example, pollens, air pollutants, viruses, animal hair, mites, and roach feces).[2]

inflammation: An immune system process that stops the progression of disease-causing microbes, often seen at the site of an injury like a cut. Signs include redness, swelling, pain, and heat.[4]

Asthma-Related Terms

inhaler/metered-dose inhaler (MDI): A device used to deliver a variety of commonly prescribed asthma medications which help ease breathing by opening up the airways.[1]

integrated pest management (IPM): Procedures developed by the U.S. Environmental Protection Agency to reduce exposure to cockroaches, rats, mice, and other pests found in a school setting.[1]

irritant: Any substance which causes inflammation or an adverse reaction on the skin or in the body. An irritant may trigger asthma or allergy symptoms, but they may not be considered an allergen. Examples of irritants include tobacco smoke, chemical fumes, insecticides, or air pollution.[1]

long-term acting medication: The standard treatment of asthma for most patients who need regular, or ongoing, medicine. These kinds of medications provide "long-term relief," by acting in a preventive way to make airways less sensitive, minimizing or reducing symptoms before they even appear.[1]

lung volume (VL): Actual volume of the lung, including the volume of the conducting airways.[2]

lymphocyte: A variety of white blood cell produced in lymphoid tissues and lymphatic glands of the body. Lymphocytes have a number of very important roles in the immune system including the production of antibodies and other substances that fight infection and disease.[2]

maximal aerobic capacity (max VO2): The rate of oxygen uptake by the body during repetitive maximal respiratory effort. Synonymous with maximal oxygen consumption.[2]

maximum breathing capacity (MBC): Maximal volume of air that can be breathed per minute by a subject breathing as quickly and as deeply as possible. This tiring lung function test is usually limited to 12–20 seconds, but given in liters (BTPS)/minute. Synonymous with maximum voluntary ventilation (MVV).[2]

maximum expiratory flow (Vmax x): Forced expiratory flow, related to the total lung capacity or the actual volume of the lung at which the measurement is made. Modifiers refer to the amount of lung volume remaining when the measurement is made. For example: Vmax 75% = instantaneous forced expiratory flow when the lung is at 75% of its total capacity. Vmax 3.0 = instantaneous forced expiratory flow when the lung volume is 3.0 liters.[2]

molds: Microscopic fungi that live on plant and animal matter. Molds can be found almost anywhere; they grow on virtually any substance when moisture is present.[2]

mucociliary transport: The process by which mucus is transported, by ciliary action, from the lungs.[2]

mucus: Often called phlegm or sputum, this slippery fluid is produced by the membranes lining the airways to aid in various body functions. Exposure to certain triggers can increase mucus production for asthma patients. The increased amount of mucus makes breathing more difficult. Mucus which is not clear may indicate a infection (unrelated to asthma) in the airways.[1]

nasopharyngeal: Relating to the nose or the nasal cavity and the pharynx (throat).[2]

nebulizer: A small, portable machine used to deliver certain asthma medications. The nebulizer is plugged into an electrical outlet. A nebulizer treatment usually takes 10–15 minutes to do.[1]

nitrogen dioxide (NO_2): A chemical that results from nitric oxide combining with oxygen in the atmosphere; a major component of photochemical smog. One of the six "criteria" pollutants for which EPA has set national ambient air quality standards. Nitrogen dioxide (NO_2) can be a byproduct of fuel-burning appliances, such as gas stoves, gas or oil furnaces, fireplaces, wood stoves and unvented kerosene or gas space heaters. NO_2 is an odorless gas that can irritate your eyes, nose, and throat and cause shortness of breath. In people with asthma, exposure to low levels of NO_2 may cause increased bronchial reactivity and make young children more susceptible to respiratory infections.[2]

outdoor air pollution: Small particles and ozone from things like exhaust from cars and factories, smoke and road dust. Outdoor air pollution may worsen chronic respiratory diseases, such as asthma.[2]

ozone: A gas that is a form of oxygen. Ozone can be good if it is high in the atmosphere because it protects us from the harmful rays of the sun. Ozone is bad when it is close to the ground because it is a major air pollutant that can cause respiratory illnesses. It results from complex chemical reactions between nitrogen dioxide and volatile organic

Asthma-Related Terms

compounds; the major component of smog. Ozone at the ground level is one of the six "criteria" pollutants for which EPA has established national ambient air quality standards.[2]

particles: Fine solids such as dust, smoke, fumes, or smog, found in the air or in emissions.[2]

particulate matter: Particles in the air, such as dust, dirt, soot, smoke, and droplets. Small have significant effects on human health. Particulate matter is one of the six "criteria" pollutants for which EPA has established national ambient air quality standards.[2]

pathogen: Any virus, microorganism, or etiologic agent causing disease.[2]

peak expiratory flow (PEF): The highest forced expiratory flow measured with a peak flow meter.[2]

peak flow meter: A small, portable hand-held device which measures how well the lungs are able to expel air, allowing asthma patients to detect airway narrowing and adjust medications accordingly. Children as young as 4-5 can learn how to use a peak flow meter.[1]

perennial: Describes something that occurs throughout the year.[5]

pneumonia: A very serious health condition where a person's lungs are filled with fluid. This makes it very hard for oxygen in the lungs to reach the blood stream.[2]

quick relief medication: Medicine taken to relieve asthma symptoms. Called "quick relief" because they can act immediately to reduce symptoms which appear suddenly.[1]

residual volume (RV): That volume of air remaining in the lungs after maximal exhalation. The method of measurement should be indicated.[2]

respiratory cycle: A respiratory cycle is constituted by the inspiration followed by the expiration of a given volume of gas, called tidal volume. The duration of the respiratory cycle is the respiratory or ventilatory period, whose reciprocal is the ventilatory frequency.[2]

respiratory virus: Illnesses affecting the airways caused by a virus. Symptoms of respiratory virus are similar to asthma symptoms. Students with asthma may experience increased asthma symptoms for some time following a respiratory virus.[1]

rhinitis: Inflammation of the nasal passages, which can cause a runny nose.[5]

risk factor: An agent that when present increases the probability of disorder expression. In asthma, there are two types of risk factors: 1) Risk factors involved in the development of asthma; these can be inherited, such as atopy, or due to environmental exposure. See "causal factors" and "contributing factors." 2) Risk factors that cause asthma exacerbation in individuals who already have the condition. These are also called triggers.[3]

RNA (ribonucleic acid): A complex molecule that is found in the cell cytoplasm and nucleus. One function of RNA is to direct the building of proteins.[4]

secondhand smoke: Secondhand smoke, also known as environmental tobacco smoke, consists of exhaled smoke from smokers and side stream smoke from the burning end of a cigarette, cigar or pipe.[2]

sensitivity/sensitization: Refers to a person's response when exposed to an allergen. For some people, repeated exposure to certain substances makes them more likely to develop an allergic reaction.[1]

sinuses: Hollow air spaces located within the bones of the skull surrounding the nose.[5]

spacer: A short tube device which can be attached to an inhaler to help the student use the inhaler more effectively.[1]

spirometry: A medical test that measures how well the lungs exhale. The information gathered during this test is useful in diagnosing certain types of lung disorders, but it is most useful when assessing for obstructive lung diseases (especially asthma and chronic obstructive pulmonary disease). In a spirometry test, a person breathes into a mouthpiece that is connected to an instrument called a spirometer. The spirometer records the amount and the rate of air that is breathed in and out over a specified time. Some of the test measurements are obtained by normal, quiet breathing, and other tests require forced inhalation or exhalation after a deep breath.[2]

sputum: Matter ejected from the lungs and windpipe through the mouth.[5]

Asthma-Related Terms

T cells: Small white blood cells (also known as T lymphocytes) that direct or directly participate in immune defenses.[4]

trachea: Commonly known as the windpipe, a cartilaginous air tube extending from the larynx (voice box) into the thorax (chest) where it divides into left and right branches.[2]

trigger: A substance or environmental condition that causes asthma or allergy symptoms to appear.[1]

upper respiratory tract: Area of the body which includes the nasal passages, mouth, and throat.[5]

vaccines: substances that contain parts of antigens from an infectious organism. By stimulating an immune response (but not disease), they protect the body against subsequent infection by that organism.[4]

vital capacity (VC): The maximum volume of air exhaled from the point of maximum inspiration.[2]

wheezing/wheeze: The whistling sound which occurs when air moves though narrowed or tightened airways. Wheezing is a classic symptom of asthma. Not all wheezing can be heard by the ears; a stethoscope may be needed to detect levels of wheezing within the lungs.[1]

Chapter 79

Directory of Asthma-Related Resources

Asthma-Related Organizations

Allergic Rhinitis and Its Impact on Asthma Workgroup
Website: http://www.whiar.com

Allergy and Asthma Network Mothers of Asthmatics
2751 Prosperity Avenue
Suite 150
Fairfax, VA 22031
Toll-Free: 800-878-4403
Fax: 703-573-7794
Website: http://www.aanma.org

Allies Against Asthma Resource Bank
University of Michigan
School of Public Health
109 S. Observatory St.
Ann Arbor, MI 48109-2029
Phone: 734-647-9047
Fax: 734-763-7379
Website: http://www.asthmaresourcebank.org
E-mail: resourcebank@umich.edu

About This Chapter: This chapter includes an list of asthma-related organizations and a list of helpful web-based documents and on-line tools. The resources in this chapter were compiled from several sources deemed reliable. The lists represent a sampling of available information; they are not complete. Inclusion does not constitute endorsement. All contact information was verified and updated in December 2005.

American Academy of Allergy, Asthma, and Immunology
611 East Wells Street
Milwaukee, WI 53202
Toll-Free: 800-822-2762
Phone: 414-272-6071
Website: http://www.aaaai.org

American Association for Respiratory Care
9425 N. MacArthur Blvd.
Suite 100
Irving, TX 75603
Phone: 972-243-2272
Fax: 972-484-2720
Website:
www.yourlunghealth.org
E-mail: info@aarc.org

American Board of Allergy and Immunology
510 Walnut Street
Suite 1701
Philadelphia, PA 19106-3699
Toll-Free: 866-264-5568
Phone: 215-592-9466
Website: http://www.abai.org
E-mail: abai@abai.org

American College of Allergy, Asthma, and Immunology
85 West Algonquin Road
Suite 550
Arlington Heights, IL 60005
Toll-Free: 800-842-7777
Phone: 847-427-1200
Fax: 847-427-1294
Website: http://www.acaai.org
E-mail: mail@acaai.org

American College of Chest Physicians
3300 Dundee Rd.
Northbrook, IL 60062-2348
Toll-Free: 800-343-2227
Phone: 847-498-1400
Website for Patient Information:
http://www.chestnet.org/patients

American Lung Association
61 Broadway, 6th Floor
New York, NY 10006
Toll-Free: 800-LUNG-USA (586-4872)
Phone: 213-315-8700
Website: http://www.lungusa.org

American Respiratory Care Foundation
9425 N. MacArthur Blvd.
Suite 100
Irving, TX 75603
Phone: 972-243-2272
Fax: 972-484-2720
Website: http://
www.arcfoundation.org
E-mail: info@arcfoundation.org

Asthma and Allergy Foundation of America
1233 20th Street, NW
Suite 402
Washington, DC 20036
Toll-Free: 800-727-8462
Phone: 202-466-7643
Website: http://www.aafa.org
E-mail: info@aafa.org

Directory of Asthma-Related Resources

Asthma and Allergy Information Association
Box 100
Toronto, ON M9W 5K9
Canada
Phone: 416-679-9521
Fax: 416-679-9524
Website: http://www.aaia.ca

Asthma and Schools
Website: http://asthmaandschools.org

Asthma Clinical Research Network
Website: http://www.acrn.org

Asthma In Canada
Website: http://www.asthmaincanada.com

Asthma Initiative of Michigan
403 Seymour
Lansing, MI 48933
Toll-Free in Michigan: 866-EZ LUNGS (395-8647)
Phone: 517-484-7206
Website: http://www.getasthmahelp.org
E-mail: info@GetAsthmaHelp.org

Asthma Partners
Toll-Free: 800-972-7863
Website: http://www.asthma.partners.org
E-mail: asthma@partners.org

Asthma Society of Canada
130 Bridgeland Avenue
Suite 425
Toronto, ON M6A 1Z4
Canada
Toll-Free in Canada: 866-787-4050
Phone: 416-787-4050
Website: http://www.asthma.ca
E-mail: info@asthma.ca

California Society for Respiratory Care
1961 Main Street
Suite 246
Watsonville, CA 95076
Phone: 888-730-CSRC (2772)
Fax: 831-763-2814
Website: http://www.csrc.org

Canadian Lung Association
3 Raymond Street
Suite 300
Ottawa, ON K1R 1A3
Canada
Toll-Free in Canada: 888-566-LUNG (5864)
Phone: 613-569-6411
Fax: 613-569-8860
Website: http://www.lung.ca/asthma
E-mail: info@lung.ca

Canadian Network for Asthma Care
16851 Mount Wolfe Rd.
Caledon, ON L7E 3P6
Canada
Phone: 905-880-1092
Fax: 905-880-9733
Website: http://www.cnac.net

Canadian Society of Allergy and Clinical Immunology
774 Echo Dr.
Ottawa ON K1S 5N8
Canada
Phone: 613-730-6272
Fax: 613-730-1116
Website: http://
www.csaci.medical.org
E-mail: csaci@rcpsc.edu

Center for Children's Health and the Environment
Mount Sinai School of Medicine
Box 1057
One Gustave Levy Place
New York, NY 10029
Phone: 212-241-7840
Fax: 212-996-0407
Website: http://
www.childenvironment.org

Centers for Disease Control and Prevention
Website: http://www.cdc.gov
Website for Asthma and Allergies: http://www.cdc.gov/health/asthma.htm

Childhood Asthma Foundation
Box 22033 Town and County Plaza
Niagara Falls, ON L2J 4J3
Canada
Toll-Free: 800-373-5696
Website: http://
www.childasthma.com
E-mail: asthmainfo@childhoodasthma.ca

Children's Asthma Network
Community Pediatric Asthma Service
South Calgary Health Centre
Cube 2270, 31 Sunpark Plaza, SE
Calgary AB T2X 3T2
Canada
Phone: 403-943-9139
Website: http://
www.calgaryhealthregion.ca/ican

Children's Hospital of Eastern Ontario
401 Smyth Road
Ottawa, ON K1H 8L1
Canada
Phone: 613-737-7600
Website: www.cheo.on.ca
E-mail: webmaster@cheo.on.ca

Cleveland Clinic
Asthma Center of Excellence
9500 Euclid Avenue
Cleveland, OH 44195
Website: http://
www.clevelandclinic.org

Consortium on Children's Asthma Camps
490 Concordia Ave.
St. Paul, MN 55103
Phone: 651-227-8014
Website: http://
asthmacamps.org/asthmacamps

Global Initiative for Asthma (GINA)
Website: http://ginasthma.com

Directory of Asthma-Related Resources

Healthy Kids: The Key to Basics
Educational Planning for Students With Asthma and Other Chronic Health Conditions
79 Elmore Street
Newton, MA 02459-1137
Phone: 617-965-9637
Website: http://www.healthy-kids.info

International Asthma Quality of Care Initiative
Website: http://www.iaqoc.com

National Asthma Education and Prevention Program
NHLBI Information Center
P.O. Box 30105
Bethesda, MD 20824-0105
Phone: 301-592-8573
Website: http://www.nhlbi.nih.gov/about/naepp

National Heart, Lung, and Blood Institute
P.O. Box 30105
Bethesda, MD 20824-0105
Phone: 301-592-8573
Website: http://www.nhlbi.nih.gov
E-mail: nhlbinfo@nhlbi.nih.gov

National Institute of Allergy and Infectious Diseases
Building 31, Room 7A-50
31 Center Drive MSC 2520
Bethesda, MD 20892-2520
Phone: 301-496-5717
Website: http://niaid.nih.gov

National Institute of Environmental Health Sciences
P.O. Box 12233
Research Triangle Park, NC 27709
Phone: 919-541-3345
Website: http://www.niehs.nih.gov

National Jewish Medical and Research Center
1400 Jackson St.
Denver, CO 80206
Toll-Free: 800-222-LUNG (5864)
Phone: 303-388-4461
Website: http://www.nationaljewish.org
E-mail: lungline@njc.org

National Lung Health Education Program
American Association for Respiratory Care
9425 MacArthur Boulevard
Irving, TX 75063
Phone: 972-910-8555
Fax: 972-484-2720
Website: http://www.nlhep.org

New York City Asthma Initiative
Website: http://www.nyc.gov/health/asthma

Northwest Asthma and Allergy Center
Toll-Free: 800-437-4055
Website: http://www.nwasthma.com
E-mail: info@nwasthma.com

Ontario Lung Association
573 King Street East, Suite 201
Toronto, ON M5A 4L3
Canada
Toll-Free in Canada: 888-972-2636
Phone: 416-864-9911
Fax: 416-864-9916
Website: http://www.on.lung.ca

Support for Asthmatic Youth (SAY)
Johns Hopkins Department of Pediatric Pulmonary
600 North Wolfe Street
Baltimore, MD 21287-2533
Phone: 410-955-2035
Website: http://www.hopkinschildrens.org/pages/clinical/support.cfm

U.S. Environmental Protection Agency
1200 Pennsylvania Ave., NW
Mail Code 6609J
Washington, DC 20460
Toll-Free: 800-438-4318
Phone: 202-343-9370
Fax: 202-343-2394
Website: http://www.epa.gov

Directory of Asthma-Related Resources

Web-Based Documents and On-Line Tools

AAIRwaves
A bi-monthly teen newsletter produced by the Asthma and Allergy Foundation of America
Website: http://www.aafa.org/subscribe.cfm?item=aairwaves

AirNow: Quality of Air Means Quality of Life
Information about air quality in states and cities, from the U.S. Environmental Protection Agency
Website: http://cfpub.epa.gov/airnow/index.cfm?action=airnow.main

Asthma and Allergies Website
Information about occupational asthma from the National Institute for Occupational Safety and Health
Website: http://www.cdc.gov/niosh/topics/asthma

Asthma and the Environment: A Strategy to Protect Children
A report from the President's Task Force on Environmental Health Risks and Safety Risks to Children
Website: http://aspe.hhs.gov/sp/asthma/appxd.pdf

Asthma Doesn't Sentence You to the Couch
Information about exercising with asthma, from Wellsource, Inc.
Website: http://vanderbiltowc.wellsource.com/dh/Content.asp?ID=376

Asthma Library
Links to videos and an article library of information about asthma, from Healthology
Website: http://aafa_as.healthology.com/focus_index.asp?f-asthma&b=aafa_as

Asthma Life Quality Text
An assessment test developed by the American College of Allergy, Asthma, and Immunology
Website: http://www.acaai.org/public/lifeQuality/lq.htm

Asthma Magazine
Website: http://www.asthmamagazine.com

Asthma Under Control
Website: http://www.asthmacontrol.com

Asthma Wizard™
Information for kids from the National Jewish Medical and Research Center
Website: http://www.nationaljewish.org/disease-info/diseases/asthma/kids/wizard-index.aspx

Asthma: A Guide for Teens with Asthma
An on-line publication from Blank Children's Hospital
Website: http://www.blankchildrens.org/documents/asthma_teens.pdf

AsthmaBusters.org
An on-line club for kids with asthma, sponsored by the American Lung Association of Nebraska
Website: http://www.asthmabusters.org

Breath of Life
An on-line exhibition related to asthma created by the National Library of Medicine
Website: http://www.nlm.nih.gov/hmd/breath/breathhome.html

Breatherville, USA™
An interactive site developed by Allergy and Asthma Network Mothers of Asthmatics
Website: http://www.aanma.org/breatherville.htm

Clinical Trials
Use this site, developed by the National Library of Medicine, to find asthma-related clinical trials (search for "Asthma").
Website: http://clinicaltrials.gov

Disease Detectives: Dr. Asthma
An educational site for kids provided by the Centers for Disease Control and Prevention
Website: http://www.bam.gov/sub_diseases/diseases_detectives_1.html

Don't Let Asthma Keep You Out of the Game
Encouragement for kids with asthma, provided by the Centers for Disease Control and Prevention
Website: http://www.bam.gov/sub_physicalactivity/physicalactivity_meetchallenge.html

Directory of Asthma-Related Resources

End Allergy and Asthma Misery: It's Worth a Shot
An online presentation about the link between asthma and allergies, provided by the American College of Allergy, Asthma, and Immunology
Website: http://www.acaai.org/powerpoint/online/slide1.html

JAMA *Asthma Information Center*
Asthma-related information and links from the producers of the *Journal of the American Medical Association*
Website: http://www.medem.com/MedLB/articleslb.cfm?sub_cat=80

Managing Asthma for Patients and Families
An educational document provided by Virtual Children's Hospital/University of Iowa
Website: http://www.vh.org/pediatric/patient/pediatrics/asthma

Mayo Clinic Health Oasis
Search for "asthma" to find information from the Mayo Clinic
Website: http://www.mayohealth.org

National Allergy Bureau
An on-line tool for information about pollen levels, provided by the American Academy of Allergy, Asthma, and Immunology
Website: http://www.aaaai.org/nab

No Attacks
A website devoted to helping asthma sufferers avoid asthma attacks, developed by the Ad Council and the U.S. Environmental Protection Agency
Website: http://www.noattacks.org

Project A: Knock the Breath out of Asthma
An interactive site for teens with asthma, developed by Teen Asthma Team (TAT)
Website: http://www.project-a.ca

What's Asthma All About?
An interactive movie by Neomedicus
Website: http://www.whatsasthma.org

Chapter 80

Health Insurance and Asthma-Related Services

Americans have insurance for asthma treatment and medical supplies. But many insurance plans have payment limits and other rules. Even if your insurance covers a treatment, getting the insurer to pay can sometimes be difficult. The information in this chapter will help you get the most from your plan and pay the least from your own pocket.

I don't have health insurance. How can I get it?

You may be eligible for a government program such as Medicaid at little or no cost. Call your state's local social services office for details. If you are not eligible for a government program, Blue Cross plans in most states have a yearly "open enrollment" period. You can't be turned down for this coverage if you pay the premium. Some states have "high-risk pool" programs in which you are assigned to one of several plans. This also requires you to pay a premium, but the state may help fund it.

Did you have coverage within the last 18 months through your own or your spouse's private employer? If so, and the employer has at least 20 workers, you can buy what's called COBRA Continuation coverage. [COBRA stands for "Consolidated Omnibus Budget Reconciliation Act, the name of the federal legislation that mandates the availability of this coverage.] You pay the plan's full premium plus a 2 percent fee.

"Health Insurance," reprinted with permission from the Asthma and Allergy Foundation of America, © 2005. All rights reserved. For additional information about asthma and related topics visit the AAFA website at http://www.aafa.org.

COBRA coverage is a better value than an individual or high-risk plan. Contact your former employer for details.

When I choose a health plan, what issues should I consider?

No specific plan is best for everyone. The three most important issues are the health services covered, the choice of providers, and the plan's cost to you. These issues are discussed in the next few answers.

You also should consider whether the plan will cover just you ("self only") or—if you have a family—them as well (a "family" plan). Finally, a plan offered through a "group" such as your employer usually will be a better value than an "individual" plan.

What should I know about coverage of asthma-related services?

Each plan has different rules for the services it covers. Most plans pay for doctor and hospital treatment for asthma if the provider is approved by the plan. But many plans limit coverage of asthma medications and medical equipment. And only a few plans—mainly "Health Maintenance Organizations"—cover preventive care.

In addition to rules specifically for asthma, plans may have rules applying to several medical conditions. Two frequent rules are preexisting condition limits and chronic condition limits.

What are preexisting and chronic condition limits?

A preexisting condition limit means that if you already have a medical condition when you sign up for a plan, the plan will limit its payments for that condition for a certain time. Some "individual" and "small group" plans have this rule, and it can be a major problem for people with asthma.

A chronic condition limit means that if a medical condition is not expected to show improvement within a certain time, then services for it won't be covered. In rare cases, this can apply to asthma.

What choice of providers do plans give me, and why is that important?

Almost every plan has a list of "approved" providers the plan will pay best, while some plans pay nothing to a "non-approved" provider. Most or all of a plan's "approved" providers are listed in its "Provider Directory." You can get a copy by asking the plan.

Health Insurance and Asthma-Related Services

Because you must pay more to use a non-approved provider, the larger the plan's approved list, the better. But provider choice isn't just about saving money. Some providers specialize in treating asthma, some are located near you, and so on. Usually, managed care plans have the fewest approved providers.

What are the types of managed-care plans and how do they limit my choice of provider?

There are three types of managed care plans: preferred provider organizations, health maintenance organizations, and "point of service" plans. A preferred provider organization (PPO) allows the patient to choose any provider, but pays approved ("preferred") providers a higher amount than non-approved providers. The plan might cover all of a PPO doctor's charge but only 80 percent of a non-PPO doctor's bill.

A health maintenance organization (HMO) pays nothing for non-emergency care if from a provider lacking a contract with the HMO. So an HMO patient has a strong financial reason to use only HMO providers. An HMO also requires you to choose a "primary care" doctor. He or she must approve referrals to "specialist" providers such as pulmonology doctors and respiratory therapists.

The third managed-care plan, called "point of service" (POS), is a cross between an HMO and a PPO. Like an HMO, it requires you to choose a primary-care doctor. Like a PPO, if you want to see a non-HMO provider, the plan will pay some amount for that care, but less than if you used an HMO provider.

Compared to traditional insurance, managed care plans are cheaper or offer more benefits. But they always have fewer choices of providers.

What out-of-pocket costs should I consider in choosing a plan?

You may have to pay four types of costs. These are:

- Premiums (periodic fees charged regardless of how many services you use).
- Deductible (yearly total amounts you must pay for one or more services before the plan will begin paying).
- Copayments (small amounts you pay each time you get a service).
- Uncovered out-of-pocket costs (your spending for services the plan doesn't cover, in contrast to premiums, deductibles and copayments).

Most plans have a "catastrophic," "stop-loss" or "hold harmless" feature that limits the total yearly amount you must pay. But that cap doesn't apply to the premium. The higher the total premium, the lower the other three types of costs.

Many people prefer to pay a higher premium to reduce their other costs. That protects them from large unexpected bills. It's especially good if you're likely to get many treatments for a major medical condition.

How can I get the best mix of covered services, provider choice, and costs?

What is best depends on your situation. Because you or a family member has asthma, it's good to have a plan with broad coverage for that condition. But you may not be able to afford a high-cost plan.

If you've long been treated by a doctor who's not contracted with any plans, you'll need to get a non-managed care plan to keep that doctor. But if you just moved to a new city, being able to see a particular provider is not as important. Your doctor's staff or a community group such as a senior citizen association can advise you what plan is best.

What is "assignment of benefits" and how can it help me?

Assignment of benefits ("assignment" for short) means your provider agrees to send a claim to your plan and accept the plan's "allowed" payment as full payment.

You don't have to pay out-of-pocket for the entire bill when you're treated. You also may save money and you don't have to mail a claim. And if the claim is denied, your provider usually can file an appeal on your behalf.

All providers contracting with managed care plans, and all Medicare and Medicaid "participating" providers must accept assignment for those plans. But some providers whose services are in high demand don't accept assignment because they can pick and choose the patients they treat. Assignment is always good financially, but it doesn't concern the quality of your care.

Should I get coverage under more than one plan?

It's not good to pay the full premium of more than one plan. The plans usually will duplicate each other but you won't be paid double. Yet sometimes having two plans makes sense.

Health Insurance and Asthma-Related Services

If you have a plan such as Medicare that has major limits, you can buy a supplemental plan such as "Medigap." If both spouses in a family have family plans, each plan may cover limits in the other.

There are three "dual coverage" rules on which plan pays first. Some plans (for example, Medigap) always pay after another plan (for example, Medicare). Read the plan's rules to determine which plan pays first.

If you and your spouse both have family plans, your plan will always pay first for your own care. Your spouse's plan will pay first for your spouse's care. After the first ("primary") plan has paid, if there's any unpaid balance, the other ("secondary") plan should be billed.

When there are two family plans and a child is treated, the "birthday rule" usually applies. The plan of the parent with the birthday earliest in the year will pay first. If the mother's birthday is January 2, and the father's is June 7, the mother's plan would pay first for the child's care. But plans in a few states use different rules.

What can I do if a plan refuses to enroll me, denies a claim or causes other problems?

Different plans have different "appeal" rules. It's important to know these rules because if you don't follow them, your problem won't be solved. In some plans, you must appeal in as little as 30 days.

You're entitled to a pamphlet summarizing your plan's rules. This "insurance policy" booklet is called an "Outline of Coverage," "Summary Benefits Plan Description," "Medicare Handbook," or similar name. You should read this. If you don't have it, you can get a copy from your plan.

Government plans such as Medicare and Medicaid give you many rights. They usually allow you to appeal several times if you disagree with a decision.

Private plans are run by insurers such as Blue Cross. Their rules are less detailed than government plans. You become eligible for a private plan if you or your spouse's employer offers it or if you pay individual premiums.

Some private plans are allowed to turn down your enrollment even if you can pay the premium. Private plans may be either "true insurance" overseen by your state government or "self-insured" plans. Self-insured plans give you fewer appeal rights. In general, plans sold to individuals and to small companies are insured plans. Those sold to large employers are self-insured. If your plan booklet does not say which type it is, contact the plan or your state's insurance commission in your state capitol.

If a claim is denied, the "Explanation of Benefits" notice you get must give a reason why. Some reasons are easier to overturn than others. If the plan says your care wasn't "medically necessary," that's a poor explanation and often can be reversed.

If your care went beyond what the plan covers, such as medications costing more than the plan's $500 yearly limit, it's unlikely the plan will reverse its decision. But it may do that if you convince the plan it would save by avoiding bigger costs. For example, asthma medication may keep you from going to the hospital. The plan doesn't have to make exceptions. When it does, that's called an "extra-contractual" benefit.

Can I see a specialist?

HMOs and POS plans require all non-emergency services from specialty providers to be pre-approved by the plan and your primary-care doctor. This also applies if you are already being treated by a specialist and you switch to a new HMO.

What if I have a medical emergency while traveling?

If you think your life could be endangered or the functioning of an organ such as your lungs permanently damaged, seek the nearest medical treatment. In most cases, your plan will pay for this care. If your condition is less serious and you are enrolled in a managed-care plan, you must call the plan's "pre-authorization" number on your insurance card and follow the plan's direction in order for the care to be paid.

Can I get my plan to pay for a second opinion?

Most plans cover second opinions for major procedures such as surgeries. For details, call your plan before getting the second opinion. If your question is about nonsurgical treatment such as prescribing one medicine rather than another, most plans won't pay for a second opinion. So ask your doctor why the specific treatment is recommended.

When I have a problem, how can I get help?

If you have a question about your plan, call the plan's customer service department, using the phone number on your enrollment card or plan brochure. Your employer's benefits office, your local labor union, or a consumer advocacy group can help.

Health Insurance and Asthma-Related Services

Your doctor or hospital office also may help, especially for a denied claim when the provider accepted assignment. And you can contact your state's Insurance Commission in your state capital.

If you follow all the rules and still have a problem, you can hire a lawyer. The lawyer can sue the plan for "breach of contract." But that is expensive and you aren't likely to win. This is why some people think the laws should be changed to give patients more rights.

Health insurance is valuable, but many problems can occur. It is important to be well informed so you can get the kind of insurance you want and pay less for it.

Chapter 81

Asthma Prescription Medications: Assistance Programs and Online Purchasing

Prescription Medication Assistance Programs

If you're unable to pay for prescription allergy and asthma medications, you might qualify for a patient assistance program. Many pharmaceutical companies provide free prescription medications to patients in need. In fact, the industry gave away nearly $1.5 billion worth of prescription medicines to 3.5 million patients in 2001.

Partnership for Prescription Assistance offers a directory of assistance programs on its website at http://www.pparx.org. Simply click on "View a list of participating programs" to learn about the programs that may be available, covered medications, eligibility requirements, and how to apply for assistance. Or call 888-4PPA-NOW (477-2669) for more information.

Be sure to ask your physician to help you complete and submit the necessary paperwork when applying for a patient assistance program.

Money-Saving Tips

- Get asthma under control. Controlled asthma costs far less than constantly wrestling with symptoms. Develop a plan with your physician for preventing attacks altogether.

This chapter includes "Prescription Medication Assistance Programs" and "Buying Prescription Medications Online," © Allergy & Asthma Network Mothers of Asthmatics (www.aanma.org). Reprinted courtesy of Allergy & Asthma Network Mothers of Asthmatics (AANMA), 800-878-4403, www.breatherville.org.

- Keep your inhaler and other medication delivery systems clean.

- Before you purchase over-the-counter (OTC) remedies, talk to your pharmacist or physician. Consumers waste a lot of money on "trial-and-error" self-medication. Some OTC products can be dangerous if mixed with prescribed medications.

- Use your inhaler, spacers, holding chambers, nebulizers, and other medication delivery systems correctly. Proper technique ensures that the medication provides maximum benefit. Ask your physician or pharmacist to review your technique periodically.

- Avoid offending asthma triggers, make environmental changes if necessary, and use a peak flow meter to help alert you to an approaching asthma flare. It takes less medication to stop an attack in its earliest stage than after symptoms worsen.

- Don't put off seeing a specialist such as an allergist or pulmonologist because you are concerned about the expense. Most often the initial expense will be offset by a reduction in emergency room and unscheduled office visits and medications. If finances are a problem, ask the physician or office manager if it is possible to establish a payment plan.

- Remember, an ounce of prevention avoids a pound of medication, side effects, and symptoms.

Buying Prescription Medications Online

With hundreds of medication-dispensing websites in business, how can you tell which sites are legitimate? The U.S. Food and Drug Administration (FDA) offers these warnings when it comes to buying medical products online:

- Check with the National Association of Boards of Pharmacy (www.nabp.net, 847-391-4406) to determine whether a website is a licensed pharmacy in good standing.

- Purchasing a medication from an illegal Web site puts you at risk. You may receive a contaminated or counterfeit product, the wrong product, an incorrect dose, or no product at all.

- Taking an unsafe or inappropriate medication puts you at risk for dangerous drug interactions and other serious health consequences.

Asthma Prescription Medications

- Getting a prescription drug by filling out a questionnaire without seeing a doctor poses serious health risks. A questionnaire does not provide sufficient information for a healthcare professional to determine if that drug is for you or safe to use, if another treatment is more appropriate, or if you have an underlying medical condition where using that drug may be harmful. The American Medical Association has determined that this practice is generally substandard medical care.

- Don't buy from sites that offer to prescribe a prescription drug for the first time without a physical exam, sell a prescription drug without a prescription, or sell drugs not approved by the FDA.

- Don't do business with sites that have no access to a registered pharmacist to answer questions.

- Avoid sites that do not identify with whom you are dealing and do not provide a U.S. address and phone number to contact if there's a problem.

- Don't purchase from foreign websites at this time because it's often illegal to import the drugs bought from these sites, the risks are greater, and there is very little the U.S. government can do if you get ripped off.

- Beware of sites that advertise a "new cure" for a serious disorder or a quick cure-all for a wide range of ailments.

- Be careful of sites that use impressive-sounding terminology to disguise a lack of good science or those that claim the government, the medical profession, or research scientists have conspired to suppress a product.

- Steer clear of sites that include undocumented case histories claiming "amazing" results.

- Talk to your healthcare professional before using any medications for the first time.

Index

Index

Index

Page numbers followed by 'n' indicate a footnote. Page numbers in *italics* indicate a table or illustration.

A

AAAAI *see* American Academy of Allergy, Asthma and Immunology
AAFA *see* Asthma and Allergy Foundation of America
AAIRwaves, Web site address 543
AANMA *see* Allergy and Asthma Network Mothers of Asthmatics
ABMS *see* American Board of Medical Specialties
Accolate (zafirlukast) *283*
AccuNeb (albuterol) *283*
ACE inhibitors, cardiac asthma *143*
acetaminophen 34, 102–3
acoustic rhinometry, aspirin-induced asthma 111
"Activity Guidelines for Youths and Adults with Asthma" (Alberta Clinical Practice Guideline) 221n
acupuncture
 asthma treatment 292, 331–36
 cortisone 29

A.D.A.M., Inc., publications
 adults 97n, 107n
 medications 281n
Adams, Kenneth 459, 461
addiction, corticosteroids 37
adolescents
 asthma 71–73
 emotional problems 373–74
adrenalin, asthma emergencies 56
adult onset asthma, overview 75–79
"Adult Onset of Asthma" (AAFA) 75n
Advair (fluticasone/salmeterol) *283*
Advil (ibuprofen) 102
aerobics, asthma 40
AeroBid (flunisolide) *123*, *283*
AeroChamber, children 60
age factor
 adult onset asthma 76, 81–87
 asthma 18
 asthma control 27
 asthma statistics 400–402
 influenza vaccine 185–86
 sinusitis 165
 see also adolescents; children; infants
AIA *see* aspirin-induced asthma
"Airborne Allergens: Something in the Air" (NIAID) 525n
"Air Filters" (AAFA) 255n

561

air filters, overview 255–60
AirNow: Quality of Air Means Quality
  of Life, Web site address 543
air purifiers, allergens 29
air quality index, described 243
airway obstruction
  asthma diagnosis 110
  described 5, 15, 58, 64
  reversal 7
airway opener medications, described
  29–30, 33
airway remodeling *see* remodeling
airways
  defined 525
  described 58, 64
  infants 58–59
Alberta Clinical Practice Guideline,
  exercise publication 221n
albuterol
  asthma treatment 30, 68, 281, *283*
  pregnancy 91
  status asthmaticus 135–38
Aleve (naproxen) 102
Alford, Gregory 481n
allergens
  adult onset asthma 75
  asthma 217–18
  childhood asthma 65–66
  defined 525
  described 58, 65
"Allergic Asthma" (AAFA) 113n
allergic asthma, overview 113–17
"Allergic Asthma A-to-Z" (AAFA)
  113n
"Allergic Asthma FAQs" (AAFA) 113n
allergic cascade, described 115
allergic process, described 100
allergic reactions
  asthma triggers 22
  defined 525
allergic response, described 99–100
allergic rhinitis
  defined 525
  fossil fuels 99–100
  overview 151–61
  pregnancy 94
Allergic Rhinitis and Its Impact
  on Asthma Workgroup, Web site
  address 537

allergies
  adult onset asthma 75–76
  air filters 259
  asthma 83
  asthma diaries 204–6
  asthma treatment 26
  defined 526
  insect stings 223
allergists
  allergy tests 218
  asthma treatment 510–14
  childhood asthma 358
  described 196
Allergy and Asthma Network
  Mothers of Asthmatics
  (AANMA)
  contact information 537
  publications
    asthma emergencies 53n
    locating physicians 195n
    school absenteeism 379n
  Web site address 198
allergy tests
  asthma diagnosis 110
  childhood asthma 358
allergy vaccination *see*
  hyposensitization
Aller Relief Chinese herb 294
Allies Against Asthma Resource
  Bank, contact information 537
alternative therapies
  allergic rhinitis 158–59
  asthma treatment 292–94
  childhood asthma 357–58
Alupent (metaproterenol) 281, *283*
alveoli
  depicted *6*
  described 4, 7, 97
Alving, Barbara 90, 467, 470
American Academy of Allergy,
  Asthma and Immunology
  (AAAAI), contact information
  538
American Association for
  Respiratory Care, contact
  information 538
American Board of Medical
  Specialties (ABMS), contact
  information 198, 538

Index

American College of Allergy, Asthma and Immunology, publications
    chickenpox 393n
    exercise 221n
American College of Chest Physicians
    aerosol therapy devices publication 497n
    contact information 538
American Lung Association
    contact information 538
    publications
        asthma attacks 49n
        childhood asthma 419n
        peak flow meters 211n
        physicians 199n
American Physiological Society, weather influences publication 237n
American Respiratory Care Foundation, contact information 538
anabolic steroids, *versus* corticosteroids 32
AnaGuard, asthma emergencies 56
anaphylactic shock, defined 526
anaphylaxis
    defined 526
    exercise 223
    food allergies 174–75
animal allergens
    asthma triggers 28, 252–53
    school settings 387–91
animal dander
    allergic response 99
    childhood asthma 362–63, 365–67
anterior rhinoscopy, allergic rhinitis 153
antibiotic medications
    allergic rhinitis 159
    asthmatic inflammation 38–39
    asthma treatment 292
    defined 526
    pneumonia 7
    sinusitis 166, 169
    status asthmaticus 138
antibodies
    defined 526
    described 65
    immunoglobulin 530

anti-cholinergics
    allergic rhinitis 158
    asthma treatment *283*, 284
    exercise-induced asthma *123*
antigens, defined 526
antihistamines
    allergic rhinitis 156–57
    cardiac asthma *143*
    described 33
    side effects 36
anti-IgE therapy 329–30
"Anti-IgE Therapy: A Revolutionary Approach to Controlling Allergy and Asthma" (Berger) 329n
anti-inflammatory medications
    asthma treatment *283*
    described 29–31, 34
    exercise-induced asthma 40, *123*
    sinusitis 169
    steroid-resistant asthma 131
antileukotrienes
    allergic rhinitis 158
    described 33–34
anxiety, asthma emergencies 55–56
approved providers, described 548–49
Apter, Andrea 295–97
Arbes, Samuel J. 477
Aristocort (triamcinolone) *283*
aristolochic acid 294
aromatherapy, asthma treatment 294
Aronow, Bruce 491
Asmanex (mometasone) *283*, 286
aspirin
    allergic rhinitis 159
    versus corticosteroids 34
    drug interactions 85
aspirin-induced asthma (AIA)
    asthma diagnosis 111
    described 102–3
assignment of benefits, described 550
asthma
    aerosol therapy devices 497–99
    causes overview 97–105
    defined 526
    described 17, 57, 64–65, 75
    diagnosis 59–60, 107–11
    overview 3–16, 17–44

asthma, continued
  rhinitis 155–56
  symptoms 23–26
  treatment overview 275–80
  see also childhood asthma
asthma action plans
  defined 526
  depicted *209*
  emergency care 370
  overview 207–10
  see also asthma management plans
Asthma and Allergies Website, Web site address 543
Asthma and Allergy Foundation of America (AAFA)
  contact information 260, 538
  publications
    adults 75n
    air filters 255n
    allergic asthma 113n
    children 63n
    corticosteroids 303n
    infants 57n
Asthma and Allergy Information Association, contact information 539
"Asthma and Flu Shots" (CDC) 183n
"Asthma and Outdoor Air Pollution" (EPA) 243n
Asthma and Schools, Web site address 539
"Asthma and Sinusitis" (Grossan) 163n
Asthma and the Environment: A Strategy to Protect Children, Web site address 543
"Asthma and Travel" (Better Health Channel) 269n
asthma attacks
  childhood asthma 354
  described 49–51, 340
  infants 57–58
  second wave 50–51
  warning signs 359–60
  see also asthma episodes
"Asthma Attacks" (American Lung Association) 49n
AsthmaBusters.org, Web site address 544

Asthma Clinical Research Network, Web site address 539
asthma control
  childhood asthma 356–58, *357*
  described 12–13
  pregnancy 92
asthma diary
  depicted *204*
  described 203–6
Asthma Doesn't Sentence You to the Couch, Web site address 543
asthma emergencies, overview 53–56
asthma episodes
  defined 526
  depicted *8*
  described 24–26
"Asthma Essentials: Glossary" (National Education Association Health Information Network) 525n
"Asthma Gene Clusters Identified" (Cincinnati Children's Hospital Medical Center) 489n
Asthma: A Guide for Teens with Asthma, Web site address 544
"Asthma in Adults" (A.D.A.M., Inc.) 97n, 107n, 281n
Asthma in Canada, Web site address 539
"Asthma in Infants" (AAFA) 57n
Asthma Initiative of Michigan, contact information 539
Asthma Library, Web site address 543
Asthma Life Quality Text, Web site address 543
Asthma Magazine, Web site address 543
asthma management
  defined 527
  described 10–11, 13–16
  pregnancy 92–94
"Asthma Management and the Allergist: Better Outcomes at Lower Cost" (Fineman; Berger) 503n
asthma management plans
  adolescents 73
  children 62, 341–43
  defined 527

Index

asthma management plans, continued
  described 13–16
  older adults 84–85
  peak flow meters 215–16
  see also asthma action plans
Asthma Partners, contact
  information 539
"Asthma Prevalence, Health Care
  Use and Mortality, 2002" (CDC)
  399n
asthma prevention, overview 45–47
asthma research
  air toxics 443–44
  allergens 476–78
  arginase enzyme 457–59
  bioaerosols 441–43
  childhood fevers 460–62
  cockroaches 478–79
  combustion-related products
    439–41
  exposure history 444–47
  genes 459–60
  genetics 466–69, 487–88, 489–91
  genetic susceptibility 447
  health status 447–50
  inner-city children 463–65
  lifestyle 450
  long-term therapy 515–22
  mold 472–73
  mouse allergens 462–63
  obesity 481–85
  pregnancy 469–72
  sinusitis 465–66
  social interventions 451–53
  socioeconomic status 450–51
  symptom-driven therapy 473–76
  treatment outcomes 503–14
"Asthma Research Results
  Highlights" (EPA) 435n
Asthma Society of Canada
  contact information 539
  medication delivery devices
    publication 313n
"Asthma Speaker's Kit for Health
  Care Professionals: Glossary"
  (CDC) 525n
asthma treatment plans *see* asthma
  action plans; asthma management
  plans

Asthma Under Control, Web site
  address 544
Asthma Wizard, Web site address 544
"Asthma: You and Your Doctor"
  (American Lung Association) 199n
atelectasis, described 7
atopy
  defined 527
  described 65, 100
Atrovent (ipratropium) *123*, *283*
Azmacort (triamcinolone) *283*

B

"Background on Food Allergies
  and Asthma" (International Food
  Information Council) 173n
bacteria
  defined 527
  sinusitis 168
B-agonists, exercise-induced asthma
  123
Ballantyne, Christine 484
basophils, defined 527
B cells, defined 527
Beasley, Richard 407n
beclomethasone 29, 31, *283*, 286
Beclovent *123*
Berger, William E. 329n, 503n
Berotec (fenoterol) 224
beta agonists
  asthma treatment 277, *283*, 287–89
  bronchodilators 311
  cardiac asthma *143*, 144
  childhood asthma 343–44
  described 281–84
  exercise-induced asthma *123*
  pregnancy 91
beta blockers, cardiac asthma *143*,
  144
Better Health Channel, travel
  concerns publication 269n
bill of rights, described 201–2
biofeedback, asthma treatment 292
bitolterol 68, 282
board certification *see* certification
Bosma, Boyd 391
Boushey, Homer 475–76

breastfeeding
  asthma 46
  childhood allergies 61
Breatherville, USA, Web site
  address 544
"Breathing Better: Action Plans Keep
  Asthma in Check" (Meadows) 207n
Breath of Life, Web site address 544
Brethaire (terbutaline) 281
Brethine (terbutaline) 281
Bricanyl (terbutaline) 281
bronchi
  defined 528
  depicted *4, 6*
  described 4, 58, 64, 525
bronchial tubes
  defined 527
  described 309–10, 525
bronchioles
  defined 527
  depicted *6*
  described 4, 58, 64, 97
bronchitis
  asthma 147–48
  defined 527
  described 5–7
  emphysema 42
bronchoconstriction
  defined 527
  described 18
  exercise-induced asthma 119–20
bronchodilators
  asthma diagnosis 110
  asthma treatment plans 15
  childhood asthma 70
  children 60
  defined 527
  described 30–31, 276
  exercise-induced asthma *123*
  overview 309–12
bronchopulmonary dysplasia,
  pulmonologists 197
bronchospasm
  bronchitis 148
  defined 527
  described 5, 15
bronchus *see* bronchi
Bronkometer (isoetharine) 282
Bronkosol (isoetharine) 282

budesonide 29, 31, 32, *283*, 287
Burkhart, Jim 473
Busse, William W. 90, 470
Buteyko breathing method 292

C

calcium supplements, osteoporosis 38
California Society for Respiratory
  Care, contact information 539
Canadian Lung Association, contact
  information 539
Canadian Network for Asthma Care,
  contact information 539
Canadian Society of Allergy and
  Clinical Immunology, contact
  information 540
"Can Asthma Be Prevented" (NHLBI)
  275n
"Can the Weather Affect My Child's
  Asthma?" (Nemours Foundation) 237n
"Can You Prevent Asthma?"
  (Children's Hospital of Eastern
  Ontario) 45n
carbon dioxide
  respiratory failure 137
  respiratory system 4
cardiac asthma, described 141–42
cascade
  described 115
  sinusitis 170
cataracts, corticosteroids 306
CAT scan *see* computed tomography
causal factors, defined 528
CDC *see* Centers for Disease Control
  and Prevention
Celebrex (celecoxib) 103
celecoxib 103
Center for Children's Health and the
  Environment, contact information
  540
Centers for Disease Control and
  Prevention (CDC)
  contact information 540
  publications
    asthma statistics 399n
    glossary 525n
    influenza 183n

Index

certification, physicians 197–98
chemicals, childhood asthma 364
chemical sensitization, defined 528
chickenpox *see* varicella
child-care settings, asthma
  management 375–76
childhood asthma
  care improvement strategies
    425–34
  coughs 347–52
  described 63–70
  emergency care 369–72
  home schooling 381–82
  statistics 419–23
  treatment overview 339–46
  see also asthma
"Childhood Asthma" (AAFA) 63n
Childhood Asthma Foundation,
  contact information 540
children
  asthma 9, 63–70
  asthma action plan 207–10
  asthma monitoring 353–58
  asthma prevention 45–47
  asthma treatment 278–79
  bedrooms 263–64
  corticosteroids 304–5
  diet and nutrition 235
  parental supervision 10
  peak flow meters 211–12, 533
  secondhand smoke 266
  weather 237–41
Children's Asthma Network,
  contact information 540
Children's Hospital of Eastern
  Ontario
  contact information 540
  publications
    asthma prevention 45n
    childhood asthma monitoring
      353n
chiropractic, childhood asthma 358
chromones
  allergic rhinitis 157–58
  described 33
chronic asthma, described 9, 18–19
chronic bronchitis
  nitrogen dioxide 253
  overview 147–49

"Chronic Care for Low-Income Children
  with Asthma: Strategies for Improvement"
  (Stanton; Dougherty) 425n
chronic condition limit, described 548
chronicity, described 13–14
chronic obstructive pulmonary
  disease (COPD)
  adult onset asthma 77
  aerosol therapy devices 497
  asthma 42, 147–49
  defined 528
  pulmonologists 197
chronic rheumatism, asthma 41
"Chronic Sinusitis Sufferers Have
  Enhanced Immune Response to
  Fungi" (NIH) 457n
Chung, Youngran 333, 334, 335
cigarette smoke *see* environmental
  tobacco smoke; secondhand smoke;
  tobacco use
cilia
  described 164
  tobacco smoke 265
Cincinnati Children's Hospital,
  publications
  asthma research 489n
  medication delivery devices 313n
Cleveland Clinic
  contact information 540
  GERD publication 179n
climates, asthma 42–43
Clinical Trials, Web site address 544
COBRA *see* Consolidated Omnibus
  Budget Reconciliation Act
"Cockroach Allergens Have Greatest
  Impact on Childhood Asthma in
  Many U.S. Cities" (NIH) 457n
cockroaches
  allergic response 99
  asthma research 478–79
  asthma triggers 250–51
  childhood asthma 363
  research 452–53
"Cockroaches and Pests" (EPA) 247n
Cohen, Martin A. 388
cold weather
  asthma diagnosis 110
  asthma trigger 28, 35, 237–38
  childhood asthma 66, 67

567

"Cold weather exercise and airway cytokine expression" (American Physiological Society) 237n
combination medications
  childhood asthma 70
  children 61
  described 30–31
Combivent (ipratropium/albuterol) 283
common cold, asthma trigger 7
common sense measures, asthma management 10
companion animals, school settings 391
computed tomography (CAT scan; CT scan)
  asthma diagnosis 111
  sinusitis 164
conditioned reflex, described 23
congestive heart failure, cardiac asthma 141–42
Consolidated Omnibus Budget Reconciliation Act (COBRA) 547–48
Consortium on Children's Asthma Camps, contact information 540
constriction, described 58, 64
contributing factors, defined 528
controllers
  asthma treatment 299–301
  described 29–30
Cook, Gretchen W. 141n, 331n
Cooke, David A. 45n, 221n, 353n, 375n
COPD *see* chronic obstructive pulmonary disease
Corsello, Philip 142, 144
Cortef (hydrocortisone) 283
corticosteroids
  allergic rhinitis 157
  asthma treatment 283, 284–87
  asthma treatment plans 15
  cardiac asthma *143*
  chickenpox 393–96
  childhood asthma 69–70
  children 60
  competitive sports 41
  described 276–77
  exercise-induced asthma 40, *123*

corticosteroids, continued
  injections 32
  osteoporosis 189–90
  overview 303–7
  pregnancy 91
  side effects 36–37
  sinusitis 168
"Corticosteroids" (AAFA) 303n
cortisone 29, *283*
Cortone (cortisone) *283*
coughing
  asthma diagnosis 108
  childhood asthma 347–52
  mucus 5
cough medicine, asthma attacks 51
cromolyn 32, 277, *283*, 289
CT scan *see* computed tomography
"Customized Program Reduces Asthma-Related Illness in Inner-City Children" (NIH) 457n
cystic fibrosis, pulmonologists 197
cytokines, allergic process 100

D

dander, defined 528
Davis, Michael S. 239
daycare settings, asthma management 375–76
daytime cough, childhood asthma 349
Decadron (dexamethasone) *283*
decongestants, allergic rhinitis 157
deoxyribonucleic acid (DNA), defined 528
dexamethasone *283*, 286
Diaz-Sanchez, David 460
diesel, defined 528
diet and nutrition
  asthma 231–35
  gastroesophageal reflux disease 181
  osteoporosis 191
  sinusitis 169–71
Disease Detectives: Dr. Asthma, Web site address 544
Diskhaler
  depicted *324*
  described 323–24

Index

"Diskhaler" (Asthma Society of Canada) 313n
Diskus
  depicted *325*
  described 324-25
"Diskus" (Asthma Society of Canada) 313n
disodium cromoglycate 157
diuretics, cardiac asthma *143*
DNA *see* deoxyribonucleic acid
"Do Hormonal Cycles Affect Asthma?" (Heilman) 493n
Dolovich, Myrna B. 498-99
Dombrowski, Mitchell 90, 471
Don't Let Asthma Keep You Out of the Game, Web site address 544
The Doser 319
Dougherty, Denise 425n
DPI *see* dry powder inhalers
drug interactions, older adults 85-86
dry powder inhalers (DPI) 314, 317
dust mites
  allergic response 99
  asthma triggers 28-29
  childhood asthma 362
  defined 528-29
  described 249
  hyposensitization 34-35
  prevention 45-46
"Dust Mites" (EPA) 247n
dust sensitivity, bedrooms 261-64
dysphonia, corticosteroids 304
dyspnea
  asthma diagnosis 107-8
  described 5, 98
  see also shortness of breath

E

"Early Fevers Associated with Lower Allergy Risk Later in Childhood" (NIH) 457n
"East Meets West: Treating Asthmatics with Acupuncture" (Cook) 331n
EIA *see* exercise-induced asthma

electronic air filters, described 257
emergency calls, described 54-55
emotional concerns
  asthma 218
  asthma emergencies 55-56
"Emotional Problems Common in Teens With Asthma" (Nemours Foundation) 373n
emphysema
  versus asthma 42
  described 148, 528
End Allergy and Asthma Misery: It's Worth a Shot, Web site address 545
environmental control measures, defined 529
Environmental Protection Agency (EPA) *see* US Environmental Protection Agency
environmental tobacco smoke
  asthma trigger 27
  children 61
  defined 529
"Enzyme May Play Unexpected Role in Asthma" (NIH) 457n
eosinophils
  allergic process 100
  asthma diagnosis 111
  steroid-resistant asthma 132
EPA (Environmental Protection Agency) *see* US Environmental Protection Agency
Epi-Pen
  asthma emergencies 56
  defined 529
ethnic factors, asthma statistics 400-402, 413-18
exacerbations
  defined 529
  described 9
  pregnancy 94
  seasonal allergic asthma 14
exercise
  asthma 218
  asthma trigger 28, 39-41
  bronchodilators 310
  childhood asthma 66-67
  osteoporosis 191
  sinusitis 169

569

exercise-induced asthma (EIA)
  defined 529
  described 39–41, 103
  overview 119–25
  treatment 279
explanation of benefits, described 552
extrinsic asthma *see* allergic asthma

F

Fabian, Denise 407n
face masks, children 60
Fauci, Anthony S. 458, 459, 461, 463
fear, asthma emergencies 55–56
fenoterol 224
fentanyl 137
FESS *see* functional endoscopic sinus surgery
FEV *see* forced expiratory volume
financial considerations
  acupuncture 335
  asthma statistics 407–11
  asthma treatment 504–10, *505*
  childhood asthma 426
  see also insurance coverage
"Finding a Good Doctor" (AANMA) 195n
Fineman, Stanley M. 503n
FIVC *see* forced inspiratory vital capacity
Flovent (fluticasone) *123, 283*
flu *see* influenza
flunisolide *283*
flu shots *see under* vaccines
fluticasone 29, 31, *283*
fluticasone/salmeterol *283*
flutter inhalation device, sinusitis 169
food allergies, asthma 173–77
Foradil (formoterol) *283*
forced expiratory volume (FEV)
  allergic rhinitis 156
  asthma diagnosis 109
  defined 529
  steroid-resistant asthma 131–32
forced inspiratory vital capacity (FIVC), defined 529

forced vital capacity (FVC), defined 529
Ford, Earl 481, 485
formoterol 30, *283*
fossil fuels, allergic response 99–100
Fredberg, Jeffrey 483
Friedman, Bernard 425n
Fromm, Robert E., Jr. 332–33
functional endoscopic sinus surgery (FESS), sinusitis 164
fungi
  allergic response 99
  defined 529
  see also molds
fungus *see* fungi
FVC *see* forced vital capacity

G

gas phase air filters, described 257
gastroenterologists, described 197
gastroesophageal reflux disease (GERD)
  asthma 104–5, 219
  diet and nutrition 234
  overview 179–81
  sinusitis 168
genes
  ADAM33 101
  asthma research 489–91
  defined 529
  GSTM1 459–60
  GSTP1 459–60
  GSTT1 459–60
  Nrf2 487–88
"Genetics Play Role In Response to Most Common Asthma Drug" (NIH) 457n
George, Maureen 295–97
GERD *see* gastroesophageal reflux disease
"GERD and Asthma" (Cleveland Clinic) 179n
GINA *see* Global Initiative for Asthma
"Global Burden of Asthma" (Masoli, et al.) 407n

Index

Global Initiative for Asthma (GINA)
   asthma overview publication 17n
   Web site address 540
glucocorticoids, steroid-resistant asthma 131–32
glucocorticosteroids 29–32, 157
   see also corticosteroids
Goldberg, Ellie 387n
grapeseed extract 293
Grossan, Murray 163n
Groth, Maritza 135n
ground level ozone, defined 530
growth factors, remodeling process 101
Gruchalla, Rebecca 479
guaifenesin 169

H

Haggerty, Catherine L. 493
Haran, Christine 295n
health insurance *see* insurance coverage
"Health Insurance" (AAFA) 547n
Health Kids: The Key to Basics, contact information 541
health maintenance organizations (HMO), described 549
heartburn, asthma 104
heart disease, asthma 141–45
"Heart Disease and Asthma: A Complex Combination" (Cook) 141n
Heilman, Erica 493n
"Help Your Child Gain Control Over Asthma" (EPA) 207n, 359n, 361n
HEPA filters *see* high efficiency particulate air filters
herbal remedies
   asthma treatment 293–94
   childhood asthma 358
heredity
   allergic asthma 118
   allergies 58
   asthma 9, 83, 101
   childhood asthma 65
   emphysema 42, 148–49
   sinusitis 166
Hershey, Gurjit K. Khurana 489–91

hidden ingredients, defined 530
high efficiency particulate air filters (HEPA filters)
   animal dander 366
   asthma triggers 28–29
   bedrooms 263
   children 61
   defined 530
   described 258
high-risk pool, described 547
histamine, defined 530
HMO *see* health maintenance organizations
home environment
   allergic asthma 118
   childhood asthma 342
   improvement 43–44
   sinusitis 166–67
homeopathy, asthma treatment 293
home schooling, childhood asthma 381–82
hormones
   asthma 101–2, 219
   asthma research 493–95
"How Asthma-Friendly Is your Child-Care Setting" (NHLBI) 375n
"How Asthma-Friendly Is Your School?" (NHLBI) 375n
"How Is Asthma Treated" (NHLBI) 275n
"How to Identify and Asthma Emergency" (AANMA) 53n
humidity
   asthma 237–38
   exercise 221–22
hybrid air filters, described 257
hydrocortisone *283*
hydrogen peroxide, asthma diagnosis 111
hyperreactive response, described 98
hypersensitivity diseases, defined 530
hypersensitivity pneumonitis, described 530
hyperventilation
   asthma 14
   asthma attacks 23
   status asthmaticus 137
hypnosis, asthma treatment 292
hyposensitization, described 26, 34–35

I

ibuprofen 102
IEP *see* individualized education programs
"If My Child Has Asthma, Can We Keep Our Pet?" (Nemours Foundation) 365n
IgE antibodies
  allergic asthma 114, 115
  allergic process 100
  allergic rhinitis 154
  childhood asthma 65
  food allergies 174
  medication 329–30
IgE inhibitors, asthma treatment 283, 329–30
IHP *see* individualized health plans
immune system
  defined 530
  food allergies 174
  immunologists 197
  inflammatory response 98
  steroid-resistant asthma 132
immunoglobulins
  allergic process 100
  defined 530
  described 65
immunologists, described 197
immunotherapy
  allergic rhinitis 160
  asthma treatment plans 16
inciters, described 20
individualized education programs (IEP), asthma management 384
individualized health plans (IHP), asthma management 389
indoor air pollutants
  defined 530
  overview 247–54
"Indoor Environmental Asthma Triggers" (EPA) 247n
inducers, described 20
induction of asthma, defined 530
infants
  asthma 57–62
  coughs 350

infections
  asthma 103–4, 218
  asthma triggers 22, 38–39
inflammation
  airway obstruction 15
  bronchitis 148
  bronchodilators 312
  defined 530
  described 17–18, 58, 64
  medications 31
inflammatory response, described 98
influenza, overview 183–88
inhalers
  defined 531
  sports activities 224–25
  see also metered dose inhalers
insects
  asthma triggers 250–51
  childhood asthma 363
insurance coverage
  air filters 260
  asthma education 342
  asthma-related services 547–53
Intal (cromolyn) *123*, 225, 283
integrated pest management (IPM), defined 531
interleukins
  allergic process 100
  remodeling process 101
  steroid-resistant asthma 132
intermittent asthma, described 7
International Asthma Quality of Care Initiative, Web site address 541
International Food Information Council, food allergies publication 173n
Internet, prescription medications 556–57
intrinsic asthma, described 116
IPM *see* integrated pest management
ipratropium *283*
ipratropium/albuterol *283*
ipratropium bromide
  allergic rhinitis 158
  asthma 68
  exercise-induced asthma *123*
  status asthmaticus 138
irritant, defined 531

isoetharine 282
isoproterenol 281
Israel, Elliot 468, 475
Isuprel (isoproterenol) 281

J

Jaakkola, Jouni 473
JAMA Asthma Information Center, Web site address 545
Johns Hopkins University, asthma research publication 487n
Johnson, Christine C. 461

K

ketamine 138
"Key Facts about Flu Vaccine" (CDC) 183n
"Key Facts about Influenza and the Influenza Vaccine" (CDC) 183n
Kiley, James 469, 474
King, Nina 458
Kita, Hirohito 465–66
Kvale, Paul A. 499

L

LAIV *see* live attenuated influenza vaccine
"Landmark Survey Reveals Asthma in Children Remains Significantly out of Control in the United States: Asthma Control in Children Falls Far Short of National Treatment Goals" (American Lung Association) 419n
larynx, depicted *4, 6*
legislation
 chronic illnesses, schools 384
 disabled students 384, 390–91
 health insurance 547–48
Lessin, Herschel 339n
leukotriene inhibitors, childhood asthma 344

leukotriene modifiers
 asthma treatment 277, *283*, 289–90
 childhood asthma 70
leukotrienes
 allergic process 100
 described 340
Leung, Donald Y. M. 131n
levalbuterol 282, *283*
lifestyles, asthma 42–44
live attenuated influenza vaccine (LAIV) 184–86
Locke-Ringer moisturizer spray, sinusitis 169
long-term acting medication, defined 531
"Long Term Effects of Asthma Therapy" (Szefler) 515n
loratadine 158
lower respiratory tract, depicted *4*
"Lung - COPD and Asthma" (National Lung Health Education Program) 147n
lungs, depicted *4, 6*
lung volume (VL), defined 531
lymphocytes, defined 531

M

"Make an Asthma Action Plan" (EPA) 207n
managed care plans, described 549
"Managing Asthma for Patients and Families" (Weinberger) 3n, 53n, 203n
Managing Asthma for Patients and Families, Web site address 545
Masoli, Matthew 407n
massage therapy
 asthma treatment 292
 childhood asthma 358
mast cells
 allergic process 100
 described 340
mast cell stabilizers
 childhood asthma 344
 exercise-induced asthma *123*
Maxair (pirbuterol) 281, *283*

Asthma Sourcebook, Second Edition

maximal aerobic capacity
  (max VO2), defined 531
maximum breathing capacity
  (MBC), defined 531
maximum expiratory flow
  (Vmax x), defined 531–32
maximum voluntary ventilation
  (MVV), described 531
max VO2 *see* maximal aerobic
  capacity
Mayo Clinic Health Oasis, Web
  site address 545
MBC *see* maximum breathing
  capacity
MDI *see* metered-dose inhalers
Meadows, Michelle 207n
mechanical air filters, described
  257
Medicaid, childhood asthma 426
Medicare, asthma services 551
medication delivery devices,
  overview 313–28
medications
  adult onset asthma 78–79
  allergic rhinitis 156–59
  assistance programs 555–56
  asthma 7, 83
  asthma control 29–35
  asthma treatment 276–77, 295–97
  asthma treatment plans 15
  asthma triggers 21
  bronchospasm 5
  cardiac asthma 142–44, *143*
  childhood asthma 68–70, 343–45
  exercise 222
  exercise-induced asthma 122, *123*
  older adults 85–86
  online ordering 556–57
  osteoporosis 189–92
  sports activities 224–25
  status asthmaticus 138–39
  see also individual medications
Medigap, described 551
Medihaler-Iso (isoproterenol) 281
meditation, asthma treatment 292
Medrol (methylprednisolone) *283*
menopause
  asthma 102
  asthma research 493–95

menstruation
  asthma 101–2, 219
  asthma research 493–95
metalloproteases 101
Metaprel (metaproterenol) 281
metaproterenol 68, 281, *283*
metered-dose inhalers (MDI)
  childhood asthma 69
  defined 531
  depicted *320*
  overview 314–22
  research 497–99
methylprednisolone 68, *283*
methylxanthine *283*
"Microbes: In Sickness and in Health"
  (NIAID) 525n
mild intermittent asthma, described
  341
mild persistent asthma, described 341
mites *see* dust mites
moderate persistent asthma,
  described 341
molds
  allergic response 99
  asthma triggers 249–50
  childhood asthma 363
  defined 532
  see also fungi
"Molds" (EPA) 247n
mometasone *283*, 286
"Monitoring My Child's Asthma"
  (Children's Hospital of Eastern
  Ontario) 353n
monoclonal antibodies, childhood
  asthma 345
montelukast 158, *283*
"More Than Half the U.S. Population
  Is Sensitive to One or More
  Allergens" (NIH) 457n
Morgan, Wayne J. 465
mucociliary transport, defined 532
mucus
  asthma attacks 49–50
  bronchitis 147–48
  defined 532
  described 58
  inflammatory response 98
  respiratory system 4–5
  sinusitis 164

Index

mucus membranes, respiratory system 4–5
MVV *see* maximum voluntary ventilation
MyPyramid Plan *232*

N

Nabel, Elizabeth G. 474
NAEPP *see* National Asthma Education and Prevention Program
naproxen 102
nasal breathing, exercise-induced asthma 122
nasal cavity, depicted *4*
nasal challenge, allergic rhinitis 154–55
nasal douching, allergic rhinitis 159
nasal endoscopy, allergic rhinitis 153
nasopharyngeal, defined 532
National Allergy Bureau, Web site address 545
National Asthma Education and Prevention Program (NAEPP)
  asthma during pregnancy 89–91
  contact information 541
"National Asthma Education and Prevention Program Resolution on Asthma Management at School" (NHLBI) 375n
National Education Association Health Information Network, glossary publication 525n
National Heart, Lung, and Blood Institute (NHLBI)
  contact information 541
  publications
    asthma treatment 275n
    childcare settings 375n
    pregnancy 89n
    school absenteeism 379n
    school settings 375n
National Institute of Allergy and Infectious Diseases (NIAID)
  contact information 541
  glossary publication 525n
National Institute of Environmental Health Sciences (NIEHS)
  contact information 541
  indoor mold publication 457n
National Institutes of Health (NIH), asthma research publications 457n
National Jewish Medical and Research Center, contact information 541
National Lung Health Education Program
  contact information 541
  COPD publication 147n
"National Study Shows 82 Percent of U.S. Homes Have Mouse Allergens" (NIH) 457n
nebulizers
  childhood asthma 343
  children 60
  defined 532
  described 314, 326–28
"Nebulizer Treatment and Cleaning" (Cincinnati Children's Hospital Medical Center) 313n
nedocromil 32, *123*, 157, 277, *283*
Nemours Foundation, publications
  childhood cough 347n
  emergency care 369n
  emotional problems 373n
  pets 365n
  weather influences 237n
"New Guidelines Conclude All Aerosol Therapy Devices Equally Effective" (American College of Chest Physicians) 497n
"New Treatment Guidelines for Pregnant Women with Asthma" (NHLBI) 89n
"New Treatment Guidelines for Pregnant Women with Asthma" (NIH) 457n
New York City Asthma Initiative, Web site address 541
NHLBI *see* National Heart, Lung, and Blood Institute
"NHLBI Study Suggests Symptom-Driven Therapy May Be Sufficient for Some Adults with Mild Persistent Asthma" (NIH) 457n

NIAID *see* National Institute of Allergy and Infectious Diseases
NIEHS *see* National Institute of Environmental Health Sciences
nighttime cough, childhood asthma 349
nitric oxide, asthma diagnosis 111
nitrogen dioxide (NO2)
  asthma trigger 253–54
  childhood asthma 363–64
  defined 532
Nitrogen Dioxide (NO2)" (EPA) 247n
NO2 *see* nitrogen dioxide
No Attacks, Web site address 545
nocturnal asthma, described 103
non-allergic asthma, described 116
nonsteroidal anti-inflammatory drugs (NSAID)
  asthma 102–3
  described 32–35
Norisodrine (isoproterenol) 281
Northwest Asthma and Allergy Center, contact information 541
NSAID *see* nonsteroidal anti-inflammatory drugs
nutrition *see* diet and nutrition

O

obesity, asthma research 481–85
occupational asthma
  described 116
  overview 127–30
Olden, Kenneth 463, 478
omalizumab *283*, 291–92, 345
Ontario Lung Association, contact information 542
open enrollment period, described 547
Orapred (prednisolone) *283*
orthodontists, described 197
osteoporosis
  corticosteroids 37–38, 285, 305–6
  overview 189–92
otolaryngologists, described 197

outdoor air pollution
  childhood asthma 364
  defined 532
  described 7–9
  overview 243–46
"Outdoor Air Pollution" (EPA) 243n
out-of-pocket costs, described 549–50
ozone
  air filters 257–59
  defined 532–33
  described 530
  research 438–39
ozone action days 243–44
ozone generators, described 257–58

P

panic, asthma emergencies 55–56
paracetamol 34
paramedics, asthma emergencies 55
particles, defined 533
particulate matter, defined 533
pathogen, defined 533
peak expiratory flow (PEF)
  allergic rhinitis 156
  asthma attacks 25
  asthma emergencies 54
  defined 533
peak expiratory flow rate (PEFR), asthma diagnosis 109
peak flow meters
  asthma attacks 26
  asthma monitoring 211–16
  asthma treatment 277–78
  childhood asthma 342–43, 355–56, 371
  defined 533
  described 116
  older adults 85
  sample chart *213*
"Peak Flow Meters" (American Lung Association) 211n
PEF *see* peak expiratory flow
PEFR *see* peak expiratory flow rate
perennial, defined 533
persistent asthma *see* chronic asthma
persistent cough, childhood asthma 349–50

576

Index

pertussis 348
pest management, described 251
pets
  asthma 44, 46
  asthma triggers 252–53
  bedrooms 264
  childhood asthma 362–63, 365–67
  children 61
  school settings 387–91
"Pets" (EPA) 247n
pharynx, depicted *4*
phlegm *see* mucus
physical activity, osteoporosis 38
physicians
  asthma care 199–202
  asthma treatment plans 13–16
  cardiac asthma 142, 145
  childhood coughing 350–51
  locating 195–98
pirbuterol 68, 281, *283*
"Plan for Attendance" (AANMA) 379n
Plaut, Marshall 465
pneumonia
  defined 533
  pulmonologists 197
point of service (POS), described 549
pollen, allergic response 99
POS *see* point of service
PPO *see* preferred provider organizations
prednisolone 32, 68, *283*
prednisone 32, 68, *123*, 131, *283*
preexisting condition limit, described 548
preferred provider organizations (PPO), described 549
pregnancy
  asthma 89–94, 102, 219
  asthma research 469–72
  asthma treatment 279
  budesonide 32
  tobacco use 266
Prelone (prednisolone) *283*
"Pressured Metered Dose Inhaler" (Asthma Society of Canada) 313n
probiotics, asthma treatment 293
Project A: Knock the Breath out of Asthma, Web site address 545

Proventil (albuterol) *123*, 281, *283*, 314–15, 318
pseudoephedrine, sinusitis 169
"Puffs, Sprays, Powders, and Mists, oh my!" (Sander) 313n
Pulmicort (budesonide) *123*, *283*, 315
pulmonary function tests, asthma diagnosis 109–10
pulmonologists
  cardiac asthma 142
  children 60
  described 197
pursed lips breathing, asthma emergencies 56

Q

"Q&A: What Is Asthma" (Global Initiative for Asthma) 17n
"Questions and Answers about Exercising With Allergies and Asthma" (American College of Allergy, Asthma and Immunology) 221n
Quibron (theophylline) *283*
"Quick Reference from the Working Group Report on Managing Asthma During Pregnancy: Recommendations for Pharmacological Treatment" (NHLBI) 89n
quick relief medication
  childhood asthma 68–69
  defined 533
QVAR (beclomethasone) *283*

R

racial factor
  allergic asthma 116
  asthma statistics *403*, 403–4, *404*, *405*, 413–18
  childhood asthma 63
refractory period
  described 225
  exercise-induced asthma 122
regulation, nitrogen dioxide 532

relaxation techniques
  asthma 43
  asthma emergencies 56
  asthma treatment 292
  exercise-induced asthma 122
relievers, described 30, 31
remodeling, described 12, 100–101
rescue medications
  versus controller medications 299–301
  emergency care 371
"Researchers Discover Gene that Determines Asthma Susceptibility by Regulating Inflammation" (Johns Hopkins University) 487n
residual volume (RV), defined 533
respiratory cycle, defined 533
respiratory failure, status asthmaticus 137
respiratory period, described 533
respiratory system
  depicted *4*
  described 525
respiratory virus
  asthma 58, 103–4
  defined 533
  see also infections
rheology, described 164
rhinitis
  asthma 151–61
  defined 534
  described 116
  see also allergic rhinitis
ribonucleic acid (RNA), defined 534
"Rights and Responsibilities of Patients with Asthma" (Weinberger) 199n
risk factors, defined 534
RNA *see* ribonucleic acid
roaches, childhood asthma 363
rofecoxib 103
Rothenberg, Marc E. 457–59
Rotrosen, Daniel 464
RV *see* residual volume

S

salbutamol 30, 281
salmeterol *283*, 287–89

Sander, Nancy 313n
Satcher, David 508
SAY *see* Support for Asthmatic Youth
Schatz, Michael 91, 472
school settings
  absenteeism 379–85
  animals 387–91
  asthma management 376–78
Schwartz, David A. 477
"Scientists Identify Genes that Regulate Allergic Responses to Diesel Fumes" (NIH) 457n
Sears, William 419
seasonal allergic asthma, described 13–14
secondhand smoke
  air filters 259
  asthma trigger 248, 265–66
  childhood asthma 66
  defined 534
"Secondhand Smoke" (EPA) 247n
second opinions, insurance coverage 552
second wave, asthma attacks 50–51
self-management, asthma 71–72
sensitivity, defined 534
sensitization
  defined 534
  described 528
Serevent (salmeterol) *123*, *283*, 287
severe persistent asthma, described 341
shortness of breath
  adult onset asthma 77
  asthma diagnosis 107–8
  childhood asthma 67
  emphysema 148
  gastroesophageal reflux disease 180
  older adults 82
  see also dyspnea
shots *see* hyposensitization; immunotherapy; vaccines
side effects
  asthma 35–36
  beta agonists 282, 288
  childhood asthma medications 68
  corticosteroids 32, 36, 69, 287, 304–7
  cromolyn 289

Index

side effects, continued
  influenza vaccine 186–87
  leukotriene modifiers 290
  peak flow meters 216
Singulair (montelukast) *283*
sinuses, defined 534
sinusitis
  asthma 105
  described 116
  overview 163–72
sleeping pills, drug interactions 85–86
Slo-bid *123*
Slo-Phyllin *123*
smooth muscle, described 4–5
social life, asthma 44
sodium cromoglycate 32
"Spacer" (Asthma Society of Canada) 313n
spacers
  childhood asthma 343
  defined 534
  depicted *322*
  described 321–22
specialists, described 196–97
Spiriva (tiotropium) *283*
spirometry
  asthma diagnosis 109–10
  defined 534
sports activities
  adolescents 73
  corticosteroids 41
  exercise guidelines 221–29
  exercise-induced asthma 124
sputum, defined 534
  see also mucus
Stanton, Mark W. 425n
statistics
  adolescents, asthma 373–74
  asthma 57, 503–4
  asthma global burden 407–11
  asthma prevalence 399–403, *400, 401, 402*
  childhood asthma 63–64, 419–23
  food allergies 173
  health care use 403–4
  influenza 183, 187–88
  older adults 81
  sinusitis 163, 164–65

"Status Asthmaticus" (Groth) 135n
status asthmaticus, overview 135–39
Stenius-Aarniala, Brita 484
steroid-resistant asthma, overview 131–33
"Steroid Resistant Asthma: Definition and Mechanisms" (Leung) 131n
steroids
  adolescents 72
  bone density 279
  childhood asthma 344–45
  described 32
  diet and nutrition 234–35
  glaucoma 501–2
  sinusitis 169
  varicella 393–96
"Sticking to the Schedule: Why People Don't Take Their Asthma Medication" (Haran) 295n
stress reduction, asthma treatment 292
stretching, described 226–27
stridor, childhood asthma 348
"Students with Chronic Illnesses: Guidance for Families, Schools, and Students" (NHLBI) 379n
"Study: Mold in Homes Doubles Risk of Asthma" (NIEHS) 457n
Sulit, Loreto G. 483
Support for Asthmatic Youth (SAY), contact information 542
surgical procedures
  allergic rhinitis 159
  sinusitis 163–64, 170
suspension, described 315
systemic corticosteroids
  see corticosteroids
Szefler, Stanley J. 515n

T

T cells
  allergic process 100
  defined 535
teenagers *see* adolescents

terbutaline 30, 68, 169, 281
tests
  adult onset asthma 77
  allergic asthma 115
  allergic rhinitis 153–55
  allergies 65
  asthma diagnosis 109–11
  food allergies 175
  infants 60
Theo-24 (theophylline) *283*
Theo-Dur *123*
theophylline
  asthma treatment *283*, 290–91
  bronchodilators 311–12
  cardiac asthma *143*
  childhood asthma 344
  described 33, 277
  exercise-induced asthma *123*
  side effects 35
  status asthmaticus 138
thrush
  corticosteroids 304
  described 69
tidal volume, described 533
tightness in chest
  adult onset asthma 76
  asthma diagnosis 108
  childhood asthma 67
  infants 59
  older adults 82
Tilade (nedocromil) 225, *283*
tiotropium *283*
tobacco use
  asthma 83, 265–67
  gastroesophageal reflux disease 181
  occupational asthma 130
  prevention 46
Tornalate (bitolterol) 282
trachea
  defined 535
  depicted *4*, *6*
  described 3, 58
travel concerns
  asthma management 269–71
  medical emergencies 552
"Treatment Of Childhood Asthma" (Lessin) 339n
triamcinolone *283*

triggers
  asthma 14, 19–22, 217–19
  avoidance 27–29
  bronchospasm 5
  childhood asthma 65–67, 342, 361–64
  defined 535
  described 117
  emergency care 370–71
  exercise-induced asthma 120
  food allergies 176–77
  indoor air pollutants 247–54
  irritants 531
  viral infections 7, 9
Trotter, J. McLean 142, 145
"Turbuhaler" (Asthma Society of Canada) 313n
Turbuhaler
  depicted *323*
  described 322–23
twins, asthma 9
twitchy airways, described 58

U

Uniphyl (theophylline) *283*
upper respiratory tract
  defined 535
  depicted *4*
US Environmental Protection Agency (EPA)
  contact information 542
  publications
    asthma action plans 207n
    asthma control 359n, 361n
    asthma research 435n
    indoor asthma triggers 247n
    outdoor air pollution 243n
"Using Your Puffer Tip Sheet" (Asthma Society of Canada) 313n

V

vaccines
  defined 535
  diphtheria-tetanus-pertussis 348
  influenza 184–88
vacuum cleaners, asthma triggers 28

Index

Vanceril *123*
varicella, corticosteroids 306, 393–96
Varon, Joseph 332, 334
vascular endothelial growth factor (VEGF), described 101
VC *see* vital capacity
VEGF *see* vascular endothelial growth factor
ventilatory frequency, described 533
ventilatory period, described 533
Ventolin (albuterol) *123*, 225, 281, *283*, 314–15, 318
Vioxx (rofecoxib) 103
viral infections
   childhood asthma 66
   described 117
vital capacity (VC)
   defined 535
   described 109
VL *see* lung volume
Vmax x *see* maximum expiratory flow

W

warming up, described 226
Wasserman, Richard L. 208
water pills *see* diuretics
weather changes
   allergic asthma 117
   asthma 218
   asthma triggers 21–22
   childhood asthma 237–41
weight control, diet and nutrition 231
"A Weighty Issue for Those with Asthma" (Alford) 481n
Weinberger, Miles 3n, 53n, 199n, 203n
"What Is a Specialist?" (AANMA) 195n
What's Asthma All About?, Web site address 545
"What to Do Until Paramedics Arrive" (AANMA) 53n
"What to Do when Animals in School Make Your Child Sick" (Goldberg) 387n
"What to Expect When Calling 9-1-1" (AANMA) 53n
wheeze, defined 535
wheezing
   adult onset asthma 76
   asthma diagnosis 107
   childhood asthma 67, 348
   defined 535
   described 7
   infants 59
   older adults 82
   steroid-resistant asthma 132
"When to Go to the ER if Your Child Has Asthma" (Nemours Foundation) 369n
whooping cough, described 348
windpipe *see* trachea
women
   adult onset asthma 76
   asthma statistics 400–402, *403*, *404*, *405*
workplace, asthma 43
   see also occupational asthma

X

Xanthine derivatives, exercise-induced asthma *123*
Xolair (omalizumab) 117, *283*, 329–30, 345
Xopenex (levalbuterol) 282, *283*

Y

"Your Child's Cough" (Nemours Foundation) 347n
"Your Doctor's Credentials" (AANMA) 195n

Z

zafirlukast *283*
Zeldin, Darryl C. 477
zileuton *283*
Zimmerman, Nives 458
Zitt, Myron J. 499
Zyflo (zileuton) *283*

Health Reference Series
COMPLETE CATALOG
List price $87 per volume. **School and library price $78 per volume.**

Adolescent Health Sourcebook

Basic Consumer Health Information about Common Medical, Mental, and Emotional Concerns in Adolescents, Including Facts about Acne, Body Piercing, Mononucleosis, Nutrition, Eating Disorders, Stress, Depression, Behavior Problems, Peer Pressure, Violence, Gangs, Drug Use, Puberty, Sexuality, Pregnancy, Learning Disabilities, and More

Along with a Glossary of Terms and Other Resources for Further Help and Information

Edited by Chad T. Kimball. 658 pages. 2002. 0-7808-0248-9.

"It is written in clear, nontechnical language aimed at general readers.... Recommended for public libraries, community colleges, and other agencies serving health care consumers."
—*American Reference Books Annual, 2003*

"Recommended for school and public libraries. Parents and professionals dealing with teens will appreciate the easy-to-follow format and the clearly written text. This could become a 'must have' for every high school teacher." —*E-Streams, Jan '03*

"A good starting point for information related to common medical, mental, and emotional concerns of adolescents." —*School Library Journal, Nov '02*

"This book provides accurate information in an easy to access format. It addresses topics that parents and caregivers might not be aware of and provides practical, useable information." —*Doody's Health Sciences Book Review Journal, Sep-Oct '02*

"Recommended reference source."
—*Booklist, American Library Association, Sep '02*

AIDS Sourcebook, 3rd Edition

Basic Consumer Health Information about Acquired Immune Deficiency Syndrome (AIDS) and Human Immunodeficiency Virus (HIV) Infection, Including Facts about Transmission, Prevention, Diagnosis, Treatment, Opportunistic Infections, and Other Complications, with a Section for Women and Children, Including Details about Associated Gynecological Concerns, Pregnancy, and Pediatric Care

Along with Updated Statistical Information, Reports on Current Research Initiatives, a Glossary, and Directories of Internet, Hotline, and Other Resources

Edited by Dawn D. Matthews. 664 pages. 2003. 0-7808-0631-X.

ALSO AVAILABLE: *AIDS Sourcebook, 1st Edition.* Edited by Karen Bellenir and Peter D. Dresser. 831 pages. 1995. 0-7808-0031-1.

AIDS Sourcebook, 2nd Edition. Edited by Karen Bellenir. 751 pages. 1999. 0-7808-0225-X.

"The 3rd edition of the *AIDS Sourcebook*, part of Omnigraphics' *Health Reference Series*, is a welcome update.... This resource is highly recommended for academic and public libraries."
—*American Reference Books Annual, 2004*

"Excellent sourcebook. This continues to be a highly recommended book. There is no other book that provides as much information as this book provides."
—*AIDS Book Review Journal, Dec-Jan 2000*

"Recommended reference source."
—*Booklist, American Library Association, Dec '99*

"A solid text for college-level health libraries."
—*The Bookwatch, Aug '99*

Cited in *Reference Sources for Small and Medium-Sized Libraries, American Library Association, 1999*

Alcoholism Sourcebook

Basic Consumer Health Information about the Physical and Mental Consequences of Alcohol Abuse, Including Liver Disease, Pancreatitis, Wernicke-Korsakoff Syndrome (Alcoholic Dementia), Fetal Alcohol Syndrome, Heart Disease, Kidney Disorders, Gastrointestinal Problems, and Immune System Compromise and Featuring Facts about Addiction, Detoxification, Alcohol Withdrawal, Recovery, and the Maintenance of Sobriety

Along with a Glossary and Directories of Resources for Further Help and Information

Edited by Karen Bellenir. 613 pages. 2000. 0-7808-0325-6.

"This title is one of the few reference works on alcoholism for general readers. For some readers this will be a welcome complement to the many self-help books on the market. Recommended for collections serving general readers and consumer health collections."
—*E-Streams, Mar '01*

"This book is an excellent choice for public and academic libraries."
—*American Reference Books Annual, 2001*

"Recommended reference source."
—*Booklist, American Library Association, Dec '00*

"Presents a wealth of information on alcohol use and abuse and its effects on the body and mind, treatment, and prevention." —*SciTech Book News, Dec '00*

"Important new health guide which packs in the latest consumer information about the problems of alcoholism." —*Reviewer's Bookwatch, Nov '00*

SEE ALSO *Drug Abuse Sourcebook, Substance Abuse Sourcebook*

583

Allergies Sourcebook, 2nd Edition

Basic Consumer Health Information about Allergic Disorders, Triggers, Reactions, and Related Symptoms, Including Anaphylaxis, Rhinitis, Sinusitis, Asthma, Dermatitis, Conjunctivitis, and Multiple Chemical Sensitivity

Along with Tips on Diagnosis, Prevention, and Treatment, Statistical Data, a Glossary, and a Directory of Sources for Further Help and Information

Edited by Annemarie S. Muth. 598 pages. 2002. 0-7808-0376-0.

ALSO AVAILABLE: Allergies Sourcebook, 1st Edition. Edited by Allan R. Cook. 611 pages. 1997. 0-7808-0036-2.

"This book brings a great deal of useful material together.... This is an excellent addition to public and consumer health library collections."
—American Reference Books Annual, 2003

"This second edition would be useful to laypersons with little or advanced knowledge of the subject matter. This book would also serve as a resource for nursing and other health care professions students. It would be useful in public, academic, and hospital libraries with consumer health collections." —E-Streams, Jul '02

Alternative Medicine Sourcebook, 2nd Edition

SEE Complementary & Alternative Medicine Sourcebook, 3rd Edition

Alzheimer's Disease Sourcebook, 3rd Edition

Basic Consumer Health Information about Alzheimer's Disease, Other Dementias, and Related Disorders, Including Multi-Infarct Dementia, AIDS Dementia Complex, Dementia with Lewy Bodies, Huntington's Disease, Wernicke-Korsakoff Syndrome (Alcohol-Reated Dementia), Delirium, and Confusional States

Along with Information for People Newly Diagnosed with Alzheimer's Disease and Caregivers, Reports Detailing Current Research Efforts in Prevention, Diagnosis, and Treatment, Facts about Long-Term Care Issues, and Listings of Sources for Additional Information

Edited by Karen Bellenir. 645 pages. 2003. 0-7808-0666-2.

ALSO AVAILABLE: Alzheimer's, Stroke & 29 Other Neurological Disorders Sourcebook, 1st Edition. Edited by Frank E. Bair. 579 pages. 1993. 1-55888-748-2.

Alzheimer's Disease Sourcebook, 2nd Edition. Edited by Karen Bellenir. 524 pages. 1999. 0-7808-0223-3.

"This very informative and valuable tool will be a great addition to any library serving consumers, students and health care workers."
—American Reference Books Annual, 2004

"This is a valuable resource for people affected by dementias such as Alzheimer's. It is easy to navigate and includes important information and resources."
—Doody's Review Service, Feb. 2004

"Recommended reference source."
—Booklist, American Library Association, Oct '99

SEE ALSO Brain Disorders Sourcebook

Arthritis Sourcebook, 2nd Edition

Basic Consumer Health Information about Osteoarthritis, Rheumatoid Arthritis, Other Rheumatic Disorders, Infectious Forms of Arthritis, and Diseases with Symptoms Linked to Arthritis, Featuring Facts about Diagnosis, Pain Management, and Surgical Therapies

Along with Coping Strategies, Research Updates, a Glossary, and Resources for Additional Help and Information

Edited by Amy L. Sutton. 593 pages. 2004. 0-7808-0667-0.

ALSO AVAILABLE: Arthritis Sourcebook, 1st Edition. Edited by Allan R. Cook. 550 pages. 1998. 0-7808-0201-2.

"... accessible to the layperson."
—Reference and Research Book News, Feb '99

Asthma Sourcebook, 2nd Edition

Basic Consumer Health Information about the Causes, Symptoms, Diagnosis, and Treatment of Asthma in Infants, Children, Teenagers, and Adults, Including Facts about Different Types of Asthma, Common Co-Occurring Conditions, Asthma Management Plans, Triggers, Medications, and Medication Delivery Devices

Along with Asthma Statistics, Research Updates, a Glossary, a Directory of Asthma-Related Resources, and More

Edited by Karen Bellenir. 609 pages. 2006. 0-7808-0866-5.

ALSO AVAILABLE: Asthma Sourcebook, 1st Edition. Edited by Annemarie S. Muth. 628 pages. 2000. 0-7808-0381-7.

"A worthwhile reference acquisition for public libraries and academic medical libraries whose readers desire a quick introduction to the wide range of asthma information." —Choice, Association of College & Research Libraries, Jun '01

"Recommended reference source."
—Booklist, American Library Association, Feb '01

"Highly recommended." —The Bookwatch, Jan '01

"There is much good information for patients and their families who deal with asthma daily."
—American Medical Writers Association Journal, Winter '01

"This informative text is recommended for consumer health collections in public, secondary school, and community college libraries and the libraries of universities with a large undergraduate population."
—American Reference Books Annual, 2001

Attention Deficit Disorder Sourcebook

Basic Consumer Health Information about Attention Deficit/Hyperactivity Disorder in Children and Adults, Including Facts about Causes, Symptoms, Diagnostic Criteria, and Treatment Options Such as Medications, Behavior Therapy, Coaching, and Homeopathy

Along with Reports on Current Research Initiatives, Legal Issues, and Government Regulations, and Featuring a Glossary of Related Terms, Internet Resources, and a List of Additional Reading Material

Edited by Dawn D. Matthews. 470 pages. 2002. 0-7808-0624-7.

"Recommended reference source."
—*Booklist, American Library Association*, Jan '03

"This book is recommended for all school libraries and the reference or consumer health sections of public libraries." —*American Reference Books Annual*, 2003

Back & Neck Sourcebook, 2nd Edition

Basic Consumer Health Information about Spinal Pain, Spinal Cord Injuries, and Related Disorders, Such as Degenerative Disk Disease, Osteoarthritis, Scoliosis, Sciatica, Spina Bifida, and Spinal Stenosis, and Featuring Facts about Maintaining Spinal Health, Self-Care, Pain Management, Rehabilitative Care, Chiropractic Care, Spinal Surgeries, and Complementary Therapies

Along with Suggestions for Preventing Back and Neck Pain, a Glossary of Related Terms, and a Directory of Resources

Edited by Amy L. Sutton. 633 pages. 2004. 0-7808-0738-3

ALSO AVAILABLE: Back & Neck Disorders Sourcebook, 1st Edition. Edited by Karen Bellenir. 548 pages. 1997. 0-7808-0202-0.

"The strength of this work is its basic, easy-to-read format. Recommended."
—*Reference and User Services Quarterly, American Library Association*, Winter '97

Blood & Circulatory Disorders Sourcebook, 2nd Edition

Basic Consumer Health Information about the Blood and Circulatory System and Related Disorders, Such as Anemia and Other Hemoglobin Diseases, Cancer of the Blood and Associated Bone Marrow Disorders, Clotting and Bleeding Problems, and Conditions That Affect the Veins, Blood Vessels, and Arteries, Including Facts about the Donation and Transplantation of Bone Marrow, Stem Cells, and Blood and Tips for Keeping the Blood and Circulatory System Healthy

Along with a Glossary of Related Terms and Resources for Additional Help and Information

Edited by Amy L. Sutton. 659 pages. 2005. 0-7808-0746-4.

ALSO AVAILABLE: Blood and Circulatory Disorders Sourcebook, 1st Edition. Edited by Karen Bellenir and Linda M. Shin. 554 pages. 1998. 0-7808-0203-9.

"Recommended reference source."
—*Booklist, American Library Association*, Feb '99

"An important reference sourcebook written in simple language for everyday, non-technical users."
—*Reviewer's Bookwatch*, Jan '99

Brain Disorders Sourcebook, 2nd Edition

Basic Consumer Health Information about Acquired and Traumatic Brain Injuries, Infections of the Brain, Epilepsy and Seizure Disorders, Cerebral Palsy, and Degenerative Neurological Disorders, Including Amyotrophic Lateral Sclerosis (ALS), Dementias, Multiple Sclerosis, and More

Along with Information on the Brain's Structure and Function, Treatment and Rehabilitation Options, Reports on Current Research Initiatives, a Glossary of Terms Related to Brain Disorders and Injuries, and a Directory of Sources for Further Help and Information

Edited by Sandra J. Judd. 625 pages. 2005. 0-7808-0744-8.

ALSO AVAILABLE: Brain Disorders Sourcebook, 1st Edition. Edited by Karen Bellenir. 481 pages. 1999. 0-7808-0229-2.

"Belongs on the shelves of any library with a consumer health collection." —*E-Streams*, Mar '00

"Recommended reference source."
—*Booklist, American Library Association*, Oct '99

SEE ALSO Alzheimer's Disease Sourcebook

Breast Cancer Sourcebook, 2nd Edition

Basic Consumer Health Information about Breast Cancer, Including Facts about Risk Factors, Prevention, Screening and Diagnostic Methods, Treatment Options, Complementary and Alternative Therapies, Post-Treatment Concerns, Clinical Trials, Special Risk Populations, and New Developments in Breast Cancer Research

Along with Breast Cancer Statistics, a Glossary of Related Terms, and a Directory of Resources for Additional Help and Information

Edited by Sandra J. Judd. 595 pages. 2004. 0-7808-0668-9.

ALSO AVAILABLE: Breast Cancer Sourcebook, 1st Edition. Edited by Edward J. Prucha and Karen Bellenir. 580 pages. 2001. 0-7808-0244-6.

"It would be a useful reference book in a library or on loan to women in a support group."
—*Cancer Forum*, Mar '03

"Recommended reference source."
—*Booklist, American Library Association*, Jan '02

"This reference source is highly recommended. It is quite informative, comprehensive and detailed in nature, and yet it offers practical advice in easy-to-read language. It could be thought of as the 'bible' of breast cancer for the consumer."
— *E-Streams, Jan '02*

"The broad range of topics covered in lay language make the *Breast Cancer Sourcebook* an excellent addition to public and consumer health library collections."
— *American Reference Books Annual 2002*

"From the pros and cons of different screening methods and results to treatment options, *Breast Cancer Sourcebook* provides the latest information on the subject."
— *Library Bookwatch, Dec '01*

"This thoroughgoing, very readable reference covers all aspects of breast health and cancer.... Readers will find much to consider here. Recommended for all public and patient health collections."
— *Library Journal, Sep '01*

SEE ALSO *Cancer Sourcebook for Women, Women's Health Concerns Sourcebook*

Breastfeeding Sourcebook

Basic Consumer Health Information about the Benefits of Breastmilk, Preparing to Breastfeed, Breastfeeding as a Baby Grows, Nutrition, and More, Including Information on Special Situations and Concerns Such as Mastitis, Illness, Medications, Allergies, Multiple Births, Prematurity, Special Needs, and Adoption

Along with a Glossary and Resources for Additional Help and Information

Edited by Jenni Lynn Colson. 388 pages. 2002. 0-7808-0332-9.

SEE ALSO *Pregnancy & Birth Sourcebook*

"Particularly useful is the information about professional lactation services and chapters on breastfeeding when returning to work.... *Breastfeeding Sourcebook* will be useful for public libraries, consumer health libraries, and technical schools offering nurse assistant training, especially in areas where Internet access is problematic."
— *American Reference Books Annual, 2003*

Burns Sourcebook

Basic Consumer Health Information about Various Types of Burns and Scalds, Including Flame, Heat, Cold, Electrical, Chemical, and Sun Burns

Along with Information on Short-Term and Long-Term Treatments, Tissue Reconstruction, Plastic Surgery, Prevention Suggestions, and First Aid

Edited by Allan R. Cook. 604 pages. 1999. 0-7808-0204-7.

"This is an exceptional addition to the series and is highly recommended for all consumer health collections, hospital libraries, and academic medical centers."
— *E-Streams, Mar '00*

"This key reference guide is an invaluable addition to all health care and public libraries in confronting this ongoing health issue."
— *American Reference Books Annual, 2000*

"Recommended reference source."
— *Booklist, American Library Association, Dec '99*

SEE ALSO *Skin Disorders Sourcebook*

Cancer Sourcebook, 4th Edition

Basic Consumer Health Information about Major Forms and Stages of Cancer, Featuring Facts about Head and Neck Cancers, Lung Cancers, Gastrointestinal Cancers, Genitourinary Cancers, Lymphomas, Blood Cell Cancers, Endocrine Cancers, Skin Cancers, Bone Cancers, Sarcomas, and Others, and Including Information about Cancer Treatments and Therapies, Identifying and Reducing Cancer Risks, and Strategies for Coping with Cancer and the Side Effects of Treatment

Along with a Cancer Glossary, Statistical and Demographic Data, and a Directory of Sources for Additional Help and Information

Edited by Karen Bellenir. 1,119 pages. 2003. 0-7808-0633-6.

ALSO AVAILABLE: *Cancer Sourcebook, 1st Edition.* Edited by Frank E. Bair. 932 pages. 1990. 1-55888-888-8.

New Cancer Sourcebook, 2nd Edition. Edited by Allan R. Cook. 1,313 pages. 1996. 0-7808-0041-9.

Cancer Sourcebook, 3rd Edition. Edited by Edward J. Prucha. 1,069 pages. 2000. 0-7808-0227-6.

"With cancer being the second leading cause of death for Americans, a prodigious work such as this one, which locates centrally so much cancer-related information, is clearly an asset to this nation's citizens and others."
— *Journal of the National Medical Association, 2004*

"This title is recommended for health sciences and public libraries with consumer health collections."
— *E-Streams, Feb '01*

"... can be effectively used by cancer patients and their families who are looking for answers in a language they can understand. Public and hospital libraries should have it on their shelves."
— *American Reference Books Annual, 2001*

"Recommended reference source."
— *Booklist, American Library Association, Dec '00*

Cited in *Reference Sources for Small and Medium-Sized Libraries*, American Library Association, 1999

"The amount of factual and useful information is extensive. The writing is very clear, geared to general readers. Recommended for all levels."
— *Choice, Association of College & Research Libraries, Jan '97*

SEE ALSO *Breast Cancer Sourcebook, Cancer Sourcebook for Women, Pediatric Cancer Sourcebook, Prostate Cancer Sourcebook*

Cancer Sourcebook for Women, 3rd Edition

Basic Consumer Health Information about Leading Causes of Cancer in Women, Featuring Facts about Gynecologic Cancers and Related Concerns, Such as Breast Cancer, Cervical Cancer, Endometrial Cancer, Uterine Sarcoma, Vaginal Cancer, Vulvar Cancer, and Common Non-Cancerous Gynecologic Conditions, in Addition to Facts about Lung Cancer, Colorectal Cancer, and Thyroid Cancer in Women

Along with Information about Cancer Risk Factors, Screening and Prevention, Treatment Options, and Tips on Coping with Life after Cancer Treatment, a Glossary of Cancer Terms, and a Directory of Resources for Additional Help and Information

Edited by Amy L. Sutton. 675 pages. 2006. 0-7808-0867-3.

ALSO AVAILABLE: Cancer Sourcebook for Women, 1st Edition. Edited by Allan R. Cook and Peter D. Dresser. 524 pages. 1996. 0-7808-0076-1.

Cancer Sourcebook for Women, 2nd Edition. Edited by Karen Bellenir. 604 pages. 2002. 0-7808-0226-8.

"An excellent addition to collections in public, consumer health, and women's health libraries."
— *American Reference Books Annual, 2003*

"Overall, the information is excellent, and complex topics are clearly explained. As a reference book for the consumer it is a valuable resource to assist them to make informed decisions about cancer and its treatments." — *Cancer Forum, Nov '02*

"Highly recommended for academic and medical reference collections." — *Library Bookwatch, Sep '02*

"This is a highly recommended book for any public or consumer library, being reader friendly and containing accurate and helpful information."
— *E-Streams, Aug '02*

"Recommended reference source."
— *Booklist, American Library Association, Jul '02*

SEE ALSO Breast Cancer Sourcebook, Women's Health Concerns Sourcebook

Cardiovascular Diseases & Disorders Sourcebook, 3rd Edition

Basic Consumer Health Information about Heart and Vascular Diseases and Disorders, Such as Angina, Heart Attacks, Arrhythmias, Cardiomyopathy, Valve Disease, Atherosclerosis, and Aneurysms, with Information about Managing Cardiovascular Risk Factors and Maintaining Heart Health, Medications and Procedures Used to Treat Cardiovascular Disorders, and Concerns of Special Significance to Women

long with Reports on Current Research Initiatives, a Glossary of Related Medical Terms, and a Directory of Sources for Further Help and Information

Edited by Sandra J. Judd. 713 pages. 2005. 0-7808-0739-1.

ALSO AVAILABLE: Cardiovascular Diseases & Disorders Sourcebook, 1st Edition. Edited by Karen Bellenir and Peter D. Dresser. 683 pages. 1995. 0-7808-0032-X.

Heart Diseases & Disorders Sourcebook, 2nd Edition. Edited by Karen Bellenir. 612 pages. 2000. 0-7808-0238-1.

"This work stands out as an imminently accessible resource for the general public. It is recommended for the reference and circulating shelves of school, public, and academic libraries."
— *American Reference Books Annual, 2001*

"Recommended reference source."
— *Booklist, American Library Association, Dec '00*

"Provides comprehensive coverage of matters related to the heart. This title is recommended for health sciences and public libraries with consumer health collections."
— *E-Streams, Oct '00*

SEE ALSO Healthy Heart Sourcebook for Women

Caregiving Sourcebook

Basic Consumer Health Information for Caregivers, Including a Profile of Caregivers, Caregiving Responsibilities and Concerns, Tips for Specific Conditions, Care Environments, and the Effects of Caregiving

Along with Facts about Legal Issues, Financial Information, and Future Planning, a Glossary, and a Listing of Additional Resources

Edited by Joyce Brennfleck Shannon. 600 pages. 2001. 0-7808-0331-0.

"Essential for most collections."
— *Library Journal, Apr 1, 2002*

"An ideal addition to the reference collection of any public library. Health sciences information professionals may also want to acquire the *Caregiving Sourcebook* for their hospital or academic library for use as a ready reference tool by health care workers interested in aging and caregiving." — *E-Streams, Jan '02*

"Recommended reference source."
— *Booklist, American Library Association, Oct '01*

Child Abuse Sourcebook

Basic Consumer Health Information about the Physical, Sexual, and Emotional Abuse of Children, with Additional Facts about Neglect, Munchausen Syndrome by Proxy (MSBP), Shaken Baby Syndrome, and Controversial Issues Related to Child Abuse, Such as Withholding Medical Care, Corporal Punishment, and Child Maltreatment in Youth Sports, and Featuring Facts about Child Protective Services, Foster Care, Adoption, Parenting Challenges, and Other Abuse Prevention Efforts

Along with a Glossary of Related Terms and Resources for Additional Help and Information

Edited by Dawn D. Matthews. 620 pages. 2004. 0-7808-0705-7.

Childhood Diseases & Disorders Sourcebook

Basic Consumer Health Information about Medical Problems Often Encountered in Pre-Adolescent Children, Including Respiratory Tract Ailments, Ear Infections, Sore Throats, Disorders of the Skin and Scalp, Digestive and Genitourinary Diseases, Infectious Diseases, Inflammatory Disorders, Chronic Physical and Developmental Disorders, Allergies, and More

Along with Information about Diagnostic Tests, Common Childhood Surgeries, and Frequently Used Medications, with a Glossary of Important Terms and Resource Directory

Edited by Chad T. Kimball. 662 pages. 2003. 0-7808-0458-9.

"This is an excellent book for new parents and should be included in all health care and public libraries."
— *American Reference Books Annual, 2004*

Colds, Flu & Other Common Ailments Sourcebook

Basic Consumer Health Information about Common Ailments and Injuries, Including Colds, Coughs, the Flu, Sinus Problems, Headaches, Fever, Nausea and Vomiting, Menstrual Cramps, Diarrhea, Constipation, Hemorrhoids, Back Pain, Dandruff, Dry and Itchy Skin, Cuts, Scrapes, Sprains, Bruises, and More

Along with Information about Prevention, Self-Care, Choosing a Doctor, Over-the-Counter Medications, Folk Remedies, and Alternative Therapies, and Including a Glossary of Important Terms and a Directory of Resources for Further Help and Information

Edited by Chad T. Kimball. 638 pages. 2001. 0-7808-0435-X.

"A good starting point for research on common illnesses. It will be a useful addition to public and consumer health library collections."
— *American Reference Books Annual 2002*

"Will prove valuable to any library seeking to maintain a current, comprehensive reference collection of health resources.... Excellent reference."
— *The Bookwatch, Aug '01*

"Recommended reference source."
— *Booklist, American Library Association, July '01*

Communication Disorders Sourcebook

Basic Information about Deafness and Hearing Loss, Speech and Language Disorders, Voice Disorders, Balance and Vestibular Disorders, and Disorders of Smell, Taste, and Touch

Edited by Linda M. Ross. 533 pages. 1996. 0-7808-0077-X.

"This is skillfully edited and is a welcome resource for the layperson. It should be found in every public and medical library." — *Booklist Health Sciences Supplement, American Library Association, Oct '97*

Complementary & Alternative Medicine Sourcebook, 3rd Edition

Basic Consumer Health Information about Complementary and Alternative Medical Therapies, Including Acupuncture, Ayurveda, Traditional Chinese Medicine, Herbal Medicine, Homeopathy, Naturopathy, Biofeedback, Hypnotherapy, Yoga, Art Therapy, Aromatherapy, Clinical Nutrition, Vitamin and Mineral Supplements, Chiropractic, Massage, Reflexology, Crystal Therapy, Therapeutic Touch, and More

Along with Facts about Alternative and Complementary Treatments for Specific Conditions Such as Cancer, Diabetes, Osteoarthritis, Chronic Pain, Menopause, Gastrointestinal Disorders, Headaches, and Mental Illness, a Glossary, and a Resource List for Additional Help and Information

Edited by Sandra J. Judd. 657 pages. 2006. 0-7808-0864-9.

ALSO AVAILABLE: Alternative Medicine Sourcebook, 1st Edition. Edited by Allan R. Cook. 737 pages. 1999. 0-7808-0200-4.

Alternative Medicine Sourcebook, 2nd Edition. Edited by Dawn D. Matthews. 618 pages. 2002. 0-7808-0605-0.

"Recommended for public, high school, and academic libraries that have consumer health collections. Hospital libraries that also serve the public will find this to be a useful resource." — *E-Streams, Feb '03*

"Recommended reference source."
— *Booklist, American Library Association, Jan '03*

"An important alternate health reference."
— *MBR Bookwatch, Oct '02*

"A great addition to the reference collection of every type of library." — *American Reference Books Annual, 2000*

Congenital Disorders Sourcebook

Basic Information about Disorders Acquired during Gestation, Including Spina Bifida, Hydrocephalus, Cerebral Palsy, Heart Defects, Craniofacial Abnormalities, Fetal Alcohol Syndrome, and More

Along with Current Treatment Options and Statistical Data

Edited by Karen Bellenir. 607 pages. 1997. 0-7808-0205-5.

"Recommended reference source."
— *Booklist, American Library Association, Oct '97*

SEE ALSO Pregnancy & Birth Sourcebook

Consumer Issues in Health Care Sourcebook

Basic Information about Health Care Fundamentals and Related Consumer Issues, Including Exams and Screening Tests, Physician Specialties, Choosing a Doctor, Using Prescription and Over-the-Counter Medications Safely, Avoiding Health Scams, Managing Common Health Risks in the Home, Care Options for

Chronically or Terminally Ill Patients, and a List of Resources for Obtaining Help and Further Information. Edited by Karen Bellenir. 618 pages. 1998. 0-7808-0221-7.

"Both public and academic libraries will want to have a copy in their collection for readers who are interested in self-education on health issues."
—*American Reference Books Annual, 2000*

"The editor has researched the literature from government agencies and others, saving readers the time and effort of having to do the research themselves. Recommended for public libraries."
—*Reference and User Services Quarterly, American Library Association, Spring '99*

"Recommended reference source."
—*Booklist, American Library Association, Dec '98*

Contagious Diseases Sourcebook

Basic Consumer Health Information about Infectious Diseases Spread by Person-to-Person Contact through Direct Touch, Airborne Transmission, Sexual Contact, or Contact with Blood or Other Body Fluids, Including Hepatitis, Herpes, Influenza, Lice, Measles, Mumps, Pinworm, Ringworm, Severe Acute Respiratory Syndrome (SARS), Streptococcal Infections, Tuberculosis, and Others

Along with Facts about Disease Transmission, Antimicrobial Resistance, and Vaccines, with a Glossary and Directories of Resources for More Information

Edited by Karen Bellenir. 643 pages. 2004. 0-7808-0736-7.

Contagious & Non-Contagious Infectious Diseases Sourcebook

Basic Information about Contagious Diseases like Measles, Polio, Hepatitis B, and Infectious Mononucleosis, and Non-Contagious Infectious Diseases like Tetanus and Toxic Shock Syndrome, and Diseases Occurring as Secondary Infections Such as Shingles and Reye Syndrome

Along with Vaccination, Prevention, and Treatment Information, and a Section Describing Emerging Infectious Disease Threats

Edited by Karen Bellenir and Peter D. Dresser. 566 pages. 1996. 0-7808-0075-3.

Death & Dying Sourcebook

Basic Consumer Health Information for the Layperson about End-of-Life Care and Related Ethical and Legal Issues, Including Chief Causes of Death, Autopsies, Pain Management for the Terminally Ill, Life Support Systems, Insurance, Euthanasia, Assisted Suicide, Hospice Programs, Living Wills, Funeral Planning, Counseling, Mourning, Organ Donation, and Physician Training

Along with Statistical Data, a Glossary, and Listings of Sources for Further Help and Information

Edited by Annemarie S. Muth. 641 pages. 1999. 0-7808-0230-6.

"Public libraries, medical libraries, and academic libraries will all find this sourcebook a useful addition to their collections."
—*American Reference Books Annual, 2001*

"An extremely useful resource for those concerned with death and dying in the United States."
—*Respiratory Care, Nov '00*

"Recommended reference source."
—*Booklist, American Library Association, Aug '00*

"This book is a definite must for all those involved in end-of-life care." —*Doody's Review Service, 2000*

Dental Care & Oral Health Sourcebook, 2nd Edition

Basic Consumer Health Information about Dental Care, Including Oral Hygiene, Dental Visits, Pain Management, Cavities, Crowns, Bridges, Dental Implants, and Fillings, and Other Oral Health Concerns, Such as Gum Disease, Bad Breath, Dry Mouth, Genetic and Developmental Abnormalities, Oral Cancers, Orthodontics, and Temporomandibular Disorders

Along with Updates on Current Research in Oral Health, a Glossary, a Directory of Dental and Oral Health Organizations, and Resources for People with Dental and Oral Health Disorders

Edited by Amy L. Sutton. 609 pages. 2003. 0-7808-0634-4.

ALSO AVAILABLE: *Oral Health Sourcebook, 1st Edition.* Edited by Allan R. Cook. 558 pages. 1997. 0-7808-0082-6.

"This book could serve as a turning point in the battle to educate consumers in issues concerning oral health."
—*American Reference Books Annual, 2004*

"Unique source which will fill a gap in dental sources for patients and the lay public. A valuable reference tool even in a library with thousands of books on dentistry. Comprehensive, clear, inexpensive, and easy to read and use. It fills an enormous gap in the health care literature." —*Reference and User Services Quarterly, American Library Association, Summer '98*

"Recommended reference source."
—*Booklist, American Library Association, Dec '97*

Depression Sourcebook

Basic Consumer Health Information about Unipolar Depression, Bipolar Disorder, Postpartum Depression, Seasonal Affective Disorder, and Other Types of Depression in Children, Adolescents, Women, Men, the Elderly, and Other Selected Populations

Along with Facts about Causes, Risk Factors, Diagnostic Criteria, Treatment Options, Coping Strategies, Suicide Prevention, a Glossary, and a Directory of Sources for Additional Help and Information

Edited by Karen Belleni. 602 pages. 2002. 0-7808-0611-5.

"*Depression Sourcebook* is of a very high standard. Its purpose, which is to serve as a reference source to the lay reader, is very well served."
—*Journal of the National Medical Association, 2004*

"Invaluable reference for public and school library collections alike." —*Library Bookwatch, Apr '03*

"Recommended for purchase."
—*American Reference Books Annual, 2003*

"Provides useful information for the general public."
—*Healthlines, University of Michigan Health Management Research Center, Sep/Oct '99*

"... provides reliable mainstream medical information ... belongs on the shelves of any library with a consumer health collection." —*E-Streams, Sep '99*

"Recommended reference source."
—*Booklist, American Library Association, Feb '99*

Dermatological Disorders Sourcebook, 2nd Edition

Basic Consumer Health Information about Conditions and Disorders Affecting the Skin, Hair, and Nails, Such as Acne, Rosacea, Rashes, Dermatitis, Pigmentation Disorders, Birthmarks, Skin Cancer, Skin Injuries, Psoriasis, Scleroderma, and Hair Loss, Including Facts about Medications and Treatments for Dermatological Disorders and Tips for Maintaining Healthy Skin, Hair, and Nails

Along with Information about How Aging Affects the Skin, a Glossary of Related Terms, and a Directory of Resources for Additional Help and Information

Edited by Amy L. Sutton. 645 pages. 2005. 0-7808-0795-2.

ALSO AVAILABLE: *Skin Disorders Sourcebook, 1st Edition.* Edited by Allan R. Cook. 647 pages. 1997. 0-7808-0080-X.

"... comprehensive, easily read reference book."
—*Doody's Health Sciences Book Reviews, Oct '97*

Diabetes Sourcebook, 3rd Edition

Basic Consumer Health Information about Type 1 Diabetes (Insulin-Dependent or Juvenile-Onset Diabetes), Type 2 Diabetes (Noninsulin-Dependent or Adult-Onset Diabetes), Gestational Diabetes, Impaired Glucose Tolerance (IGT), and Related Complications, Such as Amputation, Eye Disease, Gum Disease, Nerve Damage, and End-Stage Renal Disease, Including Facts about Insulin, Oral Diabetes Medications, Blood Sugar Testing, and the Role of Exercise and Nutrition in the Control of Diabetes

Along with a Glossary and Resources for Further Help and Information

Edited by Dawn D. Matthews. 622 pages. 2003. 0-7808-0629-8.

ALSO AVAILABLE: *Diabetes Sourcebook, 1st Edition.* Edited by Karen Bellenir and Peter D. Dresser. 827 pages. 1994. 1-55888-751-2.

Diabetes Sourcebook, 2nd Edition. Edited by Karen Bellenir. 688 pages. 1998. 0-7808-0224-1.

"This edition is even more helpful than earlier versions. . . . It is a truly valuable tool for anyone seeking readable and authoritative information on diabetes."
—*American Reference Books Annual, 2004*

"An invaluable reference." —*Library Journal, May '00*

Selected as one of the 250 "Best Health Sciences Books of 1999." —*Doody's Rating Service, Mar-Apr 2000*

Diet & Nutrition Sourcebook, 3rd Edition

Basic Consumer Health Information about Dietary Guidelines and the Food Guidance System, Recommended Daily Nutrient Intakes, Serving Proportions, Weight Control, Vitamins and Supplements, Nutrition Issues for Different Life Stages and Lifestyles, and the Needs of People with Specific Medical Concerns, Including Cancer, Celiac Disease, Diabetes, Eating Disorders, Food Allergies, and Cardiovascular Disease

Along with Facts about Federal Nutrition Support Programs, a Glossary of Nutrition and Dietary Terms, and Directories of Additional Resources for More Information about Nutrition

Edited by Joyce Brennfleck Shannon. 633 pages. 2006. 0-7808-0800-2.

ALSO AVAILABLE: *Diet & Nutrition Sourcebook, 1st Edition.* Edited by Dan R. Harris. 662 pages. 1996. 0-7808-0084-2.

Diet & Nutrition Sourcebook, 2nd Edition. Edited by Karen Bellenir. 650 pages. 1999. 0-7808-0228-4.

"This book is an excellent source of basic diet and nutrition information." —*Booklist Health Sciences Supplement, American Library Association, Dec '00*

"This reference document should be in any public library, but it would be a very good guide for beginning students in the health sciences. If the other books in this publisher's series are as good as this, they should all be in the health sciences collections."
—*American Reference Books Annual, 2000*

"This book is an excellent general nutrition reference for consumers who desire to take an active role in their health care for prevention. Consumers of all ages who select this book can feel confident they are receiving current and accurate information." —*Journal of Nutrition for the Elderly, Vol. 19, No. 4, '00*

"Recommended reference source."
—*Booklist, American Library Association, Dec '99*

SEE ALSO *Digestive Diseases & Disorders Sourcebook, Eating Disorders Sourcebook, Gastrointestinal Diseases & Disorders Sourcebook, Vegetarian Sourcebook*

Digestive Diseases & Disorders Sourcebook

Basic Consumer Health Information about Diseases and Disorders that Impact the Upper and Lower Digestive System, Including Celiac Disease, Constipation, Crohn's Disease, Cyclic Vomiting Syndrome, Diarrhea, Diverticulosis and Diverticulitis, Gallstones, Heartburn, Hemorrhoids, Hernias, Indigestion (Dyspepsia), Irritable Bowel Syndrome, Lactose Intolerance, Ulcers, and More

Along with Information about Medications and Other Treatments, Tips for Maintaining a Healthy Digestive Tract, a Glossary, and Directory of Digestive Diseases Organizations

Edited by Karen Bellenir. 335 pages. 2000. 0-7808-0327-2.

"This title would be an excellent addition to all public or patient-research libraries."
—*American Reference Books Annual, 2001*

"This title is recommended for public, hospital, and health sciences libraries with consumer health collections." —*E-Streams, Jul-Aug '00*

"Recommended reference source."
—*Booklist, American Library Association, May '00*

SEE ALSO *Diet & Nutrition Sourcebook, Eating Disorders Sourcebook, Gastrointestinal Diseases & Disorders Sourcebook*

Disabilities Sourcebook

Basic Consumer Health Information about Physical and Psychiatric Disabilities, Including Descriptions of Major Causes of Disability, Assistive and Adaptive Aids, Workplace Issues, and Accessibility Concerns

Along with Information about the Americans with Disabilities Act, a Glossary, and Resources for Additional Help and Information

Edited by Dawn D. Matthews. 616 pages. 2000. 0-7808-0389-2.

"It is a must for libraries with a consumer health section." —*American Reference Books Annual 2002*

"A much needed addition to the Omnigraphics *Health Reference Series*. A current reference work to provide people with disabilities, their families, caregivers or those who work with them, a broad range of information in one volume, has not been available until now. . . . It is recommended for all public and academic library reference collections." —*E-Streams, May '01*

"An excellent source book in easy-to-read format covering many current topics; highly recommended for all libraries." —*Choice, Association of College and Research Libraries, Jan '01*

"Recommended reference source."
—*Booklist, American Library Association, Jul '00*

Domestic Violence Sourcebook, 2nd Edition

Basic Consumer Health Information about the Causes and Consequences of Abusive Relationships, Including Physical Violence, Sexual Assault, Battery, Stalking, and Emotional Abuse, and Facts about the Effects of Violence on Women, Men, Young Adults, and the Elderly, with Reports about Domestic Violence in Selected Populations, and Featuring Facts about Medical Care, Victim Assistance and Protection, Prevention Strategies, Mental Health Services, and Legal Issues

Along with a Glossary of Related Terms and Resources for Additional Help and Information

Edited by Dawn D. Matthews. 628 pages. 2004. 0-7808-0669-7.

ALSO AVAILABLE: *Domestic Violence & Child Abuse Sourcebook, 1st Edition.* Edited by Helene Henderson. 1,064 pages. 2001. 0-7808-0235-7.

"Interested lay persons should find the book extremely beneficial. . . . A copy of *Domestic Violence and Child Abuse Sourcebook* should be in every public library in the United States."
— *Social Science & Medicine, No. 56, 2003*

"This is important information. The Web has many resources but this sourcebook fills an important societal need. I am not aware of any other resources of this type." —*Doody's Review Service, Sep '01*

"Recommended for all libraries, scholars, and practitioners." —*Choice, Association of College & Research Libraries, Jul '01*

"Recommended reference source."
—*Booklist, American Library Association, Apr '01*

"Important pick for college-level health reference libraries." —*The Bookwatch, Mar '01*

"Because this problem is so widespread and because this book includes a lot of issues within one volume, this work is recommended for all public libraries."
—*American Reference Books Annual, 2001*

Drug Abuse Sourcebook, 2nd Edition

Basic Consumer Health Information about Illicit Substances of Abuse and the Misuse of Prescription and Over-the-Counter Medications, Including Depressants, Hallucinogens, Inhalants, Marijuana, Stimulants, and Anabolic Steroids

Along with Facts about Related Health Risks, Treatment Programs, Prevention Programs, a Glossary of Abuse and Addiction Terms, a Glossary of Drug-Related Street Terms, and a Directory of Resources for More Information

Edited by Catherine Ginther. 607 pages. 2004. 0-7808-0740-5.

ALSO AVAILABLE: *Drug Abuse Sourcebook, 1st Edition.* Edited by Karen Bellenir. 629 pages. 2000. 0-7808-0242-X.

"Containing a wealth of information.... This resource belongs in libraries that serve a lower-division undergraduate or community college clientele as well as the general public."
— *Choice, Association of College and Research Libraries, Jun '01*

"Recommended reference source."
— *Booklist, American Library Association, Feb '01*

"Highly recommended." — *The Bookwatch, Jan '01*

"Even though there is a plethora of books on drug abuse, this volume is recommended for school, public, and college libraries."
— *American Reference Books Annual, 2001*

SEE ALSO *Alcoholism Sourcebook, Substance Abuse Sourcebook*

■

Ear, Nose & Throat Disorders Sourcebook

Basic Information about Disorders of the Ears, Nose, Sinus Cavities, Pharynx, and Larynx, Including Ear Infections, Tinnitus, Vestibular Disorders, Allergic and Non-Allergic Rhinitis, Sore Throats, Tonsillitis, and Cancers That Affect the Ears, Nose, Sinuses, and Throat

Along with Reports on Current Research Initiatives, a Glossary of Related Medical Terms, and a Directory of Sources for Further Help and Information

Edited by Karen Bellenir and Linda M. Shin. 576 pages. 1998. 0-7808-0206-3.

"Overall, this sourcebook is helpful for the consumer seeking information on ENT issues. It is recommended for public libraries."
— *American Reference Books Annual, 1999*

"Recommended reference source."
— *Booklist, American Library Association, Dec '98*

■

Eating Disorders Sourcebook

Basic Consumer Health Information about Eating Disorders, Including Information about Anorexia Nervosa, Bulimia Nervosa, Binge Eating, Body Dysmorphic Disorder, Pica, Laxative Abuse, and Night Eating Syndrome

Along with Information about Causes, Adverse Effects, and Treatment and Prevention Issues, and Featuring a Section on Concerns Specific to Children and Adolescents, a Glossary, and Resources for Further Help and Information

Edited by Dawn D. Matthews. 322 pages. 2001. 0-7808-0335-3.

"Recommended for health science libraries that are open to the public, as well as hospital libraries. This book is a good resource for the consumer who is concerned about eating disorders." — *E-Streams, Mar '02*

"This volume is another convenient collection of excerpted articles. Recommended for school and public library patrons; lower-division undergraduates; and two-year technical program students." — *Choice, Association of College & Research Libraries, Jan '02*

"Recommended reference source." — *Booklist, American Library Association, Oct '01*

SEE ALSO *Diet & Nutrition Sourcebook, Digestive Diseases & Disorders Sourcebook, Gastrointestinal Diseases & Disorders Sourcebook*

■

Emergency Medical Services Sourcebook

Basic Consumer Health Information about Preventing, Preparing for, and Managing Emergency Situations, When and Who to Call for Help, What to Expect in the Emergency Room, the Emergency Medical Team, Patient Issues, and Current Topics in Emergency Medicine

Along with Statistical Data, a Glossary, and Sources of Additional Help and Information

Edited by Jenni Lynn Colson. 494 pages. 2002. 0-7808-0420-1.

"Handy and convenient for home, public, school, and college libraries. Recommended."
— *Choice, Association of College and Research Libraries, Apr '03*

"This reference can provide the consumer with answers to most questions about emergency care in the United States, or it will direct them to a resource where the answer can be found."
— *American Reference Books Annual, 2003*

"Recommended reference source."
— *Booklist, American Library Association, Feb '03*

■

Endocrine & Metabolic Disorders Sourcebook

Basic Information for the Layperson about Pancreatic and Insulin-Related Disorders Such as Pancreatitis, Diabetes, and Hypoglycemia; Adrenal Gland Disorders Such as Cushing's Syndrome, Addison's Disease, and Congenital Adrenal Hyperplasia; Pituitary Gland Disorders Such as Growth Hormone Deficiency, Acromegaly, and Pituitary Tumors; Thyroid Disorders Such as Hypothyroidism, Graves' Disease, Hashimoto's Disease, and Goiter; Hyperparathyroidism; and Other Diseases and Syndromes of Hormone Imbalance or Metabolic Dysfunction

Along with Reports on Current Research Initiatives

Edited by Linda M. Shin. 574 pages. 1998. 0-7808-0207-1.

"Omnigraphics has produced another needed resource for health information consumers."
— *American Reference Books Annual, 2000*

"Recommended reference source."
— *Booklist, American Library Association, Dec '98*

■

Environmental Health Sourcebook, 2nd Edition

Basic Consumer Health Information about the Environment and Its Effect on Human Health, Including the Effects of Air Pollution, Water Pollution, Hazardous

Chemicals, Food Hazards, Radiation Hazards, Biological Agents, Household Hazards, Such as Radon, Asbestos, Carbon Monoxide, and Mold, and Information about Associated Diseases and Disorders, Including Cancer, Allergies, Respiratory Problems, and Skin Disorders

Along with Information about Environmental Concerns for Specific Populations, a Glossary of Related Terms, and Resources for Further Help and Information

Edited by Dawn D. Matthews. 673 pages. 2003. 0-7808-0632-8.

ALSO AVAILABLE: Environmentally Induced Disorders Sourcebook, 1st Edition. Edited by Allan R. Cook. 620 pages. 1997. 0-7808-0083-4.

"This recently updated edition continues the level of quality and the reputation of the numerous other volumes in Omnigraphics' **Health Reference Series.**"
— *American Reference Books Annual, 2004*

"Recommended reference source."
— *Booklist, American Library Association, Sep '98*

"This book will be a useful addition to anyone's library." — *Choice Health Sciences Supplement, Association of College and Research Libraries, May '98*

". . . a good survey of numerous environmentally induced physical disorders . . . a useful addition to anyone's library."
— *Doody's Health Sciences Book Reviews, Jan '98*

". . . provide[s] introductory information from the best authorities around. Since this volume covers topics that potentially affect everyone, it will surely be one of the most frequently consulted volumes in the *Health Reference Series.*" — *Rettig on Reference, Nov '97*

Environmentally Induced Disorders Sourcebook, 1st Edition

SEE *Environmental Health Sourcebook, 2nd Edition*

Ethnic Diseases Sourcebook

Basic Consumer Health Information for Ethnic and Racial Minority Groups in the United States, Including General Health Indicators and Behaviors, Ethnic Diseases, Genetic Testing, the Impact of Chronic Diseases, Women's Health, Mental Health Issues, and Preventive Health Care Services

Along with a Glossary and a Listing of Additional Resources

Edited by Joyce Brennfleck Shannon. 664 pages. 2001. 0-7808-0336-1.

"Recommended for health sciences libraries where public health programs are a priority."
— *E-Streams, Jan '02*

"Not many books have been written on this topic to date, and the *Ethnic Diseases Sourcebook* is a strong addition to the list. It will be an important introductory resource for health consumers, students, health care personnel, and social scientists. It is recommended for public, academic, and large hospital libraries."
— *American Reference Books Annual 2002*

"Recommended reference source."
— *Booklist, American Library Association, Oct '01*

"Will prove valuable to any library seeking to maintain a current, comprehensive reference collection of health resources. . . . An excellent source of health information about genetic disorders which affect particular ethnic and racial minorities in the U.S."
— *The Bookwatch, Aug '01*

Eye Care Sourcebook, 2nd Edition

Basic Consumer Health Information about Eye Care and Eye Disorders, Including Facts about the Diagnosis, Prevention, and Treatment of Common Refractive Problems Such as Myopia, Hyperopia, Astigmatism, and Presbyopia, and Eye Diseases, Including Glaucoma, Cataract, Age-Related Macular Degeneration, and Diabetic Retinopathy

Along with a Section on Vision Correction and Refractive Surgeries, Including LASIK and LASEK, a Glossary, and Directories of Resources for Additional Help and Information

Edited by Amy L. Sutton. 543 pages. 2003. 0-7808-0635-2.

ALSO AVAILABLE: Ophthalmic Disorders Sourcebook, 1st Edition. Edited by Linda M. Ross. 631 pages. 1996. 0-7808-0081-8.

". . . a solid reference tool for eye care and a valuable addition to a collection."
— *American Reference Books Annual, 2004*

Family Planning Sourcebook

Basic Consumer Health Information about Planning for Pregnancy and Contraception, Including Traditional Methods, Barrier Methods, Hormonal Methods, Permanent Methods, Future Methods, Emergency Contraception, and Birth Control Choices for Women at Each Stage of Life

Along with Statistics, a Glossary, and Sources of Additional Information

Edited by Amy Marcaccio Keyzer. 520 pages. 2001. 0-7808-0379-5.

"Recommended for public, health, and undergraduate libraries as part of the circulating collection."
— *E-Streams, Mar '02*

"Information is presented in an unbiased, readable manner, and the sourcebook will certainly be a necessary addition to those public and high school libraries where Internet access is restricted or otherwise problematic." — *American Reference Books Annual 2002*

"Recommended reference source."
— *Booklist, American Library Association, Oct '01*

"Will prove valuable to any library seeking to maintain a current, comprehensive reference collection of health resources. . . . Excellent reference."
— *The Bookwatch, Aug '01*

SEE ALSO *Pregnancy & Birth Sourcebook*

Fitness & Exercise Sourcebook, 2nd Edition

Basic Consumer Health Information about the Fundamentals of Fitness and Exercise, Including How to Begin and Maintain a Fitness Program, Fitness as a Lifestyle, the Link between Fitness and Diet, Advice for Specific Groups of People, Exercise as It Relates to Specific Medical Conditions, and Recent Research in Fitness and Exercise

Along with a Glossary of Important Terms and Resources for Additional Help and Information

Edited by Kristen M. Gledhill. 646 pages. 2001. 0-7808-0334-5.

ALSO AVAILABLE: *Fitness & Exercise Sourcebook, 1st Edition.* Edited by Dan R. Harris. 663 pages. 1996. 0-7808-0186-5.

"**This work is recommended for all general reference collections.**"
— *American Reference Books Annual 2002*

"**Highly recommended for public, consumer, and school grades fourth through college.**"
—*E-Streams, Nov '01*

"**Recommended reference source.**" — *Booklist, American Library Association, Oct '01*

"**The information appears quite comprehensive and is considered reliable.... This second edition is a welcomed addition to the series.**"
—*Doody's Review Service, Sep '01*

"**This reference is a valuable choice for those who desire a broad source of information on exercise, fitness, and chronic-disease prevention through a healthy lifestyle.**" —*American Medical Writers Association Journal, Fall '01*

"**Will prove valuable to any library seeking to maintain a current, comprehensive reference collection of health resources.... Excellent reference.**"
— *The Bookwatch, Aug '01*

Food & Animal Borne Diseases Sourcebook

Basic Information about Diseases That Can Be Spread to Humans through the Ingestion of Contaminated Food or Water or by Contact with Infected Animals and Insects, Such as Botulism, E. Coli, Hepatitis A, Trichinosis, Lyme Disease, and Rabies

Along with Information Regarding Prevention and Treatment Methods, and Including a Special Section for International Travelers Describing Diseases Such as Cholera, Malaria, Travelers' Diarrhea, and Yellow Fever, and Offering Recommendations for Avoiding Illness

Edited by Karen Bellenir and Peter D. Dresser. 535 pages. 1995. 0-7808-0033-8.

"**Targeting general readers and providing them with a single, comprehensive source of information on selected topics, this book continues, with the excellent caliber of its predecessors, to catalog topical information on health matters of general interest. Readable and thorough, this valuable resource is highly recommended for all libraries.**"
— *Academic Library Book Review, Summer '96*

"**A comprehensive collection of authoritative information.**" — *Emergency Medical Services, Oct '95*

Food Safety Sourcebook

Basic Consumer Health Information about the Safe Handling of Meat, Poultry, Seafood, Eggs, Fruit Juices, and Other Food Items, and Facts about Pesticides, Drinking Water, Food Safety Overseas, and the Onset, Duration, and Symptoms of Foodborne Illnesses, Including Types of Pathogenic Bacteria, Parasitic Protozoa, Worms, Viruses, and Natural Toxins

Along with the Role of the Consumer, the Food Handler, and the Government in Food Safety; a Glossary, and Resources for Additional Help and Information

Edited by Dawn D. Matthews. 339 pages. 1999. 0-7808-0326-4.

"**This book is recommended for public libraries and universities with home economic and food science programs.**" —*E-Streams, Nov '00*

"**Recommended reference source.**"
—*Booklist, American Library Association, May '00*

"**This book takes the complex issues of food safety and foodborne pathogens and presents them in an easily understood manner. [It does] an excellent job of covering a large and often confusing topic.**"
—*American Reference Books Annual, 2000*

Forensic Medicine Sourcebook

Basic Consumer Information for the Layperson about Forensic Medicine, Including Crime Scene Investigation, Evidence Collection and Analysis, Expert Testimony, Computer-Aided Criminal Identification, Digital Imaging in the Courtroom, DNA Profiling, Accident Reconstruction, Autopsies, Ballistics, Drugs and Explosives Detection, Latent Fingerprints, Product Tampering, and Questioned Document Examination

Along with Statistical Data, a Glossary of Forensics Terminology, and Listings of Sources for Further Help and Information

Edited by Annemarie S. Muth. 574 pages. 1999. 0-7808-0232-2.

"**Given the expected widespread interest in its content and its easy to read style, this book is recommended for most public and all college and university libraries.**"
— *E-Streams, Feb '01*

"**Recommended for public libraries.**"
—*Reference & User Services Quarterly, American Library Association, Spring 2000*

"**Recommended reference source.**"
—*Booklist, American Library Association, Feb '00*

"**A wealth of information, useful statistics, references are up-to-date and extremely complete. This wonderful collection of data will help students who are interested in a career in any type of forensic field. It is a great resource for attorneys who need information about types of expert witnesses needed in a particular case. It also offers useful information for fiction and nonfiction writers whose work involves a crime. A fascinating compilation. All levels." — *Choice, Association of College and Research Libraries, Jan 2000*

"There are several items that make this book attractive to consumers who are seeking certain forensic data. . . . This is a useful current source for those seeking general forensic medical answers."
—*American Reference Books Annual, 2000*

Gastrointestinal Diseases & Disorders Sourcebook, 2nd Edition

Basic Consumer Health Information about the Upper and Lower Gastrointestinal (GI) Tract, Including the Esophagus, Stomach, Intestines, Rectum, Liver, and Pancreas, with Facts about Gastroesophageal Reflux Disease, Gastritis, Hernias, Ulcers, Celiac Disease, Diverticulitis, Irritable Bowel Syndrome, Hemorrhoids, Gastrointestinal Cancers, and Other Diseases and Disorders Related to the Digestive Process

Along with Information about Commonly Used Diagnostic and Surgical Procedures, Statistics, Reports on Current Research Initiatives and Clinical Trials, a Glossary, and Resources for Additional Help and Information

Edited by Sandra J. Judd. 682 pages. 2006. 0-7808-0798-7.

ALSO AVAILABLE: Gastrointestinal Diseases & Disorders Sourcebook, 1st Edition. Edited by Linda M. Ross. 413 pages. 1996. 0-7808-0078-8.

". . . very readable form. The successful editorial work that brought this material together into a useful and understandable reference makes accessible to all readers information that can help them more effectively understand and obtain help for digestive tract problems."
— *Choice, Association of College & Research Libraries, Feb '97*

SEE ALSO Diet & Nutrition Sourcebook, Digestive Diseases & Disorders, Eating Disorders Sourcebook

Genetic Disorders Sourcebook, 3rd Edition

Basic Consumer Health Information about Hereditary Diseases and Disorders, Including Facts about the Human Genome, Genetic Inheritance Patterns, Disorders Associated with Specific Genes, Such as Sickle Cell Disease, Hemophilia, and Cystic Fibrosis, Chromosome Disorders, Such as Down Syndrome, Fragile X Syndrome, and Turner Syndrome, and Complex Diseases and Disorders Resulting from the Interaction of Environmental and Genetic Factors, Such as Allergies, Cancer, and Obesity

Along with Facts about Genetic Testing, Suggestions for Parents of Children with Special Needs, Reports on Current Research Initiatives, a Glossary of Genetic Terminology, and Resources for Additional Help and Information

Edited by Karen Bellenir. 777 pages. 2004. 0-7808-0742-1.

ALSO AVAILABLE: Genetic Disorders Sourcebook, 1st Edition. Edited by Karen Bellenir. 642 pages. 1996. 0-7808-0034-6.

Genetic Disorders Sourcebook, 2nd Edition. Edited by Kathy Massimini. 768 pages. 2001. 0-7808-0241-1.

"Recommended for public libraries and medical and hospital libraries with consumer health collections."
— *E-Streams, May '01*

"Recommended reference source."
— *Booklist, American Library Association, Apr '01*

"Important pick for college-level health reference libraries." — *The Bookwatch, Mar '01*

"Provides essential medical information to both the general public and those diagnosed with a serious or fatal genetic disease or disorder." —*Choice, Association of College and Research Libraries, Jan '97*

Head Trauma Sourcebook

Basic Information for the Layperson about Open-Head and Closed-Head Injuries, Treatment Advances, Recovery, and Rehabilitation

Along with Reports on Current Research Initiatives

Edited by Karen Bellenir. 414 pages. 1997. 0-7808-0208-X.

Headache Sourcebook

Basic Consumer Health Information about Migraine, Tension, Cluster, Rebound and Other Types of Headaches, with Facts about the Cause and Prevention of Headaches, the Effects of Stress and the Environment, Headaches during Pregnancy and Menopause, and Childhood Headaches

Along with a Glossary and Other Resources for Additional Help and Information

Edited by Dawn D. Matthews. 362 pages. 2002. 0-7808-0337-X.

"Highly recommended for academic and medical reference collections." — *Library Bookwatch, Sep '02*

Health Insurance Sourcebook

Basic Information about Managed Care Organizations, Traditional Fee-for-Service Insurance, Insurance Portability and Pre-Existing Conditions Clauses, Medicare, Medicaid, Social Security, and Military Health Care

Along with Information about Insurance Fraud

Edited by Wendy Wilcox. 530 pages. 1997. 0-7808-0222-5.

"Particularly useful because it brings much of this information together in one volume. This book will be a handy reference source in the health sciences library, hospital library, college and university library, and medium to large public library."
— *Medical Reference Services Quarterly, Fall '98*

Awarded "Books of the Year Award"
— *American Journal of Nursing, 1997*

"The layout of the book is particularly helpful as it provides easy access to reference material. A most useful addition to the vast amount of information about health insurance. The use of data from U.S. government agencies is most commendable. Useful in a library or learning center for healthcare professional students."
—Doody's Health Sciences Book Reviews, Nov '97

Health Reference Series Cumulative Index 1999

A Comprehensive Index to the Individual Volumes of the Health Reference Series, Including a Subject Index, Name Index, Organization Index, and Publication Index

Along with a Master List of Acronyms and Abbreviations

Edited by Edward J. Prucha, Anne Holmes, and Robert Rudnick. 990 pages. 2000. 0-7808-0382-5.

"This volume will be most helpful in libraries that have a relatively complete collection of the Health Reference Series." —*American Reference Books Annual, 2001*

"Essential for collections that hold any of the numerous *Health Reference Series* titles."
—*Choice, Association of College and Research Libraries, Nov '00*

Healthy Aging Sourcebook

Basic Consumer Health Information about Maintaining Health through the Aging Process, Including Advice on Nutrition, Exercise, and Sleep, Help in Making Decisions about Midlife Issues and Retirement, and Guidance Concerning Practical and Informed Choices in Health Consumerism

Along with Data Concerning the Theories of Aging, Different Experiences in Aging by Minority Groups, and Facts about Aging Now and Aging in the Future; and Featuring a Glossary, a Guide to Consumer Help, Additional Suggested Reading, and Practical Resource Directory

Edited by Jenifer Swanson. 536 pages. 1999. 0-7808-0390-6.

"Recommended reference source."
—*Booklist, American Library Association, Feb '00*

SEE ALSO Physical & Mental Issues in Aging Sourcebook

Healthy Children Sourcebook

Basic Consumer Health Information about the Physical and Mental Development of Children between the Ages of 3 and 12, Including Routine Health Care, Preventative Health Services, Safety and First Aid, Healthy Sleep, Dental Care, Nutrition, and Fitness, and Featuring Parenting Tips on Such Topics as Bedwetting, Choosing Day Care, Monitoring TV and Other Media, and Establishing a Foundation for Substance Abuse Prevention

Along with a Glossary of Commonly Used Pediatric Terms and Resources for Additional Help and Information.

Edited by Chad T. Kimball. 647 pages. 2003. 0-7808-0247-0.

"It is hard to imagine that any other single resource exists that would provide such a comprehensive guide of timely information on health promotion and disease prevention for children aged 3 to 12."
—*American Reference Books Annual, 2004*

"The strengths of this book are many. It is clearly written, presented and structured."
—*Journal of the National Medical Association, 2004*

Healthy Heart Sourcebook for Women

Basic Consumer Health Information about Cardiac Issues Specific to Women, Including Facts about Major Risk Factors and Prevention, Treatment and Control Strategies, and Important Dietary Issues

Along with a Special Section Regarding the Pros and Cons of Hormone Replacement Therapy and Its Impact on Heart Health, and Additional Help, Including Recipes, a Glossary, and a Directory of Resources

Edited by Dawn D. Matthews. 336 pages. 2000. 0-7808-0329-9.

"A good reference source and recommended for all public, academic, medical, and hospital libraries."
—*Medical Reference Services Quarterly, Summer '01*

"Because of the lack of information specific to women on this topic, this book is recommended for public libraries and consumer libraries."
—*American Reference Books Annual, 2001*

"Contains very important information about coronary artery disease that all women should know. The information is current and presented in an easy-to-read format. The book will make a good addition to any library." —*American Medical Writers Association Journal, Summer '00*

"Important, basic reference."
—*Reviewer's Bookwatch, Jul '00*

SEE ALSO Heart Diseases & Disorders Sourcebook, Women's Health Concerns Sourcebook

Heart Diseases & Disorders Sourcebook, 2nd Edition

SEE Cardiovascular Diseases & Disorders Sourcebook, 3rd Edition

Hepatitis Sourcebook

Basic Consumer Health Information about Hepatitis A, Hepatitis B, Hepatitis C, and Other Forms of Hepatitis, Including Autoimmune Hepatitis, Alcoholic Hepatitis, Nonalcoholic Steatohepatitis, and Toxic

Hepatitis, with Facts about Risk Factors, Screening Methods, Diagnostic Tests, and Treatment Options

Along with Information on Liver Health, Tips for People Living with Chronic Hepatitis, Reports on Current Research Initiatives, a Glossary of Terms Related to Hepatitis, and a Directory of Sources for Further Help and Information

Edited by Sandra J. Judd. 597 pages. 2005. 0-7808-0749-9.

Household Safety Sourcebook

Basic Consumer Health Information about Household Safety, Including Information about Poisons, Chemicals, Fire, and Water Hazards in the Home

Along with Advice about the Safe Use of Home Maintenance Equipment, Choosing Toys and Nursery Furniture, Holiday and Recreation Safety, a Glossary, and Resources for Further Help and Information

Edited by Dawn D. Matthews. 606 pages. 2002. 0-7808-0338-8.

"This work will be useful in public libraries with large consumer health and wellness departments."
— *American Reference Books Annual, 2003*

"As a sourcebook on household safety this book meets its mark. It is encyclopedic in scope and covers a wide range of safety issues that are commonly seen in the home." —*E-Streams, Jul '02*

Hypertension Sourcebook

Basic Consumer Health Information about the Causes, Diagnosis, and Treatment of High Blood Pressure, with Facts about Consequences, Complications, and Co-Occurring Disorders, Such as Coronary Heart Disease, Diabetes, Stroke, Kidney Disease, and Hypertensive Retinopathy, and Issues in Blood Pressure Control, Including Dietary Choices, Stress Management, and Medications

Along with Reports on Current Research Initiatives and Clinical Trials, a Glossary, and Resources for Additional Help and Information

Edited by Dawn D. Matthews and Karen Bellenir. 613 pages. 2004. 0-7808-0674-3.

Immune System Disorders Sourcebook, 2nd Edition

Basic Consumer Health Information about Disorders of the Immune System, Including Immune System Function and Response, Diagnosis of Immune Disorders, Information about Inherited Immune Disease, Acquired Immune Disease, and Autoimmune Diseases, Including Primary Immune Deficiency, Acquired Immunodeficiency Syndrome (AIDS), Lupus, Multiple Sclerosis, Type 1 Diabetes, Rheumatoid Arthritis, and Graves Disease

Along with Treatments, Tips for Coping with Immune Disorders, a Glossary, and a Directory of Additional Resources

Edited by Joyce Brennfleck Shannon. 671 pages. 2005. 0-7808-0748-0.

ALSO AVAILABLE: *Immune System Disorders Sourcebook.* Edited by Allan R. Cook. 608 pages. 1997. 0-7808-0209-8.

Infant & Toddler Health Sourcebook

Basic Consumer Health Information about the Physical and Mental Development of Newborns, Infants, and Toddlers, Including Neonatal Concerns, Nutrition Recommendations, Immunization Schedules, Common Pediatric Disorders, Assessments and Milestones, Safety Tips, and Advice for Parents and Other Caregivers

Along with a Glossary of Terms and Resource Listings for Additional Help

Edited by Jenifer Swanson. 585 pages. 2000. 0-7808-0246-2.

"As a reference for the general public, this would be useful in any library." —*E-Streams, May '01*

"Recommended reference source."
—*Booklist, American Library Association, Feb '01*

"This is a good source for general use."
—*American Reference Books Annual, 2001*

Infectious Diseases Sourcebook

Basic Consumer Health Information about Non-Contagious Bacterial, Viral, Prion, Fungal, and Parasitic Diseases Spread by Food and Water, Insects and Animals, or Environmental Contact, Including Botulism, E. Coli, Encephalitis, Legionnaires' Disease, Lyme Disease, Malaria, Plague, Rabies, Salmonella, Tetanus, and Others, and Facts about Newly Emerging Diseases, Such as Hantavirus, Mad Cow Disease, Monkeypox, and West Nile Virus

Along with Information about Preventing Disease Transmission, the Threat of Bioterrorism, and Current Research Initiatives, with a Glossary and Directory of Resources for More Information

Edited by Karen Bellenir. 634 pages. 2004. 0-7808-0675-1.

Injury & Trauma Sourcebook

Basic Consumer Health Information about the Impact of Injury, the Diagnosis and Treatment of Common and Traumatic Injuries, Emergency Care, and Specific Injuries Related to Home, Community, Workplace, Transportation, and Recreation

Along with Guidelines for Injury Prevention, a Glossary, and a Directory of Additional Resources

Edited by Joyce Brennfleck Shannon. 696 pages. 2002. 0-7808-0421-X.

"This publication is the most comprehensive work of its kind about injury and trauma."
—*American Reference Books Annual, 2003*

"This sourcebook provides concise, easily readable, basic health information about injuries.... This book is well organized and an easy to use reference resource suitable for hospital, health sciences and public libraries with consumer health collections."
—*E-Streams, Nov '02*

"Practitioners should be aware of guides such as this in order to facilitate their use by patients and their families."
—*Doody's Health Sciences Book Review Journal, Sep-Oct '02*

"Recommended reference source."
—*Booklist, American Library Association, Sep '02*

"Highly recommended for academic and medical reference collections."
—*Library Bookwatch, Sep '02*

Kidney & Urinary Tract Diseases & Disorders Sourcebook, 1st Edition

SEE *Urinary Tract & Kidney Diseases & Disorders Sourcebook, 2nd Edition*

Learning Disabilities Sourcebook, 2nd Edition

Basic Consumer Health Information about Learning Disabilities, Including Dyslexia, Developmental Speech and Language Disabilities, Non-Verbal Learning Disorders, Developmental Arithmetic Disorder, Developmental Writing Disorder, and Other Conditions That Impede Learning Such as Attention Deficit/ Hyperactivity Disorder, Brain Injury, Hearing Impairment, Klinefelter Syndrome, Dyspraxia, and Tourette Syndrome

Along with Facts about Educational Issues and Assistive Technology, Coping Strategies, a Glossary of Related Terms, and Resources for Further Help and Information

Edited by Dawn D. Matthews. 621 pages. 2003. 0-7808-0626-3.

ALSO AVAILABLE: *Learning Disabilities Sourcebook, 1st Edition.* Edited by Linda M. Shin. 579 pages. 1998. 0-7808-0210-1.

"The second edition of *Learning Disabilities Sourcebook* far surpasses the earlier edition in that it is more focused on information that will be useful as a consumer health resource."
—*American Reference Books Annual, 2004*

"Teachers as well as consumers will find this an essential guide to understanding various syndromes and their latest treatments. [An] invaluable reference for public and school library collections alike."
—*Library Bookwatch, Apr '03*

Named "Outstanding Reference Book of 1999."
—*New York Public Library, Feb 2000*

"An excellent candidate for inclusion in a public library reference section. It's a great source of information. Teachers will also find the book useful. Definitely worth reading."
—*Journal of Adolescent & Adult Literacy, Feb 2000*

"Readable . . . provides a solid base of information regarding successful techniques used with individuals who have learning disabilities, as well as practical suggestions for educators and family members. Clear language, concise descriptions, and pertinent information for contacting multiple resources add to the strength of this book as a useful tool."
—*Choice, Association of College and Research Libraries, Feb '99*

"Recommended reference source."
—*Booklist, American Library Association, Sep '98*

"A useful resource for libraries and for those who don't have the time to identify and locate the individual publications."
—*Disability Resources Monthly, Sep '98*

Leukemia Sourcebook

Basic Consumer Health Information about Adult and Childhood Leukemias, Including Acute Lymphocytic Leukemia (ALL), Chronic Lymphocytic Leukemia (CLL), Acute Myelogenous Leukemia (AML), Chronic Myelogenous Leukemia (CML), and Hairy Cell Leukemia, and Treatments Such as Chemotherapy, Radiation Therapy, Peripheral Blood Stem Cell and Marrow Transplantation, and Immunotherapy

Along with Tips for Life During and After Treatment, a Glossary, and Directories of Additional Resources

Edited by Joyce Brennfleck Shannon. 587 pages. 2003. 0-7808-0627-1.

"Unlike other medical books for the layperson, . . . the language does not talk down to the reader.... This volume is highly recommended for all libraries."
—*American Reference Books Annual, 2004*

Liver Disorders Sourcebook

Basic Consumer Health Information about the Liver and How It Works; Liver Diseases, Including Cancer, Cirrhosis, Hepatitis, and Toxic and Drug Related Diseases; Tips for Maintaining a Healthy Liver; Laboratory Tests, Radiology Tests, and Facts about Liver Transplantation

Along with a Section on Support Groups, a Glossary, and Resource Listings

Edited by Joyce Brennfleck Shannon. 591 pages. 2000. 0-7808-0383-3.

"A valuable resource."
—*American Reference Books Annual, 2001*

"This title is recommended for health sciences and public libraries with consumer health collections."
—*E-Streams, Oct '00*

"Recommended reference source."
—*Booklist, American Library Association, Jun '00*

Lung Disorders Sourcebook

Basic Consumer Health Information about Emphysema, Pneumonia, Tuberculosis, Asthma, Cystic Fibrosis, and Other Lung Disorders, Including Facts about Diagnostic Procedures, Treatment Strategies, Disease Prevention Efforts, and Such Risk Factors as Smoking, Air Pollution, and Exposure to Asbestos, Radon, and Other Agents

Along with a Glossary and Resources for Additional Help and Information

Edited by Dawn D. Matthews. 678 pages. 2002. 0-7808-0339-6.

"This title is a great addition for public and school libraries because it provides concise health information on the lungs."
—*American Reference Books Annual, 2003*

"Highly recommended for academic and medical reference collections." —*Library Bookwatch, Sep '02*

Medical Tests Sourcebook, 2nd Edition

Basic Consumer Health Information about Medical Tests, Including Age-Specific Health Tests, Important Health Screenings and Exams, Home-Use Tests, Blood and Specimen Tests, Electrical Tests, Scope Tests, Genetic Testing, and Imaging Tests, Such as X-Rays, Ultrasound, Computed Tomography, Magnetic Resonance Imaging, Angiography, and Nuclear Medicine

Along with a Glossary and Directory of Additional Resources

Edited by Joyce Brennfleck Shannon. 654 pages. 2004. 0-7808-0670-0.

ALSO AVAILABLE: Medical Tests, 1st Edition. Edited by Joyce Brennfleck Shannon. 691 pages. 1999. 0-7808-0243-8.

"Recommended for hospital and health sciences libraries with consumer health collections."
—*E-Streams, Mar '00*

"This is an overall excellent reference with a wealth of general knowledge that may aid those who are reluctant to get vital tests performed."
—*Today's Librarian, Jan 2000*

"A valuable reference guide."
—*American Reference Books Annual, 2000*

Men's Health Concerns Sourcebook, 2nd Edition

Basic Consumer Health Information about the Medical and Mental Concerns of Men, Including Theories about the Shorter Male Lifespan, the Leading Causes of Death and Disability, Physical Concerns of Special Significance to Men, Reproductive and Sexual Concerns, Sexually Transmitted Diseases, Men's Mental and Emotional Health, and Lifestyle Choices That Affect Wellness, Such as Nutrition, Fitness, and Substance Use

Along with a Glossary of Related Terms and a Directory of Organizational Resources in Men's Health

Edited by Robert Aquinas McNally. 644 pages. 2004. 0-7808-0671-9.

ALSO AVAILABLE: Men's Health Concerns Sourcebook, 1st Edition. Edited by Allan R. Cook. 738 pages. 1998. 0-7808-0212-8.

"This comprehensive resource and the series are highly recommended."
—*American Reference Books Annual, 2000*

"Recommended reference source."
—*Booklist, American Library Association, Dec '98*

Mental Health Disorders Sourcebook, 3rd Edition

Basic Consumer Health Information about Mental and Emotional Health and Mental Illness, Including Facts about Depression, Bipolar Disorder, and Other Mood Disorders, Phobias, Post-Traumatic Stress Disorder (PTSD), Obsessive-Compulsive Disorder, and Other Anxiety Disorders, Impulse Control Disorders, Eating Disorders, Personality Disorders, and Psychotic Disorders, Including Schizophrenia and Dissociative Disorders

Along with Statistical Information, a Special Section Concerning Mental Health Issues in Children and Adolescents, a Glossary, and Directories of Resources for Additional Help and Information

Edited by Karen Bellenir. 661 pages. 2005. 0-7808-0747-2.

ALSO AVAILABLE: Mental Health Disorders Sourcebook, 1st Edition. Edited by Karen Bellenir. 548 pages. 1995. 0-7808-0040-0.

Mental Health Disorders Sourcebook, 2nd Edition. Edited by Karen Bellenir. 605 pages. 2000. 0-7808-0240-3.

"Well organized and well written."
—*American Reference Books Annual, 2001*

"Recommended reference source."
—*Booklist, American Library Association, Jun '00*

Mental Retardation Sourcebook

Basic Consumer Health Information about Mental Retardation and Its Causes, Including Down Syndrome, Fetal Alcohol Syndrome, Fragile X Syndrome, Genetic Conditions, Injury, and Environmental Sources

Along with Preventive Strategies, Parenting Issues, Educational Implications, Health Care Needs, Employment and Economic Matters, Legal Issues, a Glossary, and a Resource Listing for Additional Help and Information

Edited by Joyce Brennfleck Shannon. 642 pages. 2000. 0-7808-0377-9.

"Public libraries will find the book useful for reference and as a beginning research point for students, parents, and caregivers."
—*American Reference Books Annual, 2001*

"The strength of this work is that it compiles many basic fact sheets and addresses for further information in

one volume. It is intended and suitable for the general public. This sourcebook is relevant to any collection providing health information to the general public."
—E-Streams, Nov '00

"From preventing retardation to parenting and family challenges, this covers health, social and legal issues and will prove an invaluable overview."
—Reviewer's Bookwatch, Jul '00

Movement Disorders Sourcebook

Basic Consumer Health Information about Neurological Movement Disorders, Including Essential Tremor, Parkinson's Disease, Dystonia, Cerebral Palsy, Huntington's Disease, Myasthenia Gravis, Multiple Sclerosis, and Other Early-Onset and Adult-Onset Movement Disorders, Their Symptoms and Causes, Diagnostic Tests, and Treatments

Along with Mobility and Assistive Technology Information, a Glossary, and a Directory of Additional Resources

Edited by Joyce Brennfleck Shannon. 655 pages. 2003. 0-7808-0628-X.

"... a good resource for consumers and recommended for public, community college and undergraduate libraries."
—American Reference Books Annual, 2004

Muscular Dystrophy Sourcebook

Basic Consumer Health Information about Congenital, Childhood-Onset, and Adult-Onset Forms of Muscular Dystrophy, Such as Duchenne, Becker, Emery-Dreifuss, Distal, Limb-Girdle, Facioscapulohumeral (FSHD), Myotonic, and Ophthalmoplegic Muscular Dystrophies, Including Facts about Diagnostic Tests, Medical and Physical Therapies, Management of Co-Occurring Conditions, and Parenting Guidelines

Along with Practical Tips for Home Care, a Glossary, and Directories of Additional Resources

Edited by Joyce Brennfleck Shannon. 577 pages. 2004. 0-7808-0676-X.

Obesity Sourcebook

Basic Consumer Health Information about Diseases and Other Problems Associated with Obesity, and Including Facts about Risk Factors, Prevention Issues, and Management Approaches

Along with Statistical and Demographic Data, Information about Special Populations, Research Updates, a Glossary, and Source Listings for Further Help and Information

Edited by Wilma Caldwell and Chad T. Kimball. 376 pages. 2001. 0-7808-0333-7.

"The book synthesizes the reliable medical literature on obesity into one easy-to-read and useful resource for the general public."
—American Reference Books Annual 2002

"This is a very useful resource book for the lay public."
—Doody's Review Service, Nov '01

"Well suited for the health reference collection of a public library or an academic health science library that serves the general population."   —E-Streams, Sep '01

"Recommended reference source."
—Booklist, American Library Association, Apr '01

" Recommended pick both for specialty health library collections and any general consumer health reference collection."   —The Bookwatch, Apr '01

Ophthalmic Disorders Sourcebook, 1st Edition

SEE Eye Care Sourcebook, 2nd Edition

Oral Health Sourcebook

SEE Dental Care & Oral Health Sourcebook, 2nd Ed.

Osteoporosis Sourcebook

Basic Consumer Health Information about Primary and Secondary Osteoporosis and Juvenile Osteoporosis and Related Conditions, Including Fibrous Dysplasia, Gaucher Disease, Hyperthyroidism, Hypophosphatasia, Myeloma, Osteopetrosis, Osteogenesis Imperfecta, and Paget's Disease

Along with Information about Risk Factors, Treatments, Traditional and Non-Traditional Pain Management, a Glossary of Related Terms, and a Directory of Resources

Edited by Allan R. Cook. 584 pages. 2001. 0-7808-0239-X.

"This would be a book to be kept in a staff or patient library. The targeted audience is the layperson, but the therapist who needs a quick bit of information on a particular topic will also find the book useful."
—Physical Therapy, Jan '02

"This resource is recommended as a great reference source for public, health, and academic libraries, and is another triumph for the editors of Omnigraphics."
—American Reference Books Annual 2002

"Recommended for all public libraries and general health collections, especially those supporting patient education or consumer health programs."
—E-Streams, Nov '01

"Will prove valuable to any library seeking to maintain a current, comprehensive reference collection of health resources.... From prevention to treatment and associated conditions, this provides an excellent survey."
—The Bookwatch, Aug '01

"Recommended reference source."
—Booklist, American Library Association, July '01

SEE ALSO Women's Health Concerns Sourcebook

Pain Sourcebook, 2nd Edition

Basic Consumer Health Information about Specific Forms of Acute and Chronic Pain, Including Muscle and Skeletal Pain, Nerve Pain, Cancer Pain, and Disorders Characterized by Pain, Such as Fibromyalgia, Shingles, Angina, Arthritis, and Headaches

Along with Information about Pain Medications and Management Techniques, Complementary and Alternative Pain Relief Options, Tips for People Living with Chronic Pain, a Glossary, and a Directory of Sources for Further Information

Edited by Karen Bellenir. 670 pages. 2002. 0-7808-0612-3.

ALSO AVAILABLE: *Pain Sourcebook, 1st Edition.*
Edited by Allan R. Cook. 667 pages. 1997. 0-7808-0213-6.

"A source of valuable information.... This book offers help to nonmedical people who need information about pain and pain management. It is also an excellent reference for those who participate in patient education."
— *Doody's Review Service, Sep '02*

"The text is readable, easily understood, and well indexed. This excellent volume belongs in all patient education libraries, consumer health sections of public libraries, and many personal collections."
— *American Reference Books Annual, 1999*

"A beneficial reference." — *Booklist Health Sciences Supplement, American Library Association, Oct '98*

"The information is basic in terms of scholarship and is appropriate for general readers. Written in journalistic style... intended for non-professionals. Quite thorough in its coverage of different pain conditions and summarizes the latest clinical information regarding pain treatment." — *Choice, Association of College and Research Libraries, Jun '98*

"Recommended reference source."
— *Booklist, American Library Association, Mar '98*

Pediatric Cancer Sourcebook

Basic Consumer Health Information about Leukemias, Brain Tumors, Sarcomas, Lymphomas, and Other Cancers in Infants, Children, and Adolescents, Including Descriptions of Cancers, Treatments, and Coping Strategies

Along with Suggestions for Parents, Caregivers, and Concerned Relatives, a Glossary of Cancer Terms, and Resource Listings

Edited by Edward J. Prucha. 587 pages. 1999. 0-7808-0245-4.

"An excellent source of information. Recommended for public, hospital, and health science libraries with consumer health collections." — *E-Streams, Jun '00*

"Recommended reference source."
— *Booklist, American Library Association, Feb '00*

"A valuable addition to all libraries specializing in health services and many public libraries."
— *American Reference Books Annual, 2000*

Physical & Mental Issues in Aging Sourcebook

Basic Consumer Health Information on Physical and Mental Disorders Associated with the Aging Process, Including Concerns about Cardiovascular Disease, Pulmonary Disease, Oral Health, Digestive Disorders, Musculoskeletal and Skin Disorders, Metabolic Changes, Sexual and Reproductive Issues, and Changes in Vision, Hearing, and Other Senses

Along with Data about Longevity and Causes of Death, Information on Acute and Chronic Pain, Descriptions of Mental Concerns, a Glossary of Terms, and Resource Listings for Additional Help

Edited by Jenifer Swanson. 660 pages. 1999. 0-7808-0233-0.

"This is a treasure of health information for the layperson." — *Choice Health Sciences Supplement, Association of College & Research Libraries, May 2000*

"Recommended for public libraries."
—*American Reference Books Annual, 2000*

"Recommended reference source."
— *Booklist, American Library Association, Oct '99*

SEE ALSO *Healthy Aging Sourcebook*

Podiatry Sourcebook

Basic Consumer Health Information about Foot Conditions, Diseases, and Injuries, Including Bunions, Corns, Calluses, Athlete's Foot, Plantar Warts, Hammertoes and Clawtoes, Clubfoot, Heel Pain, Gout, and More

Along with Facts about Foot Care, Disease Prevention, Foot Safety, Choosing a Foot Care Specialist, a Glossary of Terms, and Resource Listings for Additional Information

Edited by M. Lisa Weatherford. 380 pages. 2001. 0-7808-0215-2.

"Recommended reference source."
— *Booklist, American Library Association, Feb '02*

"There is a lot of information presented here on a topic that is usually only covered sparingly in most larger comprehensive medical encyclopedias."
— *American Reference Books Annual 2002*

Pregnancy & Birth Sourcebook, 2nd Edition

Basic Consumer Health Information about Conception and Pregnancy, Including Facts about Fertility, Infertility, Pregnancy Symptoms and Complications, Fetal Growth and Development, Labor, Delivery, and the Postpartum Period, as Well as Information about Maintaining Health and Wellness during Pregnancy and Caring for a Newborn

Along with Information about Public Health Assistance for Low-Income Pregnant Women, a Glossary, and Directories of Agencies and Organizations Providing Help and Support

Edited by Amy L. Sutton. 626 pages. 2004. 0-7808-0672-7.

ALSO AVAILABLE: Pregnancy & Birth Sourcebook, 1st Edition. Edited by Heather E. Aldred. 737 pages. 1997. 0-7808-0216-0.

"A well-organized handbook. Recommended."
— Choice, Association of College and Research Libraries, Apr '98

"Recommended reference source."
— Booklist, American Library Association, Mar '98

"Recommended for public libraries."
— American Reference Books Annual, 1998

SEE ALSO Congenital Disorders Sourcebook, Family Planning Sourcebook

Prostate Cancer Sourcebook

Basic Consumer Health Information about Prostate Cancer, Including Information about the Associated Risk Factors, Detection, Diagnosis, and Treatment of Prostate Cancer

Along with Information on Non-Malignant Prostate Conditions, and Featuring a Section Listing Support and Treatment Centers and a Glossary of Related Terms

Edited by Dawn D. Matthews. 358 pages. 2001. 0-7808-0324-8.

"Recommended reference source."
— Booklist, American Library Association, Jan '02

"A valuable resource for health care consumers seeking information on the subject. . . . All text is written in a clear, easy-to-understand language that avoids technical jargon. Any library that collects consumer health resources would strengthen their collection with the addition of the *Prostate Cancer Sourcebook*."
— American Reference Books Annual 2002

Prostate & Urological Disorders Sourcebook

Basic Consumer Health Information about Urogenital and Sexual Disorders in Men, Including Prostate and Other Andrological Cancers, Prostatitis, Benign Prostatic Hyperplasia, Testicular and Penile Trauma, Cryptorchidism, Peyronie Disease, Erectile Dysfunction, and Male Factor Infertility, and Facts about Commonly Used Tests and Procedures, Such as Prostatectomy, Vasectomy, Vasectomy Reversal, Penile Implants, and Semen Analysis

Along with a Glossary of Andrological Terms and a Directory of Resources for Additional Information

Edited by Karen Bellenir. 631 pages. 2005. 0-7808-0797-9.

Public Health Sourcebook

Basic Information about Government Health Agencies, Including National Health Statistics and Trends, Healthy People 2000 Program Goals and Objectives, the Centers for Disease Control and Prevention, the Food and Drug Administration, and the National Institutes of Health

Along with Full Contact Information for Each Agency

Edited by Wendy Wilcox. 698 pages. 1998. 0-7808-0220-9.

"Recommended reference source."
— Booklist, American Library Association, Sep '98

"This consumer guide provides welcome assistance in navigating the maze of federal health agencies and their data on public health concerns."
— SciTech Book News, Sep '98

Reconstructive & Cosmetic Surgery Sourcebook

Basic Consumer Health Information on Cosmetic and Reconstructive Plastic Surgery, Including Statistical Information about Different Surgical Procedures, Things to Consider Prior to Surgery, Plastic Surgery Techniques and Tools, Emotional and Psychological Considerations, and Procedure-Specific Information

Along with a Glossary of Terms and a Listing of Resources for Additional Help and Information

Edited by M. Lisa Weatherford. 374 pages. 2001. 0-7808-0214-4.

"An excellent reference that addresses cosmetic and medically necessary reconstructive surgeries. . . . The style of the prose is calm and reassuring, discussing the many positive outcomes now available due to advances in surgical techniques."
— American Reference Books Annual 2002

"Recommended for health science libraries that are open to the public, as well as hospital libraries that are open to the patients. This book is a good resource for the consumer interested in plastic surgery."
— E-Streams, Dec '01

"Recommended reference source."
— Booklist, American Library Association, July '01

Rehabilitation Sourcebook

Basic Consumer Health Information about Rehabilitation for People Recovering from Heart Surgery, Spinal Cord Injury, Stroke, Orthopedic Impairments, Amputation, Pulmonary Impairments, Traumatic Injury, and More, Including Physical Therapy, Occupational Therapy, Speech/ Language Therapy, Massage Therapy, Dance Therapy, Art Therapy, and Recreational Therapy

Along with Information on Assistive and Adaptive Devices, a Glossary, and Resources for Additional Help and Information

Edited by Dawn D. Matthews. 531 pages. 1999. 0-7808-0236-5.

"This is an excellent resource for public library reference and health collections."
— American Reference Books Annual, 2001

"Recommended reference source."
— Booklist, American Library Association, May '00

Respiratory Diseases & Disorders Sourcebook

Basic Information about Respiratory Diseases and Disorders, Including Asthma, Cystic Fibrosis, Pneumonia, the Common Cold, Influenza, and Others, Featuring Facts about the Respiratory System, Statistical and Demographic Data, Treatments, Self-Help Management Suggestions, and Current Research Initiatives

Edited by Allan R. Cook and Peter D. Dresser. 771 pages. 1995. 0-7808-0037-0.

"Designed for the layperson and for patients and their families coping with respiratory illness. . . . an extensive array of information on diagnosis, treatment, management, and prevention of respiratory illnesses for the general reader." — *Choice, Association of College and Research Libraries, Jun '96*

"A highly recommended text for all collections. It is a comforting reminder of the power of knowledge that good books carry between their covers."
— *Academic Library Book Review, Spring '96*

"A comprehensive collection of authoritative information presented in a nontechnical, humanitarian style for patients, families, and caregivers." — *Association of Operating Room Nurses, Sep/Oct '95*

SEE ALSO Lung Disorders Sourcebook

■

Sexually Transmitted Diseases Sourcebook, 3rd Edition

Basic Consumer Health Information about Chlamydial Infections, Gonorrhea, Hepatitis, Herpes, HIV/AIDS, Human Papillomavirus, Pubic Lice, Scabies, Syphilis, Trichomoniasis, Vaginal Infections, and Other Sexually Transmitted Diseases, Including Facts about Risk Factors, Symptoms, Diagnosis, Treatment, and the Prevention of Sexually Transmitted Infections

Along with Updates on Current Research Initiatives, a Glossary of Related Terms, and Resources for Additional Help and Information

Edited by Amy L. Sutton. 629 pages. 2006. 0-7808-0824-X.

ALSO AVAILABLE: *Sexually Transmitted Diseases Sourcebook, 1st Edition.* Edited by Linda M. Ross. 550 pages. 1997. 0-7808-0217-9.

Sexually Transmitted Diseases Sourcebook, 2nd Edition. Edited by Dawn D. Matthews. 538 pages. 2001. 0-7808-0249-7.

"Recommended for consumer health collections in public libraries, and secondary school and community college libraries."
— *American Reference Books Annual 2002*

"Every school and public library should have a copy of this comprehensive and user-friendly reference book."
— *Choice, Association of College & Research Libraries, Sep '01*

"This is a highly recommended book. This is an especially important book for all school and public libraries." — *AIDS Book Review Journal, Jul-Aug '01*

"Recommended reference source."
— *Booklist, American Library Association, Apr '01*

"Recommended pick both for specialty health library collections and any general consumer health reference collection." — *The Bookwatch, Apr '01*

■

Skin Disorders Sourcebook, 1st Edition

SEE *Dermatological Disorders Sourcebook, 2nd Edition*

■

Sleep Disorders Sourcebook, 2nd Edition

Basic Consumer Health Information about Sleep and Sleep Disorders, Including Insomnia, Sleep Apnea, Restless Legs Syndrome, Narcolepsy, Parasomnias, and Other Health Problems That Affect Sleep, Plus Facts about Diagnostic Procedures, Treatment Strategies, Sleep Medications, and Tips for Improving Sleep Quality

Along with a Glossary of Related Terms and Resources for Additional Help and Information

Edited by Amy L. Sutton. 567 pages. 2005. 0-7808-0745-6.

ALSO AVAILABLE: *Sleep Disorders Sourcebook, 1st Edition.* Edited by Jenifer Swanson. 439 pages. 1998. 0-7808-0234-9.

"This text will complement any home or medical library. It is user-friendly and ideal for the adult reader."
— *American Reference Books Annual, 2000*

"A useful resource that provides accurate, relevant, and accessible information on sleep to the general public. Health care providers who deal with sleep disorders patients may also find it helpful in being prepared to answer some of the questions patients ask."
— *Respiratory Care, Jul '99*

"Recommended reference source."
— *Booklist, American Library Association, Feb '99*

■

Smoking Concerns Sourcebook

Basic Consumer Health Information about Nicotine Addiction and Smoking Cessation, Featuring Facts about the Health Effects of Tobacco Use, Including Lung and Other Cancers, Heart Disease, Stroke, and Respiratory Disorders, Such as Emphysema and Chronic Bronchitis

Along with Information about Smoking Prevention Programs, Suggestions for Achieving and Maintaining a Smoke-Free Lifestyle, Statistics about Tobacco Use, Reports on Current Research Initiatives, a Glossary of Related Terms, and Directories of Resources for Additional Help and Information

Edited by Karen Bellenir. 621 pages. 2004. 0-7808-0323-X.

Sports Injuries Sourcebook, 2nd Edition

Basic Consumer Health Information about the Diagnosis, Treatment, and Rehabilitation of Common Sports-Related Injuries in Children and Adults

Along with Suggestions for Conditioning and Training, Information and Prevention Tips for Injuries Frequently Associated with Specific Sports and Special Populations, a Glossary, and a Directory of Additional Resources

Edited by Joyce Brennfleck Shannon. 614 pages. 2002. 0-7808-0604-2.

ALSO AVAILABLE: *Sports Injuries Sourcebook, 1st Edition.* Edited by Heather E. Aldred. 624 pages. 1999. 0-7808-0218-7.

"This is an excellent reference for consumers and it is recommended for public, community college, and undergraduate libraries."
— *American Reference Books Annual, 2003*

"Recommended reference source."
— *Booklist, American Library Association, Feb '03*

Stress-Related Disorders Sourcebook

Basic Consumer Health Information about Stress and Stress-Related Disorders, Including Stress Origins and Signals, Environmental Stress at Work and Home, Mental and Emotional Stress Associated with Depression, Post-Traumatic Stress Disorder, Panic Disorder, Suicide, and the Physical Effects of Stress on the Cardiovascular, Immune, and Nervous Systems

Along with Stress Management Techniques, a Glossary, and a Listing of Additional Resources

Edited by Joyce Brennfleck Shannon. 610 pages. 2002. 0-7808-0560-7.

"Well written for a general readership, the *Stress-Related Disorders Sourcebook* is a useful addition to the health reference literature."
— *American Reference Books Annual, 2003*

"I am impressed by the amount of information. It offers a thorough overview of the causes and consequences of stress for the layperson. . . . A well-done and thorough reference guide for professionals and nonprofessionals alike."
— *Doody's Review Service, Dec '02*

Stroke Sourcebook

Basic Consumer Health Information about Stroke, Including Ischemic, Hemorrhagic, Transient Ischemic Attack (TIA), and Pediatric Stroke, Stroke Triggers and Risks, Diagnostic Tests, Treatments, and Rehabilitation Information

Along with Stroke Prevention Guidelines, Legal and Financial Information, a Glossary, and a Directory of Additional Resources

Edited by Joyce Brennfleck Shannon. 606 pages. 2003. 0-7808-0630-1.

"This volume is highly recommended and should be in every medical, hospital, and public library."
— *American Reference Books Annual, 2004*

Substance Abuse Sourcebook

Basic Health-Related Information about the Abuse of Legal and Illegal Substances Such as Alcohol, Tobacco, Prescription Drugs, Marijuana, Cocaine, and Heroin; and Including Facts about Substance Abuse Prevention Strategies, Intervention Methods, Treatment and Recovery Programs, and a Section Addressing the Special Problems Related to Substance Abuse during Pregnancy

Edited by Karen Bellenir. 573 pages. 1996. 0-7808-0038-9.

"A valuable addition to any health reference section. Highly recommended."
— *The Book Report, Mar/Apr '97*

". . . a comprehensive collection of substance abuse information that's both highly readable and compact. Families and caregivers of substance abusers will find the information enlightening and helpful, while teachers, social workers and journalists should benefit from the concise format. Recommended."
— *Drug Abuse Update, Winter '96/'97*

SEE ALSO *Alcoholism Sourcebook, Drug Abuse Sourcebook*

Surgery Sourcebook

Basic Consumer Health Information about Inpatient and Outpatient Surgeries, Including Cardiac, Vascular, Orthopedic, Ocular, Reconstructive, Cosmetic, Gynecologic, and Ear, Nose, and Throat Procedures and More

Along with Information about Operating Room Policies and Instruments, Laser Surgery Techniques, Hospital Errors, Statistical Data, a Glossary, and Listings of Sources for Further Help and Information

Edited by Annemarie S. Muth and Karen Bellenir. 596 pages. 2002. 0-7808-0380-9.

"Large public libraries and medical libraries would benefit from this material in their reference collections."
— *American Reference Books Annual, 2004*

"Invaluable reference for public and school library collections alike."
— *Library Bookwatch, Apr '03*

Thyroid Disorders Sourcebook

Basic Consumer Health Information about Disorders of the Thyroid and Parathyroid Glands, Including Hypothyroidism, Hyperthyroidism, Graves Disease, Hashimoto Thyroiditis, Thyroid Cancer, and Parathyroid Disorders, Featuring Facts about Symptoms, Risk Factors, Tests, and Treatments

Along with Information about the Effects of Thyroid Imbalance on Other Body Systems, Environmental Factors That Affect the Thyroid Gland, a Glossary, and a Directory of Additional Resources

Edited by Joyce Brennfleck Shannon. 599 pages. 2005. 0-7808-0745-6.

Transplantation Sourcebook

Basic Consumer Health Information about Organ and Tissue Transplantation, Including Physical and Financial Preparations, Procedures and Issues Relating to Specific Solid Organ and Tissue Transplants, Rehabilitation, Pediatric Transplant Information, the Future of Transplantation, and Organ and Tissue Donation Along with a Glossary and Listings of Additional Resources

Edited by Joyce Brennfleck Shannon. 628 pages. 2002. 0-7808-0322-1.

"Along with these advances [in transplantation technology] have come a number of daunting questions for potential transplant patients, their families, and their health care providers. This reference text is the best single tool to address many of these questions. . . . It will be a much-needed addition to the reference collections in health care, academic, and large public libraries."
— *American Reference Books Annual, 2003*

"Recommended for libraries with an interest in offering consumer health information." — *E-Streams, Jul '02*

"This is a unique and valuable resource for patients facing transplantation and their families."
— *Doody's Review Service, Jun '02*

Traveler's Health Sourcebook

Basic Consumer Health Information for Travelers, Including Physical and Medical Preparations, Transportation Health and Safety, Essential Information about Food and Water, Sun Exposure, Insect and Snake Bites, Camping and Wilderness Medicine, and Travel with Physical or Medical Disabilities Along with International Travel Tips, Vaccination Recommendations, Geographical Health Issues, Disease Risks, a Glossary, and a Listing of Additional Resources

Edited by Joyce Brennfleck Shannon. 613 pages. 2000. 0-7808-0384-1.

"Recommended reference source."
— *Booklist, American Library Association, Feb '01*

"This book is recommended for any public library, any travel collection, and especially any collection for the physically disabled."
—*American Reference Books Annual, 2001*

Urinary Tract & Kidney Diseases & Disorders Sourcebook, 2nd Edition

Basic Consumer Health Information about the Urinary System, Including the Bladder, Urethra, Ureters, and Kidneys, with Facts about Urinary Tract Infections, Incontinence, Congenital Disorders, Kidney Stones, Cancers of the Urinary Tract and Kidneys, Kidney Failure, Dialysis, and Kidney Transplantation Along with Statistical and Demographic Information, Reports on Current Research in Kidney and Urologic Health, a Summary of Commonly Used Diagnostic Tests, a Glossary of Related Terms, and a Directory of Resources for Additional Help and Information

Edited by Ivy L. Alexander. 649 pages. 2005. 0-7808-0750-2.

ALSO AVAILABLE: *Kidney & Urinary Tract Diseases & Disorders Sourcebook, 1st Ed.* Edited by Linda M. Ross. 602 pages. 1997. 0-7808-0079-6.

Vegetarian Sourcebook

Basic Consumer Health Information about Vegetarian Diets, Lifestyle, and Philosophy, Including Definitions of Vegetarianism and Veganism, Tips about Adopting Vegetarianism, Creating a Vegetarian Pantry, and Meeting Nutritional Needs of Vegetarians, with Facts Regarding Vegetarianism's Effect on Pregnant and Lactating Women, Children, Athletes, and Senior Citizens Along with a Glossary of Commonly Used Vegetarian Terms and Resources for Additional Help and Information

Edited by Chad T. Kimball. 360 pages. 2002. 0-7808-0439-2.

"Organizes into one concise volume the answers to the most common questions concerning vegetarian diets and lifestyles. This title is recommended for public and secondary school libraries." — *E-Streams, Apr '03*

"Invaluable reference for public and school library collections alike." — *Library Bookwatch, Apr '03*

"The articles in this volume are easy to read and come from authoritative sources. The book does not necessarily support the vegetarian diet but instead provides the pros and cons of this important decision. The *Vegetarian Sourcebook* is recommended for public libraries and consumer health libraries."
— *American Reference Books Annual, 2003*

Women's Health Concerns Sourcebook, 2nd Edition

Basic Consumer Health Information about the Medical and Mental Concerns of Women, Including Maintaining Health and Wellness, Gynecological Concerns, Breast Health, Sexuality and Reproductive Issues, Menopause, Cancer in Women, the Leading Causes of Death and Disability among Women, Physical Concerns of Special Significance to Women, and Women's Mental and Emotional Health Along with a Glossary of Related Terms and Directories of Resources for Additional Help and Information

Edited by Amy L. Sutton. 748 pages. 2004. 0-7808-0673-5.

ALSO AVAILABLE: *Women's Health Concerns Sourcebook, 1st Edition.* Edited by Heather E. Aldred. 567 pages. 1997. 0-7808-0219-5.

"Handy compilation. There is an impressive range of diseases, devices, disorders, procedures, and other physical and emotional issues covered . . . well organized, illustrated, and indexed." —*Choice, Association of College and Research Libraries, Jan '98*

SEE ALSO *Breast Cancer Sourcebook, Cancer Sourcebook for Women, Healthy Heart Sourcebook for Women, Osteoporosis Sourcebook*

■

Workplace Health & Safety Sourcebook

Basic Consumer Health Information about Workplace Health and Safety, Including the Effect of Workplace Hazards on the Lungs, Skin, Heart, Ears, Eyes, Brain, Reproductive Organs, Musculoskeletal System, and Other Organs and Body Parts

Along with Information about Occupational Cancer, Personal Protective Equipment, Toxic and Hazardous Chemicals, Child Labor, Stress, and Workplace Violence

Edited by Chad T. Kimball. 626 pages. 2000. 0-7808-0231-4.

"As a reference for the general public, this would be useful in any library." —*E-Streams, Jun '01*

"Provides helpful information for primary care physicians and other caregivers interested in occupational medicine. . . . General readers; professionals."
— *Choice, Association of College & Research Libraries, May '01*

"Recommended reference source."
—*Booklist, American Library Association, Feb '01*

"Highly recommended." —*The Bookwatch, Jan '01*

■

Worldwide Health Sourcebook

Basic Information about Global Health Issues, Including Malnutrition, Reproductive Health, Disease Dispersion and Prevention, Emerging Diseases, Risky Health Behaviors, and the Leading Causes of Death

Along with Global Health Concerns for Children, Women, and the Elderly, Mental Health Issues, Research and Technology Advancements, and Economic, Environmental, and Political Health Implications, a Glossary, and a Resource Listing for Additional Help and Information

Edited by Joyce Brennfleck Shannon. 614 pages. 2001. 0-7808-0330-2.

"Named an Outstanding Academic Title." —*Choice, Association of College & Research Libraries, Jan '02*

"Yet another handy but also unique compilation in the extensive Health Reference Series, this is a useful work because many of the international publications reprinted or excerpted are not readily available. Highly recommended." —*Choice, Association of College & Research Libraries, Nov '01*

"Recommended reference source."
—*Booklist, American Library Association, Oct '01*

Teen Health Series
Helping Young Adults Understand, Manage, and Avoid Serious Illness

List price $65 per volume. **School and library price $58 per volume.**

Alcohol Information for Teens
Health Tips about Alcohol and Alcoholism
Including Facts about Underage Drinking, Preventing Teen Alcohol Use, Alcohol's Effects on the Brain and the Body, Alcohol Abuse Treatment, Help for Children of Alcoholics, and More

Edited by Joyce Brennfleck Shannon. 370 pages. 2005. 0-7808-0741-3.

Allergy Information for Teens
Health Tips about Allergic Reactions Such as Anaphylaxis, Respiratory Problems, and Rashes
Including Facts about Identifying and Managing Allergies to Food, Pollen, Mold, Animals, Chemicals, Drugs, and Other Substances

Edited by Karen Bellenir. 400 pages. 2006. 0-7808-0799-5.

Asthma Information for Teens
Health Tips about Managing Asthma and Related Concerns
Including Facts about Asthma Causes, Triggers, Symptoms, Diagnosis, and Treatment

Edited by Karen Bellenir. 386 pages. 2005. 0-7808-0770-7.

"It is so clearly written and well organized that even hesitant readers will be able to find the facts they need, whether for reports or personal information.... A succinct but complete resource."
— *School Library Journal, Sep '05*

Cancer Information for Teens
Health Tips about Cancer Awareness, Prevention, Diagnosis, and Treatment
Including Facts about Frequently Occurring Cancers, Cancer Risk Factors, and Coping Strategies for Teens Fighting Cancer or Dealing with Cancer in Friends or Family Members

Edited by Wilma R. Caldwell. 428 pages. 2004. 0-7808-0678-6.

"Recommended for school libraries, or consumer libraries that see a lot of use by teens."
— *E-Streams, May 2005*

"A valuable educational tool."
— *American Reference Books Annual, 2005*

"Young adults and their parents alike will find this new addition to the *Teen Health Series* an important reference to cancer in teens."
— *Children's Bookwatch, February 2005*

Diabetes Information for Teens
Health Tips about Managing Diabetes and Preventing Related Complications
Including Information about Insulin, Glucose Control, Healthy Eating, Physical Activity, and Learning to Live with Diabetes

Edited by Sandra Augustyn Lawton. 400 pages. 2006. 0-7808-0811-8.

Diet Information for Teens, 2nd Edition
Health Tips about Diet and Nutrition
Including Facts about Dietary Guidelines, Food Groups, Nutrients, Healthy Meals, Snacks, Weight Control, Medical Concerns Related to Diet, and More

Edited by Karen Bellenir. 426 pages. 2006. 0-7808-0820-7.

ALSO AVAILABLE: *Diet Information for Teens, 1st Edition.* Edited by Karen Bellenir. 399 pages. 2001. 0-7808-0441-4.

"Full of helpful insights and facts throughout the book. ... An excellent resource to be placed in public libraries or even in personal collections."
— *American Reference Books Annual 2002*

"Recommended for middle and high school libraries and media centers as well as academic libraries that educate future teachers of teenagers. It is also a suitable addition to health science libraries that serve patrons who are interested in teen health promotion and education."
— *E-Streams, Oct '01*

"This comprehensive book would be beneficial to collections that need information about nutrition, dietary guidelines, meal planning, and weight control.... This reference is so easy to use that its purchase is recommended."
— *The Book Report, Sep-Oct '01*

"This book is written in an easy to understand format describing issues that many teens face every day, and then provides thoughtful explanations so that teens can make informed decisions. This is an interesting book

that provides important facts and information for today's teens."
—Doody's Health Sciences Book Review Journal, Jul-Aug '01

"A comprehensive compendium of diet and nutrition. The information is presented in a straightforward, plain-spoken manner. This title will be useful to those working on reports on a variety of topics, as well as to general readers concerned about their dietary health."
—School Library Journal, Jun '01

Drug Information for Teens, 2nd Edition

Health Tips about the Physical and Mental Effects of Substance Abuse

Including Information about Marijuana, Inhalants, Club Drugs, Stimulants, Hallucinogens, Opiates, Prescription and Over-the-Counter Drugs, Herbal Products, Tobacco, Alcohol, and More

Edited by Sandra Augustyn Lawton. 460 pages. 2006. 0-7808-0862-2.

ALSO AVAILABLE: *Drug Information for Teens, 1st Edition.* Edited by Karen Bellenir. 452 pages. 2002. 0-7808-0444-9.

"A clearly written resource for general readers and researchers alike." —*School Library Journal*

"The chapters are quick to make a connection to their teenage reading audience. The prose is straightforward and the book lends itself to spot reading. It should be useful both for practical information and for research, and it is suitable for public and school libraries."
—*American Reference Books Annual, 2003*

"Recommended reference source."
—*Booklist, American Library Association, Feb '03*

"This is an excellent resource for teens and their parents. Education about drugs and substances is key to discouraging teen drug abuse and this book provides this much needed information in a way that is interesting and factual." —*Doody's Review Service, Dec '02*

Eating Disorders Information for Teens

Health Tips about Anorexia, Bulimia, Binge Eating, and Other Eating Disorders

Including Information on the Causes, Prevention, and Treatment of Eating Disorders, and Such Other Issues as Maintaining Healthy Eating and Exercise Habits

Edited by Sandra Augustyn Lawton. 337 pages. 2005. 0-7808-0783-9.

Fitness Information for Teens

Health Tips about Exercise, Physical Well-Being, and Health Maintenance

Including Facts about Aerobic and Anaerobic Conditioning, Stretching, Body Shape and Body Image, Sports Training, Nutrition, and Activities for Non-Athletes

Edited by Karen Bellenir. 425 pages. 2004. 0-7808-0679-4.

"This book will be a great addition to any public, junior high, senior high, or secondary school library."
—*American Reference Books Annual, 2005*

Learning Disabilities Information for Teens

Health Tips about Academic Skills Disorders and Other Disabilities That Affect Learning

Including Information about Common Signs of Learning Disabilities, School Issues, Learning to Live with a Learning Disability, and Other Related Issues

Edited by Sandra Augustyn Lawton. 337 pages. 2005. 0-7808-0796-0.

Mental Health Information for Teens

Health Tips about Mental Health and Mental Illness

Including Facts about Anxiety, Depression, Suicide, Eating Disorders, Obsessive-Compulsive Disorders, Panic Attacks, Phobias, Schizophrenia, and More

Edited by Karen Bellenir. 406 pages. 2001. 0-7808-0442-2.

"In both language and approach, this user-friendly entry in the *Teen Health Series* is on target for teens needing information on mental health concerns." —*Booklist, American Library Association, Jan '02*

"Readers will find the material accessible and informative, with the shaded notes, facts, and embedded glossary insets adding appropriately to the already interesting and succinct presentation."
—*School Library Journal, Jan '02*

"This title is highly recommended for any library that serves adolescents and parents/caregivers of adolescents." —*E-Streams, Jan '02*

"Recommended for high school libraries and young adult collections in public libraries. Both health professionals and teenagers will find this book useful."
—*American Reference Books Annual 2002*

"This is a nice book written to enlighten the society, primarily teenagers, about common teen mental health issues. It is highly recommended to teachers and parents as well as adolescents."
—*Doody's Review Service, Dec '01*

Sexual Health Information for Teens

Health Tips about Sexual Development, Human Reproduction, and Sexually Transmitted Diseases

Including Facts about Puberty, Reproductive Health, Chlamydia, Human Papillomavirus, Pelvic Inflammatory Disease, Herpes, AIDS, Contraception, Pregnancy, and More

Edited by Deborah A. Stanley. 391 pages. 2003. 0-7808-0445-7.

"This work should be included in all high school libraries and many larger public libraries. . . . highly recommended."
— *American Reference Books Annual 2004*

"Sexual Health approaches its subject with appropriate seriousness and offers easily accessible advice and information."
— *School Library Journal, Feb. 2004*

Skin Health Information for Teens

Health Tips about Dermatological Concerns and Skin Cancer Risks

Including Facts about Acne, Warts, Hives, and Other Conditions and Lifestyle Choices, Such as Tanning, Tattooing, and Piercing, That Affect the Skin, Nails, Scalp, and Hair

Edited by Robert Aquinas McNally. 429 pages. 2003. 0-7808-0446-5.

"This volume, as with others in the series, will be a useful addition to school and public library collections."
— *American Reference Books Annual 2004*

"This volume serves as a one-stop source and should be a necessity for any health collection."
— *Library Media Connection*

Sports Injuries Information for Teens

Health Tips about Sports Injuries and Injury Protection

Including Facts about Specific Injuries, Emergency Treatment, Rehabilitation, Sports Safety, Competition Stress, Fitness, Sports Nutrition, Steroid Risks, and More

Edited by Joyce Brennfleck Shannon. 405 pages. 2003. 0-7808-0447-3.

"This work will be useful in the young adult collections of public libraries as well as high school libraries."
— *American Reference Books Annual 2004*

Suicide Information for Teens

Health Tips about Suicide Causes and Prevention

Including Facts about Depression, Risk Factors, Getting Help, Survivor Support, and More

Edited by Joyce Brennfleck Shannon. 368 pages. 2005. 0-7808-0737-5.

Health Reference Series

Adolescent Health Sourcebook
AIDS Sourcebook, 3rd Edition
Alcoholism Sourcebook
Allergies Sourcebook, 2nd Edition
Alternative Medicine Sourcebook, 2nd Edition
Alzheimer's Disease Sourcebook, 3rd Edition
Arthritis Sourcebook, 2nd Edition
Asthma Sourcebook
Attention Deficit Disorder Sourcebook
Back & Neck Sourcebook, 2nd Edition
Blood & Circulatory Disorders Sourcebook, 2nd Edition
Brain Disorders Sourcebook, 2nd Edition
Breast Cancer Sourcebook, 2nd Edition
Breastfeeding Sourcebook
Burns Sourcebook
Cancer Sourcebook, 4th Edition
Cancer Sourcebook for Women, 2nd Edition
Cardiovascular Diseases & Disorders Sourcebook, 3rd Edition
Caregiving Sourcebook
Child Abuse Sourcebook
Childhood Diseases & Disorders Sourcebook
Colds, Flu & Other Common Ailments Sourcebook
Communication Disorders Sourcebook
Congenital Disorders Sourcebook
Consumer Issues in Health Care Sourcebook
Contagious & Non-Contagious Infectious Diseases Sourcebook
Contagious Diseases Sourcebook
Death & Dying Sourcebook
Dental Care & Oral Health Sourcebook, 2nd Edition
Depression Sourcebook
Diabetes Sourcebook, 3rd Edition
Diet & Nutrition Sourcebook, 2nd Edition
Digestive Diseases & Disorder Sourcebook
Disabilities Sourcebook
Domestic Violence Sourcebook, 2nd Edition
Drug Abuse Sourcebook, 2nd Edition
Ear, Nose & Throat Disorders Sourcebook
Eating Disorders Sourcebook
Emergency Medical Services Sourcebook
Endocrine & Metabolic Disorders Sourcebook
Environmentally Health Sourcebook, 2nd Edition
Ethnic Diseases Sourcebook
Eye Care Sourcebook, 2nd Edition
Family Planning Sourcebook
Fitness & Exercise Sourcebook, 2nd Edition
Food & Animal Borne Diseases Sourcebook
Food Safety Sourcebook
Forensic Medicine Sourcebook
Gastrointestinal Diseases & Disorders Sourcebook
Genetic Disorders Sourcebook, 2nd Edition
Head Trauma Sourcebook
Headache Sourcebook
Health Insurance Sourcebook
Health Reference Series Cumulative Index 1999
Healthy Aging Sourcebook
Healthy Children Sourcebook
Healthy Heart Sourcebook for Women